Handbook on Medical Student Evaluation and Assessment

Handbook on Medical Student Evaluation and Assessment

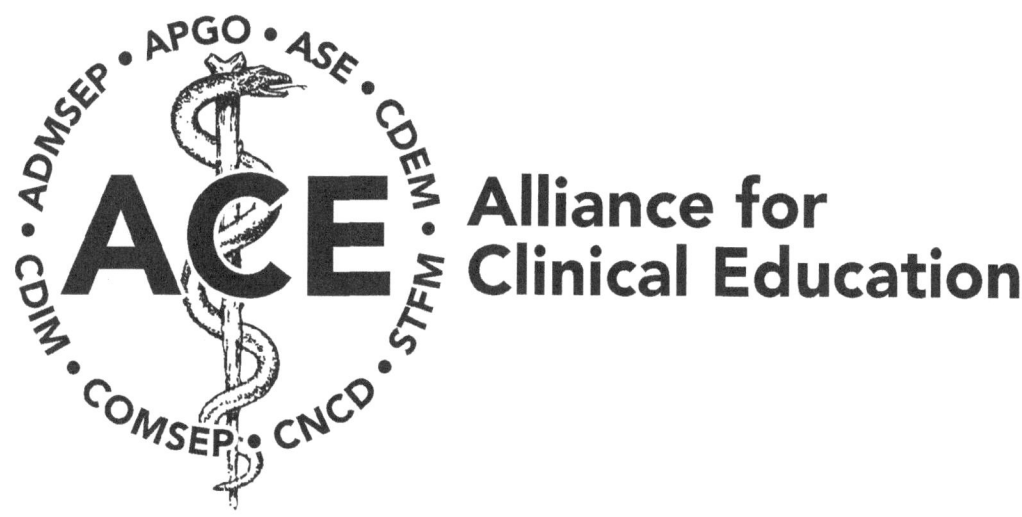 Alliance for Clinical Education

Louis N. Pangaro, M.D.
William C. McGaghie, Ph.D.
Editors

>> North Syracuse, New York <<
<< Gegensatz Press >>
>> 2015 <<

Cataloging in publication:

Alliance for Clinical Education
        Handbook on medical student evaluation and assessment / Alliance for Clinical Education ; Louis N. Pangaro, William C. McGaghie, editors.
        xiv, 274 p. : ill. ; 26 cm.
        Includes bibliographical references and index.
        ISBN 978-1-62130-730-3 (paperback)
        ISBN 978-1-62130-731-0 (Kindle e-book)
        ISBN 978-1-62130-733-4 (Smashwords e-book)
        ISBN 978-1-62130-732-7 (Ingram e-book)
1. Medicine - Study and teaching. 2. Clinical competence - Evaluation. 3. Medical students.
[DNLM: 1. Educational Measurement - handbooks. 2. Education, Medical - handbooks. 3. Educational Measurement - methods. W 18 A436h 2015]
I. Pangaro, Louis N. II. McGaghie, William C. III. Title. IV. Title: ACE handbook on medical student evaluation and assessment.
        R 837.A2 A436 H236 2015   610.76 - dc22   AACR2
Library of Congress Control Number 2014954211

First edition, first printing. Printed in the United States of America.

Copyright © 2015 by the Alliance for Clinical Education.

All rights reserved. Except for brief quotations in book reviews, no part of this book may be reproduced or transmitted in any form, or by any means, without the prior written permission of the copyright holder.

The guillemets, or two pairs of opposing chevrons, dark on the lower cusps and light on the upper, are a trademark of Gegensatz Press.

Distributed to the trade worldwide by:
Gegensatz Press
108 Deborah Lane
North Syracuse, NY 13212-1931
<www.gegensatzpress.com>

BISAC subject heading: MED024000 MEDICAL / Education & Training
Designed by Eric v.d. Luft. Printed on acid-free paper. ∞

Contents

Foreword   vii
Ronald M. Harden, O.B.E., M.D., F.R.C.P. (Glas.), F.R.C.S. (Ed.), F.R.C.P.C.

Preface   ix
Louis N. Pangaro, M.D.; William C. McGaghie, Ph.D.

Contributors   xii

Section One   1

1. Introduction   1
William C. McGaghie, Ph.D.

2. A Primer of Evaluation Terminology: Definitions and Important Distinctions in Evaluation   13
Louis N. Pangaro, M.D.

3. System Approaches to Student Assessment   27
Louis N. Pangaro, M.D.

4. Sharing Student Performance Information Across Courses and Clerkships   43
Lynn M. Cleary, M.D.

5. Using Pre-Clerkship Variables to Identify High-Risk Students   49
Jeffrey S. LaRochelle, M.D., M.P.H.; Gerald D. Denton, M.D., M.P.H.

6. Assessment in the Post-Clerkship Year   59
Meenakshy K. Aiyer, M.B.B.S.; Matthew Joseph Mischler, M.D.

Section Two   71

7. Introduction to Section Two: Integrating Assessment Methods with Blueprints   71
Louis N. Pangaro, M.D.

8. Descriptive Evaluations and Clinical Performance Evaluations in the Workplace   77
Rechell G. Rodriguez, M.D.; Paul A. Hemmer, M.D., M.P.H.

9. Direct Observation of Students' Clinical Skills   97
Eric Holmboe, M.D.

10. Evaluating Medical Procedures: Evaluation and Transfer to the Bedside   113
Jeffrey H. Barsuk, M.D., M.S.; Eytan Szmuilowicz, M.D.

11. Assessing Clinical Reasoning   127
Steven Durning, M.D.; Joseph Rencic, M.D.;
Lambert Schuwirth, M.D.

12. The Search for a Meaningful Evaluation of Professionalism   147
Emily E. Anderson, Ph.D., M.P.H.; Mark Kuczewski, Ph.D.

13. Feedback   163
Lisa E. Leggio, M.D.; T. Andrew Albritton, M.D.

Section Three   175

14. Introduction to Section Three: Structured Assessments for Clerkships   175
William C. McGaghie, Ph.D.

15. Clerkship Examinations   177
Thomas Sisson, M.D.; Cyril Grum, M.D.

16. Writing Multiple Choice Questions   191
Ruth-Marie E. Fincher, M.D.; Robert R. Nesbit, Jr., M.D.

17. Standardized Patient-Based Assessment of Clinical Skills in Clerkships   201
Michael Ainsworth, M.D.; Karen Szauter, M.D.

18. Assessment Using Simulation Technologies   209
Keith F. Muccino, S.J., M.D.; Viva Jo Siddall, M.S., M.S., R.R.T., R.C.P., C.C.M.E.-P.

19. Designing and Setting Standards in Clerkship Examinations   229
Julia Corcoran, M.D., M.H.P.E.

20. Converting Evaluations into Grades   239
Michael Battistone, M.D.

21. Legal Aspects of Assigning Failing Grades   251
Thomas Jamieson, M.D., J.D.; Paul A. Hemmer, M.D., M.P.H.; Louis N. Pangaro, M.D.

22. Conclusions   263
William C. McGaghie, Ph.D.; Louis N. Pangaro, M.D.

Index   271

Foreword

The clinical teacher has multiple roles to play as information provider, facilitator of learning, role model, curriculum or course planner, developer of learning resources and experiences, and assessor of students' competence. Of these, the role of assessor is probably the most important and one of the most difficult. The student can find alternative approaches to learning but has to accept the assessment system imposed on him or her. The Alliance for Clinical Education is to be congratulated on producing a sequel to the *Guidebook for Clerkship Directors*, specifically on the subject of assessment. What we assess and how we assess it demonstrates to the student what we value and has a profound effect on their behavior and approach to learning. There is no better way of raising standards and the quality of our education program than through appropriate and effective assessment with feedback to the student and teacher. The importance of assessment to determine whether a student is fit to pass from one phase of an education program to the next, or on completion of the program to practice as a doctor is obvious. Working with the OSCE, I found that assessment can also be a powerful instrument for learning - assessment *for* learning and assessment *as* learning, as well as assessment *of* learning. Through assessment the teacher shares with the student a concept of quality, what matters, and the standard that needs to be achieved. This *Handbook* addresses these issues and introduces readers to their role as assessors of students' competence.

What do we expect of our teachers in relation to assessment? We certainly expect them to have basic skills in relation to the assessment of students in different contexts using a range of instruments such as multiple choice questions, OSCEs, work-based assessments, and the use of simulation and new technologies. But as teachers we are more than technicians with some basic knowledge of what to do. As professionals we should understand why we are doing it and appreciate some of the principles underpinning how we assess our students. This *Handbook* meets these demands. It provides useful descriptions, topics, and guidelines relating to a wide range of different approaches to assessment, about which as teachers we should be familiar. But it does much more. It helps readers to understand the process of assessment and how to approach important challenges such as the use of assessment to identify high-risk students and the problems associated with assigning failing grades.

This *Handbook* provides a theoretical and practical insight into assessment. It challenges us to think about what it is we are assessing. Traditionally, emphasis has been on the assessment of history taking skills, physical examination, and practical procedures. Very much in line with the move to an outcome or competency-based approach to education and competency-based assessment, the text also encourages us to look at how we assess learning domains such as clinical reasoning and professionalism.

Traditionally we have tended to look at each assessment of a student as an isolated event and not with a broader vision of the assessment as part of an overall program. This *Handbook* has the potential to make an important contribution to assessment by encouraging a greater use to be made of the information gained about a student in an assessment across the interfaces of the different curriculum phases. This sharing of assessment information about a student across the different elements in the education program resonates powerfully with the concept of a smoother continuum of education across the different phases of education, a theme very much on today's agenda in medical education.

Returning to my opening comment - assessment of students is important. We are seeing significant changes taking place in medical education and in how students are assessed. While as teachers we may not always adopt the latest teaching method or educational strategy, to fail to understand how we can best assess our students and not to do it in an appropriate manner is a lost opportunity with potentially serious consequences. To paraphrase John Dewey - "If we assess today's students as we assessed yesterday's, we rob them of tomorrow." This book provides readers with an insight into how they can assess students more effectively and efficiently in the context of the changes in medical education. It can serve as a springboard for us to examine our own assessment practices.

Ronald M. Harden, O.B.E., M.D., F.R.C.P. (Glas.),
F.R.C.S. (Ed.), F.R.C.P.C.
Professor of Medical Education (Emeritus)
University of Dundee
General Secretary of AMEE and Editor of *Medical Teacher*

Preface

The Alliance for Clinical Education (ACE) *Handbook on Medical Student Evaluation and Assessment* is written to provide practical guidance for course and clerkship directors working in clinical education. Although the focus is undergraduate medical education, we realize that there are many interns in the first postgraduate year whose readiness for supervised clinical practice may need to be improved, or at least verified. The chapters in this book reflect both evidence and opinion drawn from experience working with undergraduate medical students and with residents in graduate medical education.

The *Handbook* is a sequel to the successful *Guidebook for Clerkship Directors* from the Alliance for Clinical Education, now in its fourth edition (2012). Over the first three editions of the *Guidebook*, its chapter on evaluation of medical students became broader in scope and deeper in scholarship; i.e., it grew much longer! Assessment and evaluation continue to be among the most important and complex problems faced by medical clinical teachers and clinical academic leaders, i.e., course directors, clerkship directors, program directors, and associate deans. The scope of the *Guidebook* also increased dramatically over successive editions. Consequently the ACE directors realized that the length of the student evaluation chapter could not be sustained. The ACE leadership, the editors of the *Guidebook*, and the publisher, Gegensatz Press, asked us to provide a fuller version, a new book, not just expanded, but in more depth, and updated since the publication of the 2012 *Guidebook*. This volume is a book-length extension of the writing about assessment and evaluation of medical students that was previously presented in a single chapter.

We prepared this book for colleagues who are looking for a comprehensive approach and practical guidance to address problems of medical student evaluation and assessment with a focus on students who are on a growth curve, i.e., they not at the point for a final judgment about readiness for independent practice. It is not our intention to compete with recent books that focus on residents or have a theoretical orientation. Consistent with the interdisciplinary mission of the Alliance, the chapter authors and literature cited come from all medical practice specialties.

There is no more important statement about what we think of ourselves as a medical profession than our student evaluation practices. Rigorous medical student evaluation gives confidence to future patients of our trainees and establishes fairness for students and their teachers about what we ask of them. Hence our motto: "Evaluation is professionalism."

This book-length treatment about medical student assessment and evaluation provides more depth than the student evaluation chapter found in the fourth edition of the 2012 *Guidebook*. The goal of this *Handbook* is practical advice. The intent is to give readers evidence-based guidance. However, rigorous and useful evidence is not always available, and the varied settings of medical education research studies may limit their generalizability. Therefore, we provide a set of evidence and experience-based principles for the issues addressed in the twenty-two chapters. Most physicians will be comfortable with this approach because they use principles of physiology and basic reasoning to solve clinical problems every day when scientific evidence is not always available.

The *Handbook* is structured in three sections. The first section (Chapters 1-6) begins with a general introduction to the purposes and methods of evaluation (Chapter 1) by Dr. McGaghie, and continues with a primer of evaluation terms (Chapter 2) and a discussion of systems of assessment in medical education (Chapter 3), both by Dr. Pangaro. A discussion of shared information across the interfaces of courses and clerkships, both horizontally and vertically, leads to the chapters on sharing student performance information across courses and clerkships (Chapter 4, by Dr. Cleary) and using pre-clerkship variables to identify high-risk students (Chapter 5, by Drs. LaRochelle and Denton). Section One concludes with a discussion about medical student assessment in the post-clerkship year(s) (Chapter 6, by Drs. Aiyer and Mischler).

Section Two (Chapters 7-13) covers medical student assessment methods that are used in the clinical workplace, and which are critical to formative evaluation. The section begins with a discussion of integrating methods (Chapter 7, by Dr. Pangaro). In Chapter 8, Drs. Rodriguez and Hemmer discuss descriptive evaluations and clinical performance evaluations in the workplace. Dr. Holmboe discusses direct observation of student clinical skills in Chapter 9. Chapter 10, by Drs. Barsuk and Szmuilowicz, covers evaluating medical procedures and transfer to the bedside. Drs. Durning, Rencic, and Schuwirth present state-of-the-art information on assessing clinical reasoning in Chapter 11. Drs. Anderson and Kuczewski, specialists in ethics and humanities, write about the evaluation of professionalism in Chapter 12. Section Two concludes with Chapter 13, on feedback, by Drs. Leggio and Allbritton.

Section Three (Chapters 14-22) deals with standardized, summative assessments, especially the use of examinations at the end of a clinical experience (Chapter 14, by Dr. McGaghie). Chapter 15 on clerkship examinations, by Drs. Sisson and Grum, covers written examinations prepared at individual medical schools and obtained from external sources, e.g., the National Board of Medical Examiners (NBME). Drs. Fincher and Nesbit present a tutorial on writing multiple choice questions in Chapter 16. Use of standardized patients and OSCEs for assessment of clinical skills in clerkships is covered by Drs. Ainsworth and Szauter in Chapter 17. Assessments with other forms of simulation technology are discussed by Dr. Muccino and Ms. Siddall in Chapter 18. Three final chapters follow: on designing and setting standards for clerkship examinations by Dr. Corcoran (Chapter 19); converting evaluations into grades (Chapter 20) by Dr. Battistone; and legal aspects of assigning failing grades (Chapter 21) by Drs. Jamieson, Hemmer, and Pangaro.

A concluding Chapter 22 by the editors comments on future directions for educational practice and research, research approaches that will be needed, and the required infrastructure.

Acknowledgments: We thank Susan Cox, M.D., President of the Alliance for Clinical Education; Bruce Morgenstern, M.D., Editor-in-Chief of the fourth edition of the *Guidebook for Clerkship Directors*; and Gary Beck, Ph.D., Executive Director of the Alliance, for their editorial assistance and support throughout the project.

Colleagues in our own institutions have provided much help throughout the writing and editing process. We are indebted to the F. Edward Hébert School of Medicine of the Uniformed Services University of the Health Sciences, "America's medical school," and to the Ralph P. Leischner, Jr., M.D. Institute for Medical Education at the Loyola University of Chicago Stritch School of Medicine for supporting this work.

Louis N. Pangaro, Bethesda, Maryland
William C. McGaghie, Maywood, Illinois
September 2014

Contributors

Michael A. Ainsworth, M.D.
Professor of Internal Medicine
Vice Dean for Academic Affairs
University of Texas Medical Branch, Galveston, Texas

Meenakshy K. Aiyer, M.B.B.S., F.A.C.P.
Associate Professor of Clinical Medicine
Associate Dean for Academic Affairs
University of Illinois College of Medicine at Peoria, Peoria, Illinois

T. Andrew Albritton, M.D.
Professor of Medicine
Senior Associate Dean for Curriculum
Medical College of Georgia at Georgia Regents University, Augusta, Georgia

Emily E. Anderson, Ph.D., M.P.H.
Assistant Professor
Neiswanger Institute for Bioethics
Loyola University of Chicago
Stritch School of Medicine, Maywood, Illinois

Jeffrey H. Barsuk, M.D., M.S., S.F.H.M.
Associate Professor of Medicine
Department of Medicine
Director of Simulation and Patient Safety
Northwestern University Feinberg School of Medicine, Chicago, Illinois

Michael J. Battistone, M.D.
Associate Professor
Department of Medicine
University of Utah School of Medicine, Salt Lake City, Utah

Lynn M. Cleary, M.D.
Professor of Medicine
Vice President for Academic Affairs
State University of New York Upstate Medical University, Syracuse, New York

Julia Corcoran, M.D., M.H.P.E.
Associate Professor of Surgery
Northwestern University Feinberg School of Medicine, Chicago, Illinois

G. Dodd Denton, M.D., M.P.H.
Associate Professor of Medicine
Primary Care Clerkship Director
University of Queensland, Brisbane, Australia
Ochsner Clinical School, New Orleans, Louisiana

Steven J. Durning, M.D., Ph.D., F.A.C.P.
Professor of Medicine and Pathology
Director, Introduction to Clinical Reasoning Course
F. Edward Hébert School of Medicine
Uniformed Services University of the Health Sciences, Bethesda, Maryland

Ruth-Marie E. Fincher, M.D.
Professor of Medicine and Vice Dean for Academic Affairs Emerita
Medical College of Georgia at Georgia Regents University, Augusta, Georgia

Cyril M. Grum, M.D.
Professor and Senior Associate Chair for Undergraduate Medical Education
Department of Internal Medicine
University of Michigan Medical School, Ann Arbor, Michigan

Paul A. Hemmer, M.D., M.P.H.
Professor and Vice Chair, Educational Programs, Department of Medicine
F. Edward Hébert School of Medicine
Uniformed Services University of the Health Sciences, Bethesda, Maryland

Eric Holmboe, M.D., F.A.C.P., F.R.C.P.
Senior Vice President, Milestone Development and Evaluation
Accreditation Council for Graduate Medical Education
Adjunct Professor of Medicine
Yale University, New Haven, Connecticut
Adjunct Professor of Medicine
Uniformed Services University of the Health Sciences, Bethesda, Maryland

Thomas W. Jamieson, M.D.
Medical Consultation and Review, Department of Veterans Affairs
Office of Inspector General
Office of Healthcare Inspections, Washington, D.C.

Mark Kuczewski, Ph.D.
The Fr. Michael I. English, S.J., Professor of Medical Ethics
Chair, Department of Medical Education
Loyola University of Chicago
Stritch School of Medicine, Maywood, Illinois

Jeff LaRochelle, M.D., M.P.H.
Associate Professor of Medicine
F. Edward Hébert School of Medicine
Uniformed Services University of the Health Sciences, Bethesda, Maryland

Lisa Engen Leggio, M.D.
Associate Professor of Pediatrics
Director of Pediatric Student Education
Medical College of Georgia at Georgia Regents University, Augusta, Georgia

William C. McGaghie, Ph.D.
Director, Ralph P. Leischner, Jr., M.D. Institute for Medical Education
Professor of Medical Education
Loyola University Chicago
Stritch School of Medicine, Maywood, Illinois

Matthew Mischler, M.D.
Clinical Assistant Professor of Medicine
Clerkship Director, M3 and M4 Internal Medicine
OSF Saint Francis Medical Center
University of Illinois College of Medicine at Peoria, Peoria, Illinois

Keith F. Muccino, S.J., M.D.
Associate Dean for Clinical Performance and Assistant Professor of Medicine
Loyola University of Chicago
Stritch School of Medicine, Maywood, Illinois

Robert R. Nesbit, Jr., M.D., F.A.C.S.
Professor Emeritus of Surgery
Director of Medical Student Education (Surgery)
Medical College of Georgia at Georgia Regents University, Augusta, Georgia

Louis N. Pangaro, M.D., M.A.C.P.
Professor and Chairman, Department of Medicine (MED)
F. Edward Hébert School of Medicine
Uniformed Services University of the Health Sciences, Bethesda, Maryland

Joseph Rencic, M.D.
Associate Professor of Medicine
Tufts Medical Center, Boston, Massachusetts

Rechell G. Rodriguez, M.D., F.A.C.P.
Associate Clerkship Director
Associate Professor of Medicine
F. Edward Hébert School of Medicine
Uniformed Services University of the Health Sciences, Bethesda, Maryland

Lambert Schuwirth, M.D., Ph.D.
Professor of Medical Education
Director of the Prideaux Centre for Health Professions Education
Flinders University, Adelaide, Australia
Professor of Innovative Assessment
Maastricht University, Maastricht, Netherlands

Viva Jo Siddall, M.S., M.S., R.R.T., R.C.P., C.C.M.E.-P.
Medical Educator II Research Coordinator
Loyola University Chicago
Stritch School of Medicine, Maywood, Illinois

Thomas H. Sisson, M.D.
Professor of Medicine
Department of Internal Medicine
University of Michigan Medical School, Ann Arbor, Michigan

Karen Szauter, M.D.
Professor
Department of Internal Medicine and Office of Clinical Simulation
University of Texas Medical Branch, Galveston, Texas

Eytan Szmuilowicz, M.D.
Director, Section of Palliative Medicine
Assistant Professor of Medicine
Northwestern University Feinberg School of Medicine, Chicago, Illinois

Section One

Chapter 1
Introduction

William C. McGaghie, Ph.D.

The terms "evaluation" and "assessment" frequently have negative connotations for learners engaged in a program of study. Evaluations and assessments can be strong motivators that channel learner thinking and behavior, with the potential of adverse consequences for those who fall short. Such learner perceptions contrast with faculty intent, where evaluation is considered a tool needed to boost medical student competence and, for medical educators, to protect the public. Nonetheless, learners often perceive the stakes to be high and evaluation to be a source of anxiety. Evaluation in medical education can have an upside, especially as both learners and teachers acknowledge that the goal is to produce superb clinicians. When educational evaluation data are seen and used as a tool, not as a weapon, the outlook becomes improvement and mastery rather than enforcement. This outlook also changes the psychological climate toward constructive progress instead of apprehension.[1,2]

This introduction provides a four-part overview and sets a point of departure for the twenty-one chapters that follow, organized as three sections. Much of this amplifies work published nearly three decades ago.[3] The foundation material was published previously in the chapter on medical student evaluation in the *ACE Guidebook for Clerkship Directors* - fourth edition - (Gegensatz Press, 2012). This has now been expanded and updated to report new developments.

1.1. Purposes of Learner Evaluation

There are at least eight purposes of learner evaluation in medical education: (a) accreditation, (b) assess competence, (c) document learner experience, (d) gauge academic progress, (e) predict performance, (f) generate feedback for improvement, (g) assign grades, and (h) judge program effectiveness. Each of these purposes is addressed in many ways throughout the remaining sections and chapters. They are all important, but for different reasons.

1.1.1. Accreditation

Undergraduate medical education in the United States is governed by the Liaison Committee on Medical Education (LCME) which imposes detailed requirements for learner evaluation that medical education programs must fulfill just to stay in business.[4] Cyclic accreditation reviews assure that, once met, a medical education program's learner evaluation criteria and standards do not erode, and do in fact evolve.

1.1.2. Assess Competence

Assessment of medical student competence is a basic responsibility for all programs of clinical medical education. Such assessments represent accomplishment benchmarks, tangible signs of medical student progress along the educational continuum. They depend, of course, on *a priori* statements of cognitive, procedural, or affective learning goals; high performance standards; and measurement methods that yield reliable data about student achievement. Medical educators realize that sound competence assessments can also provide focussed feedback to students and feedback about educational program effectiveness for faculty and administration.

Competence assessments external to a clerkship are also imposed in the form of standardized "board" examinations. With few exceptions at this point in time, clerkship-level medical students have successfully passed USMLE Step 1 and are beginning preparation for Step 2 and its clinical component (Step 2 CS) involving standardized patients (SPs).

1.1.3. Document Learner Experience

Most clerkship directors and residency program directors struggle to document and especially manage student exposure to a variety of clinical problems.[5] This is an important task to ensure adequate compliance with the LCME Standard 6.2, Required Clinical Experiences.[4] The growing use of SPs (see Chapter 17) and other forms of medical simulation (see Chapter 18) can complement contact with real patients and increase uniformity of exposure within the clinical curriculum.

1.1.4. Gauge Academic Progress

Educational evaluations are used to gauge and monitor student academic progress at frequent intervals. Medical students are expected to advance through the medical clinical curriculum on a "critical path," achieving successive program goals, both within individual clerkships and across the clerkship timetable. Wide deviations from that path are a source of concern for clerkship directors and may require remediation.

1.1.5. Predict Performance

Today's educational evaluations are often used to forecast performance on future assessments. The success of educational forecasts usually stems from the similarity of the skills being assessed, congruence of measurement methods, and the time span between the measurements (shorter is better for prediction). The conventional wisdom that "the best way to predict future behavior is to rely on one's current and past behavior" is correct.[6] Rigorous evaluations that produce reliable data give teachers and medical learners a window to future performance. The question of whether this information should be passed to future clerkships is addressed in Chapter 4.

1.1.6. Generate Feedback for Improvement

Medical learners are usually eager to discuss their educational experiences and are anxious to find ways to boost their fund of knowledge or improve their clinical skills. "Performance feedback" is a term that is widely used to describe information that gives learners knowledge of results about their study and clinical work. Given *specific feedback* about their progress or deficits, medical students can either move to new areas of clinical practice or take steps to improve marginal performance (see Chapter 13).

An educational program needs to have three basic features before useful feedback can be given to learners. First, the program needs to have clear goals that represent a graduated set of milestones for medical students. Second, the program needs to have a means to collect, store, and routinely retrieve reliable data that learners and their teachers can use for educational feedback. Third, the program needs faculty who are willing to take time to review candidly the evaluative data with students tied to clerkship goals. Chapter 3 deals with what the education system provides to ensure the utility and consistency of evaluation and feedback.

1.1.7. Assign Grades

Clerkships usually operate inside a university environment. Academic tradition holds that variation in student achievement is acknowledged by the administrative action of assigning low and high grades. One of the toughest everyday responsibilities that clerkship directors face is translating data about student performance into medical school grades to fulfill university expectations (see Chapters 20 and 21).

Grades assign value to medical student work. As discussed in the lexicon of evaluation in Chapter 2, grades can be given in a normative way ("on the curve") to compare students against their peers or in ways that compare all students against a fixed achievement standard. Fair and impartial grade assignment is a necessary condition of clerkship education.

1.1.8. Judge Program Effectiveness

Learner evaluation data, including local knowledge tests and board examination scores, results of objective structured clinical examinations (OSCEs) and SP-based clinical exams, measures of professionalism, and tests using medical simulations, can be employed in a variety of ways to judge the effectiveness of a medical education program. Quality improvement (QI) is another outcome when medical student performance data are used to judge clerkship effectiveness.

1.2. Evaluation Goals

Clerkship directors are expected to articulate the evaluation goals and the domains that are being assessed when designing medical student evaluation. The Accreditation Council for Graduate Medical Education (ACGME) has identified six competencies for evaluation of postgraduate learning outcomes: practice-based learning and improvement, patient care, professionalism, interpersonal and communication skills, medical knowledge, and systems-based practice.[7] Many medical schools have also adopted these six categories to frame and manage student assessment. Other frameworks are also in use, including the Canadian CanMEDS Physician Competency Framework[8] and the Scottish Doctors Learning Outcomes.[9] The features and uses of a variety of frameworks for learner assessment in medicine are summarized in a recent report.[10] Many would agree that a distillate of five equally weighted goals from these frameworks should focus undergraduate medical student evaluation. These five goals are: (a) professional knowledge, (b) technical and procedural skills, (c) professionalism, (d) professional relationships, and (e) physician-patient relationships. Each evaluation goal is addressed by different measures of medical student achievement.

1.2.1. Professional Knowledge

Medical knowledge assessment is done via internal (e.g., course, clerkship, see Chapter 15) and external (e.g., USMLE Steps 1 and 2) evaluations that rely mainly on multiple choice questions (MCQs) (see Chapter 16). The primacy of these tests demonstrates that knowledge acquisition is a basic goal of undergraduate medical education.

1.2.2. Technical and Procedural Skills

Assessment of medical student technical and procedural proficiency has grown in frequency and sophistication over the past decade. Measures are now available that permit objective evaluation of such skills as cardiac auscultation,[11] ACLS maneuvers,[1,2] and the female pelvic examination.[12,13] Most of these measures rely on simulation technology embodied in SPs or medical simulators[14] (see Chapters 17 and 18).

1.2.3. Professionalism

Professionalism is expressed in each young physician's character, reliability, honesty, ability to keep confidences, and other nonacademic qualities that embody "the good doctor" (see Chapter 12).

Teaching and evaluating student professionalism has become one of the highest priorities of U.S. medical schools. Assessing professionalism is difficult to do with precision.[15,16] However, such assessments are essential because, "Unprofessional behavior in medical school is associated with subsequent disciplinary action by a state medical board."[17]

1.2.4. Professional Relationships

A fourth evaluation goal is professional relationships. This goal goes beyond personal integrity to embrace respect for other members of the health care team, administrative staff, and other colleagues. Professional relationships are currently addressed infrequently in undergraduate medical education, while its profile is rising in graduate and continuing medical education (GME, CME). Received clinical wisdom, in addition to the literature on patient safety,[18,19] teach that clinical patient care is no longer a solitary activity. Instead, nearly all patient care is now delivered by teams of clinicians having different credentials and skills.[20,21] The emerging educational goal is how to turn a team of experts into an expert team.

1.2.5. Physician-Patient Relationships

The doctor-patient relationship is the hallmark of effective clinical practice. Recent threats to doctor-patient relationships include time pressures due to the managed care environment, social class differences, ethnic differences, and communication lapses.

1.3. Matching Evaluation Goals and Tools

A persistent problem in evaluation and grading of medical students is matching evaluation goals and tools. Many different tools are available, ranging from long, standardized tests such as the MCAT to simulations, OSCEs, and short, bedside encounters. Some evaluation tools are highly quantitative and objective, whereas others are qualitative and subjective. Each type of measure has a place in medical learner evaluation. However, the decision to select and use evaluation tools should be based on a clear understanding of one's evaluative purpose and context.

Table 1. Evaluation Methods Commonly Used in Medical Education

Method	Description	Advantages	Problems
1. Descriptive evaluation[22]	Gives a clear portrait of student status and achievements. Highly individualized; underscores the uniqueness of each medical learner in light of clerkship goals.	Requires in-depth faculty knowledge of each student. A qualitative, clinical snapshot of student performance on the clerkship. Works best with faculty group consensus.	Reliability is a concern without rater training and checks for rater bias. Are results consistent and reproducible?
2. Records of clinical encounters[5]	Case-by-case documentation of (a) clinical problems seen; and (b) decisions made about each problem.	Long-run formulation of learner practice profile. Helps identify clinical problems where more experience is needed. Best managed using computer database. Useful for gaining hospital privileges after training.	Requires high degree of learner compliance.
3. Formal (external) examinations[23,24]	Long, standardized examinations covering large bodies of medical content; often composed of separate disciplinary subtests.	Usually high-quality exams that give a general portrait of an examinee's fund of knowledge.	Test content may not match local educational objectives exactly. Not useful to pinpoint specific learning deficits. High monetary costs.
4. Local (internal) examinations[25]	Examinations written by local faculty for use in courses or clerkships.	Can be created to match local teaching emphases closely ; exams unite instruction and evaluation.	Quality can suffer if faculty are disinterested or unschooled in test development. Major cost is faculty time.
5. Simulations[26,27]	Static models, mannequins, computer-based and virtual reality approximations of clinical encounters with patients. May be used for individual or team evaluation.	Lifelike approach to evaluating learner skills and clinical reasoning. Enjoyed by clinicians; also excellent for instruction.	Simulations vary greatly in fidelity to genuine patient care problems. Scoring rules to capture clinical performance are difficult to derive. Generalization of performance across cases needs to be better established.

Table 1 (continued from previous page)

6. Objective structured clinical examination[28]	Examinees rotate through a series of stations where, in about five minutes each, they are questioned, asked to interpret clinical data, perform a procedure, or otherwise show proficiency with clinical materials.	Concrete, realistic approach to evaluating discrete clinical skills among learners. Requires prompt responses to real clinical material. Bluffing is unlikely.	Faculty involvement and cooperation is essential; tight management is needed to operate effectively.
7. Checklists[29-31]	Step-by-step "yes-no" or "right-wrong" protocols used to assess either skill at a clinical procedure (e.g., ACLS) or at preparing a clinical product (e.g., a sterile tray).	Useful to evaluate specific procedures and products. Little guesswork once checklist items and their order are agreed on.	Can appear simplistic unless procedures and products are critical. Use may require much faculty time. Rater training is essential.
8. Rating scales[29,32]	General assessments, often of learner character or noncognitive professional qualities, based on the rater's memory rather than direct observation of specific events.	Allows evaluators to quantify important qualitative factors that underlie good clinical care.	Frequent "halo" effect (leniency) meaning low ratings are rare.
9. Oral examinations[33]	Face-to-face learner-evaluator encounters where learners are questioned about clinical subjects; sometimes used to gauge if learners can withstand stress.	Historically grounded, have been used for medical learner evaluation for over 3,000 years. Encourage student-faculty interaction.	Notoriously unreliable approach to learner evaluation. Unstandardized; subject to capricious evaluator behavior.
10. Anecdotal records[34,35]	Dean's letters, faculty letters of recommendation.	Highly personalized approach to description of learner achievement and frequently, learner readiness to pursue more advanced training.	"Halo" effect is common. Frequently difficult to interpret as recipients try to "read between the lines."

Table 1 (continued on next page)

11. Chart (record) reviews[36]	Faculty-learner case discussions based on data contained in patient charts and recent progress notes.	High relevance due to grounding in real clinical work. No or low cost; straightforward, immediate feedback about patient management.	Cases selected should be representative of the learner's experience or practice, not chosen because they are unusual.
12. Standardized patients (SPs)[28]	Laypersons are trained and calibrated to present patient health problems uniformly. SPs frequently record data about learner performance.	Very high realism. SPs can record reliable data and give leaners excellent feedback. Especially useful to evaluate skills in physical diagnosis and interviewing.	SP training and calibration takes time. Careful management of the evaluation plan is needed.
13. Video reviews[37]	Learner-faculty review and critique of video recorded encounters involving the learner and patients.	Very high realism; allows mutual assessment of patient management and learner's interpersonal skill and professional qualities.	Can be "highly charged." Some learners need time to "desensitize" from seeing or hearing themselves on video recordings.
14. Educational prescription contracts, personal learning plans[38]	Written agreement between learner and evaluator about learner's educational goals for a specified period of time.	Clear specification of learner's educational intentions and outcome measures. States educational criteria and standards. Notes what support faculty will provide.	Some learners and faculty are reluctant to express expectations for one another.
15. Portfolios[39,40]	Maintenance of a tangible cumulative record of clinical, scholarly, or professional accomplishments. May contain products like publications, records of site visits, data on teaching skill, or other material.	Detailed accounting of student's nonacademic accomplishments using hard evidence from material products.	Requires high degree of learner compliance. Must specify inclusion and exclusion criteria for eligible entries. Should not duplicate educational transcript.
16. 360 degree evaluation[41,42]	Evaluation of a medical learner using rating data from a variety of sources, e.g., self, peers, supervisors, nursing staff, patients.	Broad array of data sources presents a rich portrait of the learner's perceived competence. Allows normative comparisons using different data sets.	Cumbersome and difficult to manage without a computer or Web-based system. Requires high compliance from different data sources.

Table 1 describes sixteen common evaluation methods in medical education. The table also contains a short comment about the advantages of each method and a statement about potential problems associated with using each procedure. At least one citation is given for each method to encourage further reading by those who seek more detailed information.

No single evaluation method yields useful data for all purposes. Academic physicians need to think hard about their reasons for wanting to assess a student's knowledge, procedural skill, self-confidence, honesty, dependability, or any other clinically relevant characteristic. Only after identifying the purpose of the evaluation (e.g., educational diagnosis, technical proficiency, overall performance on a rotation) should the clerkship director select a measurement tool that will produce meaningful data to inform the needed decisions.

1.4. Evaluation and Learner Motivation

Medical educators know that examinations shape and drive student behavior. Today's medical students often live from test to test, usually viewing each evaluation experience as a trial rather than an opportunity. The evaluations that students encounter are to them an operational definition of the curriculum because, no matter what is presented or discussed, passing tests defines life in medical school. This issue was raised over fifty years ago by George Miller in his famous book, *Teaching and Learning in Medical School*,[43] and in fact was noted about British medical education in the nineteenth century.[44]

The origins of assessment-driven behavior are not hard to detect, as discussed by Good.[45] She astutely describes the widespread and high-level culture of "evaluation apprehension" in the medical profession. Left unchecked, this apprehension can have bad effects, such as needless competition; reduced student cooperation; defensiveness; attempts at one-upmanship; and reliance on expensive extracurricular commercial test preparation courses that have no tangible benefits.[46] The challenge to medical educators is to craft and use evaluation and grading methods that truly are tools for formative and summative student improvement, not weapons that intimidate. The following sections and chapters of this book provide blueprints to fulfill that goal.

References

1. Wayne DB, Butter J, Siddall VJ, et al. Simulation-based training of internal medicine residents in advanced cardiac life support protocols: A randomized trial. Teach Learn Med 2005;17(3):210-216.
2. Wayne DB, Butter J, Siddall VJ, et al. Mastery learning of advanced cardiac life support skills by internal medicine residents using simulation technology and deliberate practice. J Gen Intern Med 2006;21(3):251-256.

3. McGaghie WC. Evaluation of learners. In: McGaghie WC, Frey JJ, eds. Handbook for the Academic Physician. New York: Springer, 1986: 125-146.
4. LCME. Functions and Structure of a Medical School: Standards for Accreditation of Medical Education Programs Leading to the M.D. Degree. Washington, DC: Liaison Committee on Medical Education, June 2013.
5. Stahl JE, Balasubramanian HJ, Gao X, et al. Balancing clinical experience in outpatient residency training. Med Decis Making 2014;34(4):464-472.
6. Greenburg DL, Durning SJ, Cohen DLK, et al. Identifying medical students likely to exhibit poor professionalism and knowledge during internship. J Gen Intern Med 2007;22(12):1711-1717.
7. ACGME. Common Program Requirements. Chicago: Accreditation Council for Graduate Medical Education, July 2013.
8. Frank JR, ed. The Royal College of Physicians and Surgeons of Canada. The CanMEDS 2005 Physician Competency Framework. <fhs.mcmaster.ca/pathres/resident_resources/documents/CanMEDS2005_e.pdf>. Accessed February 7, 2015.
9. Scottish Deans' Medical Curriculum Group. The Scottish Doctor: Learning Outcomes for the Medical Undergraduate in Scotland: A Foundation for Competent and Reflective Practitoners - third edition - Dundee, Scotland: Association for Medical Education in Europe Office, April 2008.
10. Pangaro LN, ten Cate O. Frameworks for learner assessment in medicine: AMEE guide no. 78. Med Teach. 2013;35(6):e1197-e1210.
11. Butter J, McGaghie WC, Cohen ER, et al. Simulation-based mastery learning improves cardiac auscultation skills in medical students. J Gen Intern Med 2010;25(8):780-785.
12. Pugh CM, Srivastava S, Shavelson R, et al. The effect of simulator use on learning and self-assessment: The case of Stanford University's e-pelvis simulator. Stud Health Technol Inform 2001;81:396-400.
13. Pugh CM, Youngblood P. Development and validation of assessment measures for a newly developed physical examination simulator. J Am Med Inform Assoc 2001;9(5):448-460.
14. Issenberg SB, McGaghie WC, Petrusa ER, et al. Features and uses of high-fidelity medical simulations that lead to effective learning: A BEME systematic review. Med Teach 2005;27(1):10-28.
15. Stern DT, ed. Measuring Medical Professionalism. New York: Oxford University Press, 2006.
16. Hemmer PA, Hawkins RE, Jackson JL, Pangaro LN. Assessing how well three evaluation methods detect deficiencies in medical students' professionalism in two settings of an internal medicine clerkship. Acad Med. 2000;75(2):167-173.
17. Papadakis MA, Hodgson CS, Teherani A, Kohatsu ND. Unprofessional behavior in medical school is associated with subsequent disciplinary action by a state medical board. Acad Med 2004;79(3):244-249.
18. Bogner MS, ed. Human Error in Medicine - second edition - Boca Raton, FL: CRC, 2014.
19. Kohn LT, Corrigan JM, Donaldson MS, eds. Institute of Medicine. Committee on Quality of Health Care in America. To Err is Human: Building a Safer Health System. Washington, DC: National Academies Press, 2000.
20. Siassakos D, Fox R, Bristowe K, et al. What makes maternity teams effective and safe? Lessons from a series of research on teamwork, leadership and team training. Acta Obstet Gynecol Scand 2013;92(11):1239-1243.

21. Neily J, Mills PD, Young-Xu Y, et al. Association between implementation of a medical team training program and surgical mortality. JAMA 2010;304(15):1693-1700.
22. Battistone MJ, Milne C, Sande MA, et al. The feasibility and acceptability of implementing formal evaluation sessions and using descriptive vocabulary to assess student performance on a clinical clerkship. Teach Learn Med 2002;14(1):5-10.
23. Case SM, Swanson DB. Constructing Written Test Questions for the Basic and Clinical Sciences - third edition - Philadelphia: National Board of Medical Examiners, 2000.
24. Juul D. Evaluation of knowledge acquisition. In: McGaghie WC, ed. International Best Practices for Evaluation in the Health Professions. London: Radcliffe, 2013: 127-138.
25. Jozefowicz RF, Koeppen BM, Case S, et al. The quality of in-house medical school examinations. Acad Med 2002;77(2):156-161.
26. McGaghie WC, Issenberg SB, Petrusa ER, Scalese RJ. A critical review of simulation-based medical education research: 2003-2009. Med Educ 2010;44(1): 50-63.
27. McGaghie WC, Issenberg SB, Barsuk JH, Wayne DB. A critical review of simulation-based mastery learning with translational outcomes. Med Educ 2014;48(4):375-385.
28. Boursicot K, Etheridge L, Setna Z, et al. Clinical competence assessment. In: McGaghie WC, ed. International Best Practices for Evaluation in the Health Professions. London: Radcliffe, 2013: 97-125.
29. Adler MD, Vozenilek JA, Trainor JL, et al. Comparison of checklist and anchored global rating instrument for performance rating of simulated pediatric emergencies. Sim Healthc 2011;6(1):18-24.
30. Stufflebeam DL. Guidelines for Developing Evaluation Checklists: The Checklist Development Checklist (CDC). Western Michigan University Evaluation Center, July 2000. <www.wmich.edu/evalctr/archive_checklists/guidelines_cdc.pdf>. Accessed April 2, 2015.
31. Hales B, Terblanche M, Fowler R, Sibbald W. Development of medical checklists for improved quality of patient care. Int J Qual Health Care 2008;20(1):22-30.
32. Williams RG, Klamen DA, McGaghie WC. Cognitive, social, and environmental sources of bias in clinical performance ratings. Teach Learn Med 2003;15(4): 270-292.
33. Tekian A, Yudkowsky R. Oral examinations. In: Downing SM, Yudkowsky R, eds. Assessment in Health Professions Education. New York: Routledge, 2009: 269-285.
34. Edmond M, Roberson M, Hasan N. The dishonest dean's letter: An analysis of 532 dean's letters from 99 U.S. medical schools. Acad Med 1999;74(9):1033-1035.
35. Lurie SJ, Lambert DR, Nofziger AC, et al. Relationship between peer assessment during medical school, dean's letter rankings, and ratings by internship directors. J Gen Intern Med 2007;22(1):13-16.
36. Payne N, Corbett E, Bradley E, et al. Pediatric chart review and case presentation OSCE (objective structured clinical examination). 2007. <www.mededportal.org/publication/570>. Accessed February 7, 2015.
37. Ericsson KA. Necessity is the mother of invention: Video recording firsthand perspectives of critical medical procedures to make simulated training more effective. Acad Med 2014;89(1):17-20.
38. Challis M. Personal learning plans: AMEE guide no. 19. Med Teach 2000;22(3): 225-236.

39. Tekian A, Yudkowsky R. Assessment portfolios. In: Downing SM, Yudkowsky R., eds. Assessment in Health Professions Education. New York: Routledge, 2009: 287-304.
40. Searle NS, Teal CR, Richards BF, et al. A standards-based, peer-reviewed teaching award to enhance a medical school's teaching environment and inform the promotions process. Acad Med 2012;87(7):870-876.
41. Kaplan SH, Ware JE. The patient's role in health care and quality assessment. In: Goldfield N, Nash DB, eds. Providing Quality Care: The Challenge to Clinicians. Philadelphia: American College of Physicians, 1989: 25-68.
42. Center for Creative Leadership. 360 by Design Facilitator's Guide. <www.ccl.org/leadership/pdf/assessments/360bdfacguide.pdf>. Accessed February 7, 2015.
43. Miller GE, ed. Teaching and Learning in Medical School. Cambridge, MA: Harvard University Press, 1961.
44. Newman C. The Evolution of Medical Education in the Nineteenth Century. London: Oxford University Press, 1957.
45. Good MJD. American Medicine: The Quest for Competence. Berkeley: University of California Press, 1995.
46. McGaghie WC, Downing SM, Kubilius R. What is the impact of commercial test preparation courses on medical examination performance? Teach Learn Med 2004;16(2):202-211.

Chapter 2
A Primer of Evaluation Terminology: Definitions and Important Distinctions in Evaluation

Louis N. Pangaro, M.D.

Through a series of definitions and distinctions, this chapter provides a lexicon for key terms and issues in evaluation and assessment. The purpose is to provide clinical educators with a quick reference to terms that guide the practical decisions to be made in clerkships. Since terms are sometimes used differently in different contexts, and by different authors, etymologies may be provided for root usage in the "embryology" of the term. Etymologies are based principally on *The Compact Edition of the Oxford English Dictionary* (Oxford: Clarendon Press, 1971).

The foundation material was published previously in the chapter on medical student evaluation in the *ACE Guidebook for Clerkship Directors* - fourth edition - (Gegensatz Press, 2012). This has now been expanded and updated to report new developments.

The following definitions and distinctions are discussed:

1. Evaluation vs. Grading vs. Assessment; Evaluative Judgments.
2. Formative vs. Summative Evaluation.
3. Process vs. Product (Outcome) Measurements; Baseline Measurements.
4. Dichotomous vs. Scalar Grading.
5. Normative vs. Fixed Standards (Criterion-Based).
6. Compensatory vs. "Weakest-Link" Models.
7. Descriptive vs. Quantitative Methods ("Subjective" and "Objective").
8. Analytic vs. Synthetic Approaches; Developmental Approaches.
9. Competence vs. Performance
10. "Competencies" and "Milestones."
11. Reliability and Validity; Feasibility.
12. Curriculum vs. Syllabus.

2.1. Evaluation vs. Grading vs. Assessment; Evaluative Judgments

Evaluation, rooted in "value" and derived from the Latin *valere* ("to be strong"), indicates a judgment of how well a student's strengths correspond to the "values" of the concerned communities, including the department, the school, and the profession. *Grading* implies assigning a label to the level of performance achieved, and derives from the Latin word *gradus,* or step. Grading within a medical school is, effectively, an administrative action classifying the level of performance achieved. Since *evaluation* implies values, words are needed to convey the meaning, such as an explicit or implied description *in words* of how a student is performing. *Grade,* however, implies a concise classification that can be expressed with letters, terms, or even numbers, i.e.: A, B, C, D, etc.; Honors, High Pass, Pass, Low Pass, Fail, Incomplete, Withdrawal; 96%, 76%, etc., of the level achieved.

Assessment is sometimes used to embrace the entire process of evaluation and grading. It comes from a Latin term meaning "to set a tax," and implies someone sitting in judgment. (The term *assessor* meant someone who "sat at" or "next to" a judge's bench). However, it can also be used to refer to the process of measuring something (an "assay," such as a radio-immunoassay) or of acquiring direct observations about a learner ("sitting next to" a student). The term *assessment,* then, combines the quantitative and qualitative aspects of gathering data for evaluation.

Judgments are part of all our key processes - evaluation, grading, and even clinical reasoning. There is typically a side-to-side comparison between what one observes (the actual) and what one expects to see (the ideal, or the standard; see below). In the diagnostic reasoning process, there is a side-to-side comparison between a patient's findings and the pattern compatible with a given diagnosis.

To judge (*juger* in Old French, from Latin *iudicare*, "to say that something is just or correct") is to decide how closely an assessment of the student's performance fits with what is expected for that level of training. In other words, it is an educational diagnosis or classification of how well the student is doing. As noted below, the assessments that are input into the judgment may be numerical or descriptive, but in either case, the process depends upon some prior judgment of what is expected.

The primary judgment made in the process of evaluation is whether the observations made of a student's performance meet an expected standard of performance. The confidence in the individual judgment must be sufficient for feedback and for aggregate judgments for grading. The primary judgment made in the process of grading is whether the student or resident may advance to the next step in training. The confidence in this judgment must be sufficient to meet an institutional standard for high-stakes decisions, and must be defensible.

While there is some flexibility, perhaps even disagreement, on which terms are used for which part of the process, it can be useful to construct a sequence in which, together, the terms establish a rhythm (assessment-evaluation-grading), and constitute a three-phase process that corresponds to the familiar rhythm of clinical medicine; this rhythm, in turn, reflects the classical sequence of observation-reflection-action. In this sequence, grading would be an administrative action, and feedback would be an educational action (see Table 2).

Table 2. The Rhythm of the Evaluation Process

Educational Process	Aristotle (*De Anima* = Περι Ψυχης = *On the Soul, passim*)	Clinical Process
Assessment = Making observations about learners.	Observation Sensation αισθησις	History and Physical
Evaluation = Determining learner's success for expected level.	Reflection Thought διανοια	Diagnosis
Grading/Feedback = Taking an action. Grading: an administrative/societal action. Feedback: an educational action.	Action Activity ενεργεια	Therapy

Practically, decisions about who is asked to evaluate a student, and who gets to "grade," have to be decided in each school and in each setting, and teachers' responses often depend on how they see the consequences of their role in this process (see Chapter 20). Grades are often submitted to the registrar's office as terse summative letters (A, B, C, etc.) or steps (Honors, High, Pass, etc); and these reductions of performance into a single letter or word can be seen by teachers and students as categorical judgments on the student as a person. Hence, the grading framework used will dictate a choice of terms that can affect what teachers are willing to contribute to grading.

2.2. Formative vs. Summative Evaluation

Formative evaluation is done to "form" or "shape" the subsequent performance of a learner, specifically by generating and providing feedback. It is done *during* an experience, and can be done by teachers as frequently as time will allow, but it should also be done formally at specified times, for instance, halfway through an experience. The Latin root, *forma*, can mean "shape," but also "beauty," implying a standard of comparison, a judgment linked to some agreed-upon expectation. This is understood in definitions of feedback, which is the "action arm" of formative evaluation.[1]

Summative evaluation is done at the end of a unit of time, typically at the end of the clerkship, and "sums" up the student's performance. Whereas formative evaluation is done primarily for the sake of the student and for continued learning, summative evaluation fulfills our responsibility to society, pronouncing the student ready for the next level of training. Summative evaluation often includes a *grade* as well as narrative description of performance and recommendations for improvement. A grade without comment would provide only minimal guidance to a student, and would not help the student improve subsequent performance. Therefore, it is recommended that a grade (classification label) always be accompanied by an evaluation (description in words).

2.3. Process vs. Product (Outcome) Measurements; Baseline Measurements

This distinction is meant to capture the difference between (1) the curriculum that students experience (process) and (2) their achievements (products, outcomes). The concept has been described as the process-product paradigm.[2] Process measurements could include documentation that students have actually completed clerkship tasks (e.g., number of patients seen, number of procedures done), while product measurements include typical, end-of-clerkship assessments (e.g., National Board of Medical Examiners subject exams). Often educational research tries to document the relationships between what we do to students (process), and how they are changed by this experience (product). Since research shows that much of what individual students actually achieve depends as much on their personal characteristics as on the formal curriculum, it is useful to document their "baseline" status, i.e., what they bring to the clerkship, by having pre-clerkship measurements such as pre-clerkship GPA or USMLE Step 1 scores[3,4] (see Chapter 5).

2.4. Dichotomous vs. Scalar Grading

Dichotomous grading (etymologically from Greek, "cutting into two") divides a group of students into those who pass and those who fail. *Polytomous* ("cutting into many parts") or, more commonly, *scalar* (*scala* = "steps," in Italian) grading recognizes a broader spectrum of student performance by providing a series of steps for assigning grades, such as Honors, High Pass, Pass, Low Pass, Fail, or the equivalent letter grades, A, B, C, D, F. Continuous grading would refer to a series of numbers in small intervals, such as 88%, 87%, 86%, etc. Generally speaking, dichotomous grading fulfills our responsibility to society by determining whether or not a learner is ready to advance to the next level. Scalar and continuous grading helps faculty and students compare performances among students, and may also help graduate program directors to rank their applicants. For quantitative assessments (such as multiple choice examinations or OSCEs), the conversion from an exam score to a final grade can be straightforward, even if the cut points are arbitrary. However, students and teachers have had an ongoing concern about the lack of clarity in how descriptive assessments from teachers are converted into a stepwise grading system (such as Honors, High Pass, etc.).

One simple method of addressing this problem is to categorize teachers' observations about a student's performance in stepwise levels, such as: second-year, third-year, fourth-year, internship - or: "reporter," "interpreter," "manager," "educator."[5,6]

2.5. Normative vs. Fixed Standards (Criterion-Based)

Normative grading is "relative." It assigns grades to students' performance by comparing them with a group, the "norm" (Latin, *norma* = "standard" or "rule"), such as a contemporary peer group. This comparison group could be a national reference, such as all students taking a certifying examination, or a local group of students taking a clerkship at the same time of year. Normative grading can be done in a mathematical way, generating a "curve," with grade rankings based on distance above or below the mean score. Normative grading is often done less formally, with half the students in the middle (for example, a grade of High Pass), a quarter receiving Pass, and a quarter receiving Honors. In any case, the essence of normative grading is to compare students with each other. Comparing a student with him/herself to gauge progress can be called *ipsative* (*ipse* = "self").

What is often called *criterion-based* grading sets mastery standards for each grading level (Pass, High Pass, etc) and is more "absolute," less relative, than norm-referenced methods. Basically, criterion-based grading is really *fixed-standard grading*, in which experts first decide what the tested domain will be (the criterion, the "what") and then what will be expected standards of proficiency (fixed standards, the "how much?"). This approach depends upon a prior judgment of what has "content validity" (see below). For example, in the domain of manual skill in suturing, the fixed standard is the degree of proficiency that must be achieved - adequacy of wound closure, the number of sutures used, and the time taken to close the wound. The examiner then decides whether the "criteria" have been met, and how well. (*Crites* means a "judge" in Greek.)

Choice of a criterion-based or fixed-standard system is one of the most difficult choices made in a clerkship, and has powerful consequences for grading decisions. In a fixed or absolute standard system, a group of three students working with a single teacher could *all* receive grades of either Pass or Honors, depending on the criteria they met. But in a normative system, they compete against each other (see Chapter 20 for a more in-depth discussion).

Another consequence of a fixed-standard grading system is that it would typically yield more grades at the upper end of the grading spectrum *at the end* of an academic year, when students would typically perform better; while a normative grading system would try to assign the same number of Honors grades at the start as at the end of the year. This highlights the difference between evaluation and grading. At the start of the year, performance as a strong "interpreter" might lead to a grade of Honors, but at the end of the year only to a grade of High Pass.

In practice, most clerkship directors agree that the dichotomous Pass/Fail decision should be based on criteria, rather than an arbitrary failing of a certain percentage of students in each clerkship for each year. It is the distinction between Honors, High Pass, Pass, etc. that is more problematic. Each institution, or perhaps each clerkship, has to decide which is fairer to patients and society (ranking students based on mastery of certain criteria) or fairer to students (assuring equal distribution of grades, irrespective of the time of year a student takes the clerkship).

2.6. Compensatory vs. "Weakest-Link" Models

A *compensatory* grading system *averages* aspects of a student's performance across several parameters to yield a final grade. For instance, a high score on a multiple choice final examination plus a failing clinical evaluation might calculate to a grade of Pass; it "compensates" (Latin, "balances"). A *non-compensatory* ("weakest link") approach would conclude that the student is not better than his/her lowest level of competence in a core area of evaluation. For instance, an excellent examination score would not compensate for poor professionalism, or vice versa. Therefore, a student with unacceptable performance in any domain of evaluation could not receive a passing final grade. Generally speaking, clerkships must determine which aspects of performance are so important that deficiencies in any cannot be compensated for by proficiency in others.

2.7. Descriptive vs. Quantitative Methods ("Subjective" and "Objective")

Descriptive methods of evaluation describe a student's performance using words. The process depends on an adequate and accepted vocabulary for what is observed, yielding a generally understood narrative of a student's performance.

Quantitative methods try to convert observations of a student's performance on a measurement scale that can yield a numerical score. Most summative grades are a combination of the two methods. A survey by the Clerkship Directors in Internal Medicine (CDIM) revealed that, on average, 63% of the clerkship grade was derived from narrative clinical evaluations and the remainder was from final examination scores.[7]

There is a tendency to refer to quantified examinations as "objective" (outside the self, therefore impersonal and unbiased; German *objektiv*), and narrative evaluations as "subjective" (existing in the mind or person, therefore assumed to idiosyncratic). However, these terms can be quite misleading. In comparison to descriptive evaluations, a multiple choice examination is dispassionate (not caring, for instance, about how confidently a student speaks), has a single "grader" (the scoring device), and its precision and reliability are more easily calculated. However, we should not confuse objectivity with reliability; and "objectification" has been called a better term for MCQs or OSCEs.[8] In any case, objectivity (or objectification) does not mean that an assessment itself has validity. Each step in creating an MCQ, decisions about what to test, and the wording of each item, involves judgments that reflect the opinions of teachers.[9]

Unspoken assumptions in the process of converting teachers' evaluations into grades often lead students to regard teachers' evaluations as subjective and arbitrary. Many students protest a lower-than-desired grade by arguing that a high score on a multiple choice test is "objective" (and therefore valid) and that the narrative evaluation describing unprofessional behavior is "subjective" (and therefore not valid). Yet, descriptive methods can achieve a level of reliability (see below) and validity that is sufficient for high-stakes decisions.[10,11] Both assessment methods have a role in assessment and in determining summative grades; one is not inherently more valuable than the other, so the commonly used terms "subjective" and "objective" - which undervalue the former - should be avoided if possible.

2.8. Analytic vs. Synthetic Approaches; Developmental Approaches

Analysis in Greek means a "loosening," a "taking apart," or a "dissolution." Traditional evaluation theory analyzes or "breaks up" a student's performance into several components: attitudes, skills, and knowledge (ASK).[12] Each component can be assessed by tools appropriate for each domain. For instance, multiple choice tests might be used to assess knowledge, and SPs can assess history-taking skills.

A "synthetic" approach "puts things together" and asks how the student's abilities in several domains come together to achieve a level of proficiency. The RIME scheme[5] introduces a vocabulary for synthetic evaluation of students' clinical skills. This describes development in clinical skills from "reporter" to "interpreter" to "manager" to "educator" (RIME) in which each task requires *all three* facets of the analytic model. For instance, a reliable "reporter" must combine skill in physical examination technique with the knowledge of what to look for in the patient at hand, and also with respect for the patient's privacy. The ability to communicate findings honestly and accurately must be combined with a sense of duty to fulfill one's responsibilities each day. While there is a developmental aspect to this, it does not imply that all students go sequentially through stages of development. Rather, the RIME scheme is intended as a "razor" defining a level of performance below which the learner should not fall.

Recently there has been initiative to apply analytic competency approaches to medical students. In the CanMEDS[13] framework the analytic approach (of six contributory roles, such as "scholar," "communicator" and "advocate") supports the dominance of "medical expert" at the primary role, which may be seen as a synthesis of all the roles. In the ACGME framework for assessment, three of the "competencies" fit the analytic model: professionalism, interpersonal skill, knowledge; and three are synthetic: patient care, system-based practice, and practice-based learning and improvement. Clerkship and program directors can resolve any uncertainty for faculty by seeing patient care as the *central*, synthetic competency in the ACGME framework, toward which the others are supportive.

It is important to recognize framework hybrids. For instance, the ACGME competencies have an overall analytic approach, in which knowledge, skills, and attitudes are incorporated in the first three competencies. However, patient care, system-based practice, and practice-based learning each requires a synthesis of domains for success.

Analytic and synthetic approaches are complementary. For instance, the RIME synthetic vocabulary offers an initial assessment framework for organizing observations about a learner's development toward independence in the domain of patient care (or as a medical expert). A teacher who recognizes that a student is an effective reporter, but not yet an interpreter, should then switch to an analytic approach in order to determine what will help the student take the next step. For example, if there is a problem moving from reporter to interpreter, does the student need to acquire more knowledge, to practice the skill of differential diagnosis, or to become more confident? Analytic and synthetic approaches reinforce each other.

The ACGME approach is intended to reach a dichotomous decision about competence at the point when a resident leaves training, and moves into unsupervised practice; therefore, it minimizes the developmental approach. However, the recent shift to assessment primarily through "milestones" (see below) that are based on a progressive movement from beginner to proficient to expert.[14] Clerkship students are in the transition from pre-clinical status to internship, and some developmental aspect is usually required in framing the evaluation system.

2.9. Competence vs. Performance

These terms have complementary meanings, but their meanings are sometimes used interchangeably, and educators should pay careful attention to how the terms are being used in a specific context. In the more common use of the terms, "competence" is what a student has the ability to do at certain times or under test conditions (in this sense, related to the Latin etymology of the word, "to strive with" or "to compete"), and "performance" is what a student does consistently on a daily basis, even when not being watched. This distinction is best reflected in the "know-can-do" description of levels of accomplishment as described in Miller's triangle; that is, the student "knows what to do," "can apply it," "can do it successfully under test conditions," and "*does* do it" regularly. Alternatively phrased, the student "knows how," "shows how" and "does." So, the distinction between competence and performance also highlights two differences, one in the setting - *in vitro* (a simulation center) or *in vivo* (actual practice), and another in process (whether the person is being observed or is *aware* of being observed).

However, these terms can also be used meaningfully in *exactly the reverse senses*, in which "performance" refers to a display ("shows how") while being observed (i.e., performing for an audience or being "on stage") in test conditions; and "competence" denotes all the attributes to function independently. In this less conventional use of the terms, competence can actually never be demonstrated until it is actually achieved in practice, in a sustained, independent way.

In practice, competence is defined in many ways and embodies many frameworks. In the analytic model, competence is proficiency in tasks in each of the contributing domains (knowledge, skills, and attitudes). In a developmental model, competence can be described in relation to the steps above it (intuitive expertise) and below it (proficiency).[15]

In the synthetic model, competence is putting all the necessary characteristics and qualities together for each patient in a sustained way. The *definition of competence* in a profession, in this model, is the ability to give to every situation which a professional might face all that properly belongs to that situation, and no more.[16] This means that a competent person first has to make the decision about what a situation requires. Since the efficiency and judgment needed to exclude unnecessary effort implies a level that is beyond most students, it may not be appropriate to use the term "competence" for students at all.

Do clerkship directors judge that a learner is "competent" (or has "competence") when proficiency is achieved in each of several "competencies," or must they all be brought to bear, consistently, in the care of individual patients? Actual practice situations are truly *in vivo*, and have the complexity of authentic decision making. *In vitro* tests, such as clinical skills examinations, focus on clinical "performance" and have often narrowed down the task for the learner. While use of the analytic method to create an assessment method for some single aspect of competence is useful for a student at the undergraduate level, it has more problems when applied to a resident about to begin unsupervised practice.

Clerkship directors therefore typically use a variety of quantitative methods to assess aspects of competence (written examinations, direct observations of interviewing skill, etc.) and rely on summary observations of teachers to see whether they can put things together.

2.10. "Competencies" and "Milestones"

The term "competency" came into common use with the introduction by the ACGME of the six "general competencies" in 1999, which were to guide the teaching and assessment of those in graduate education.[17] The six items do not together *equal* "competence," but all are part of the characteristics and detailed skills sets expected to be present in a resident ready for independent practice. In a sense the "competencies" do not describe competence, but facilitate measurement; i.e., they constitute a framework with which program directors can assess proficiency, competency by competency, with a toolbox of methods for each. This fits quite well with facilitating the ACGME Outcome Project,[25] which is intended to link processed-in-training to product (outcomes) at the end of training or in subsequent practice. Presentation and explanation of the competencies has been emphasized less since ACGME introduced the Next Accreditation System (NAS) in 2007.[18]

The "competencies" were intended to benchmark the final level of proficiency achieved by each resident, so they do not contain an explicitly developmental aspect. Clerkship directors have therefore debated their utility for medical students. The question was largely rendered moot by the influence of the strong forces of regulation of the ACGME and the endorsement of the Association of American Medical Colleges (AAMC). Therefore, clerkship directors must articulate what would be expected of starting and finishing third-year students and finishing fourth-year students. Similarly, program directors must make expectations clear for interns and PGY-2 residents. Since 2007 the ACGME and American Board of Medical Specialties (ABMS) have been working together to remedy the problem by specifying developmental "milestones" for residents.[19]

Milestones[19] are observable tasks that *combine* knowledge, skills, and attitudes, and therefore may be seen as synthetic. Each milestone may be associated with several of the ACGME competencies, but their advantage is that they allow faculty observers to focus on the task rather than the framework. This combination of different domains means that milestones are a synthetic approach.[13] Because they constitute criteria, which have higher standards of performance as trainees approach independent practice, they also require setting developmental standards, and thus work better than the "competencies" for those who work with learners at different levels of training.

2.11. Reliability and Validity; Feasibility

Reliability is the consistency, replicability, stability, or reproducibility of results. ("Rely" comes from the Latin *religare*, "to tie back," "to bind," "to connect.") Downing states: "In its most straightforward definition, reliability refers to the reproducibility of assessment data or scores, over time or occasions."[20] Reliability is the probability that a repetition of an assessment will yield the same result. Since this is rarely perfect, i.e., 100% reproducible, reliability is the amount of the observed variance that is due to the student (true score variance) rather than to the test and everything else (error variance), and is usually expressed as a decimal figure between 0 and 1.0. High reliability suggests that the "signal" (what we want to measure) is sufficiently greater than the "noise" (problems inherent in the assessment method), so that we can consider the results reproducible, or at least representative. For licensure or certification examinations, at least 90% of the variance should be true score variance (a reliability figure of 0.9). For school-based end-of-course or clerkship examination, which must be passed to advance in the curriculum, a figure of 0.8 is recommended.[20]

Validity is the confidence that we have measured what we wanted to measure, what we "value" (similar in etymology to "evaluation").[21] The validity of a test means that we are entitled to have confidence in the conclusions or inferences that we reach about the achievement (or competence) of a student based on this *specific* administration of the examination, rather than from the test in and of itself.[22]

There are several ways to establish that inferences drawn from a test are justified, and that each one depends upon the assumptions made in establishing the evidence. These underlying assumptions may be referred to as "constructs," and in this sense all arguments for validity are constructs in which we postulate that the data set in question has an important relationship to other information or data sets. Thus, in the current unitary theory of validity,[23] *all* validity may be considered to be *"construct" validity* in which the results are consistent with reasonable theory (e.g., experts perform better than novices).[23]

It may be helpful for clerkship directors to be aware of terms that have previously been used to label some common constructs. *Content validity* reflects whether a particular assessment reflects enough of the domain you want to assess, and assumes that this can be a judgment of experts, or by comparison with some list of external standards, such as from the core curricula available from clerkship groups, e.g., CDIM, Society of Teachers of Family Medicine (STFM), etc. *Face validity* refers to a judgment that the assessment method seems to experts to be appropriate for the competency in question. For instance, use of a multiple choice test to assess interpersonal skills would not have face validity. *Criterion/concurrent validity* is more numerical, and is based on the construct that the results of the assessment method should agree - usually expressed as a correlation coefficient - with other appropriate measures of students' performance. *Predictive validity* refers to the assumption (construct) that the results of one assessment measure are important, or verified, insofar as they are reflected in subsequent performance. This too is best demonstrated with mathematical methods, such as correlations or linear regression. *Consequential validity* is a term applied to a belief that the social effects of an evaluation system are important, and perhaps essential as a basis for interpreting the examination's usefulness.[23] For students, and perhaps for clerkship directors, one consequence of grades might be a student's choice of what GME specialty to apply to.

Clerkship directors are referred to the excellent articles by Downing,[20] Cook and Beckman,[24] and Cizek[23] on these subjects. The essential point is that a test or assessment is not *in itself* valid or not. The conclusions that are drawn from a particular data set are valid, or not, for the situation and specific set of students. One must be careful to examine both the data and the underlying assumptions when reaching such judgments.

Feasibility (from the French *faire*, "to do") addresses whether an assessment can actually be conducted in your own clerkship setting. Time to prepare and conduct the assessment, money to support the development, and space all contribute to feasibility. Feasibility is often the rate-limiting step in deciding how we evaluate our students. To some extent, *acceptability* to students and faculty is another aspect of feasibility. For students, their acceptance may be contingent upon perceived fairness, or upon cost in time and money. For faculty, simplicity of use and perhaps being distanced from legal implications would be the priorities. Nonetheless, it is preferable to develop reliable and valid tools, then try to make them work.

2.12. Curriculum vs. Syllabus

To some extent, what we measure and reward with a grade will determine what students learn, as in the common formulation, "Assessment drives the curriculum." The list of topics or skills that we wish students to master is the "syllabus" (a term derived from a corrupt Latin reading of a Greek word which meant "label"), and the methods we use to help students master this list are, collectively, the "curriculum" (that is, the "horse race" that we put students through, from the Latin *currere*, "to run," as in the word "current"). This distinction has implications for evaluation. If each of a school's clinical clerkships has a different list of topics to master, these are typically knowledge-based, and will require an emphasis on multiple choice tests to establish content mastery. On the other hand, if schools wish to have common goals across clerkships, then these must be process-based, such as skills in interviewing and physical examination, in differential diagnosis, and in rapid mastery of the necessary knowledge to go beyond collecting facts to interpreting them. In this approach, "curriculum" for third-year students might be seen as an invitation to move from reporter to interpreter; the basic strategy for clinical teachers would be to have a clear expectation that a student will offer a reasonable opinion.

Most clerkships accept a responsibility to be both discipline-specific (proficiency in the unique syllabus of subjects not taught elsewhere) and interdisciplinary (emphasizing common expectations which will lead to a successful performance in residency). As a consequence, the clerkship's blueprint for evaluation might identify, explicitly, the methods to assess both the discipline-specific and the interdepartmental goals.

Disclaimer

The opinions herein are the author's own, and do not represent the Uniformed Services University or the Department of Defense.

Additional Resources

Holmboe ES, Hawkins RE, eds. Practical Guide to the Evaluation of Clinical Competence. Philadelphia: Mosby, 2008.
McGaghie WC, ed. International Best Practices for Evaluation in the Health Professions. London: Radcliffe, 2013.
Pangaro LN, ten Cate O. Frameworks for learner assessment in medicine: AMEE guide no. 78. Med Teach 2013;35(6):e1197-e1210.
Schuwirth LWT, van der Vleuten CPM, General overview of the theories used in assessment: AMEE guide no. 57, Med Teach 2011;33(10):783-797.

References

1. van de Ridder JM, Stokking KM, McGaghie WC, ten Cate OT. What is feedback in clinical education? Med Educ. 2008;42(2):189-197.
2. Gage, NL. Hard Gains in the Soft Sciences: The Case of Pedagogy. Bloomington, IN: Phi Delta Kappa, Center on Evaluation and Research, 1985.
3. Durning SJ, Pangaro LN, Denton GD, et al. Intersite consistency as a measurement of programmatic evaluation in a medicine clerkship with multiple, geographically separated sites. Acad Med. 2003;78(10 Suppl):S36-S38.
4. Durning SJ, Hemmer PA, Pangaro LN. The structure of program evaluation: An approach for evaluating a course, clerkship, or components of a residency or fellowship training program. Teach Learn Med. 2007;19(3):308-318.
5. Pangaro LN. A new vocabulary and other innovations for improving descriptive in-training evaluations. Acad Med 1999;74(11):1203-1207.

6. Battistone MJ, Milne C, Sande MA, et al. The feasibility and acceptability of implementing formal evaluation sessions and using descriptive vocabulary to assess student performance on a clinical clerkship. Teach Learn Med 2002;14(1):5-10.
7. Hemmer PA, Papp KK, Mechaber AJ, Durning SJ. Evaluation, grading, and use of the RIME vocabulary on internal medicine clerkships: Results of a national survey and comparison to other clinical clerkships. Teach Learn Med 2008;20(2):118-126.
8. Norman GR, van der Vleuten CPM, De Graaff E. Pitfalls in the pursuit of objectivity: Issues of validity, efficiency and acceptability. Med Educ 1991;25(2):119-126.
9. Case SM, Swanson DB. Constructing Written Test Questions for the Basic and Clinical Sciences - third edition - Philadelphia: National Board of Medical Examiners, 2000.
10. Roop SA, Pangaro LN. Effect of clinical teaching on student performance during a medicine clerkship. Am J Med. 2001;110(3):205-209.
11. Lavin B, Pangaro LN. Internship ratings as a validity outcome measure for an evaluation system to identify inadequate clerkship performance. Acad Med 1998;73(9):998-1002.
12. Pangaro LN, ten Cate O. Frameworks for learner assessment in medicine: AMEE guide no. 78. Med Teach. 2013;35(6):e1197-e1210.
13. Frank JR, Snell LS, ten Cate O, et al. Competency-based medical education: Theory to practice. Med Teach 2010;32(8):638-645.
14. Nasca TJ, Philibert I, Brigham T, Flynn TC. The next GME accreditation system: Rationale and benefits. N Engl J Med 2012;366(11):1051-1056.
15. Carraccio CL, Benson BJ, Nixon LJ, Derstine PL. From the educational bench to the clinical bedside: Translating the Dreyfus developmental model to the learning of clinical skills. Acad Med 2008;83(8):761-767.
16. Pangaro LN. Investing in descriptive evaluation: A vision for the future of assessment. Med Teach 2000;22(5):478-481.
17. ACGME Outcome Project. General Competencies. <dconnect.acgme.org/outcome/comp/compMin.asp>. Accessed February 5, 2015.
18. ACGME. Program and Institutional Accreditation. Milestones. <www.acgme.org/acgmeweb/tabid/430/ProgramandInstitutionalAccreditation/NextAccreditationSystem/Milestones.aspx>. Accessed April 6, 2015.
19. American Board of Internal Medicine. Milestones Framework. <www.abim.org/milestones/public>. Accessed April 6, 2015.
20. Downing SM. Reliability: On the reproducibility of assessment data. Med Educ 2004;38(9):1006-1012.
21. Downing SM. Validity: On meaningful interpretation of assessment data. Med Educ 2003;37(9):830-837.
22. Downing SM, Haladyna TM. Validity threats: Overcoming interference with proposed interpretations of assessment data. Med Educ. 2004;38(3):327-333.
23. Cizek GJ. Defining and distinguishing validity: Interpretations of score meaning and justifications of test use. Psychol Methods 2012;17(1):31-43.
24. Cook DA, Beckman TJ. Current concepts in validity and reliability for psychometric instruments: Theory and application. Amer J Med 2006;119(2):166.e7-e16.
25. Gordon P, Tomasa L, Kerwin J. ACGME Outcomes [sic] Project: Selling our expertise. Fam Med 2004;36(3):164-167.

Chapter 3
System Approaches to Student Assessment

Louis N. Pangaro, M.D.

The assessment of individual students is most effective when placed in a supportive system of evaluation. The assessment system has several roles in facilitating:

- planning and coordinating the use of specific assessment methods;
- establishing a network for data retrieval, analysis, and feedback into the process;
- providing the resources needed to support assessment within the medical school curriculum.

This chapter will provide specific context for the following three chapters of the *Handbook*, which deal with the flow of information across the administrative boundaries of clerkships and courses: Chapter 4, "Sharing Student Performance Information Across Courses and Clerkships"; Chapter 5, "Using Pre-Clerkship Variables to Identify High-Risk Students"; and Chapter 6, on post-clerkship assessment. These chapters discuss the use of information about student assessments across the interfaces of curricular phases. This present chapter also provides general background for the remaining chapters of the *Handbook*, dealing with assessment methods and summative evaluation.

The educational systems and system structure, and the processes of communication and conversation *within* the medical school, especially at the level of departments, are typically responsible for the assessment of students in courses and clerkships. Although the prime interest is the assessment of students as individuals, the broader issues of program evaluation and educational research[1] are essential contexts for this discussion. At the student (or teacher) level, the system provides a basic curriculum for all students (or faculty development for all teachers), and individual assessments and feedback for both students and teachers. At the program level, the system provides evaluation and feedback to course directors about group performance, and to chairs or deans about mission success and the adequacy of resources.

3.1. What is a "System"?

A "system" (etymologically from Greek, *systema* = "things standing together") may be understood as a connected group of elements (structure) and processes (function), which together can achieve more than the individual items on their own.[2] It is *function* - especially in processes of communication and feedback - which creates the "value added" by the "system" to its structures (courses and curricular offices). Though not visually explicit in most organizational diagrams, it is the feedback loops that allow the process to be improved and optimized, and perhaps even to succeed. At all "interfaces"[2] between the elements of the system, these communication loops convey - sometimes explicitly, sometime tacitly - what the organization is all about, what it is trying to optimize.

There are other ways of describing systems, such as in terms of specific elements that work together over time (horizontal models) to "produce" something, in our case, a student ready for supervised practice; or alternatively in an organization that is vertical and hierarchical, specifying the control elements. In the rest of this chapter we will review a horizontal quality model, borrowed from industry,[3] to illustrate communications across phases of the curriculum over time; then we will review a vertical model depicting a series of up-and-down conversations between layers in an educational system.[4]

These different models - horizontal over time, and vertical in terms of control - often contain similar elements arranged in different ways according to the perspective taken, and none should be seen as either right or wrong. Systems can be described in terms of their elements, how these communicate, achieve their goals, and monitor their outputs, whether and how they self-regulate (or self-correct), and whether their organizational processes are simple, complicated, or complex.[5] It is important to emphasize that there is not a single "correct" model to describe a comprehensive educational system, any more than there is a correct choice between anatomy and physiology. The utility of the approach depends on the question being asked, or the problem to be solved.

3.2. Horizontal Models from a Quality Management Perspective

We will look at the elements of a system, horizontally, as a temporal sequence designed to achieve a specific outcome. The 1960s "process-product paradigm"[6] of Gage provides one initial model for relating actions in a social science context, such as teaching, to subsequent desired outcomes, such as learning: what the teacher does (the process) results in what the student learns (the product). Working in quality improvement for health care, Donabedian in 1980 expanded this approach, and proposed a "structure-process-output" model.[7] Table 3.1 provides the basic elements of this model.

This can be further expanded into an Outcomes Logic Model[8] (see Figure 3.1), which will schematically represent how planned work is to lead to intended results. The structural elements are inputs/resources, activities (process) and their immediate products (outputs), short and intermediate results (outcomes) and ultimate benefits (impact), and these can later be populated with the specifics of an educational assessment system (see Table 3.2).

Table 3.1. The Donabedian Model for Health Care Quality Improvement
(Adapted from: Health Research and Services Administration. Quality Improvement. <www.hrsa.gov/quality/toolbox/methodology/qualityimprovement/>. Accessed February 6, 2015)

Structure	Process	Output
People		Care delivered
Infrastructure	What is done	Health improved
Materials	How it is done	Patient satisfaction
Technology		
Information		

Figure 3.1. The Outcomes Logic Model

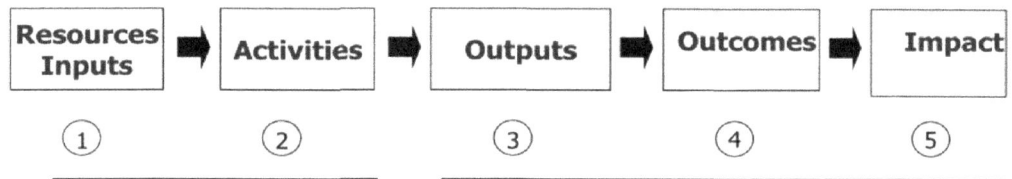

Your Planned Work — Your Intended Results

Table 3.2. Horizontal System Model:
Examples of Elements within the Outcome Logic Model

INPUT	ACTIVITIES/PROCESSES	OUTCOMES	IMPACT
Resources	Curriculum	Learning	Improved care, health
Hardware (inputs) • Students • Teachers • Patients • Facility Software (resources) • Mental Models • Goals and Objectives • Syllabus • Educational Scholarship	• Instructional Methods (lecture, small groups, clinical attachments) • Faculty Development • Faculty Calibration	• Assessments of individuals • Evaluation of curriculum or curricular elements	Improved Practice • Quality • Safety • Efficiency Decrease in Patients' • Disease • Death • Disability • Disaffection
	• Environment • Program Evaluation	• Success in GME • Licensing	
	OUTPUTS		
	Work produced by students: • H&Ps • Progress Notes	• Accreditation • Program Improvement	

In brief, for:

- *"Inputs"*: We can mean what must be available as substrate for the ongoing processes of instruction and assessment. In addition to people and things ("hardware"), the inputs may include the principles, and the goals and objectives of the curriculum.
- *"Activities"* include instructional methods for students and faculty development for teachers. The *activity* of instruction yields immediate *outputs,* documenting the process which has occurred, such as the number of teaching sessions attended, the number of patients seen, or clinical diagnoses studied. The *activity* of assessment (multiple choice tests, teachers' evaluations, etc.) yields an immediate *output* reflecting what the student has learned.
- *"Outcomes"* of the system may include the students' eventual readiness for future responsibilities (as a final year student, or in the first year of postgraduate training).
- The *"impact"* of the undergraduate system, should time and resources allow, could be the care of patients given during the GME period.

In this way the horizontal model allows us to group elements of curriculum and assessment into where they lie as "phases" of the process, although it should be said at once that these phases are more conceptual, rather than a true time sequence; it places the system elements as a stream of activity sequence that produces a product. As noted by Donabedian,[10] this may be better explained as an unbroken chain of antecedent means, followed by intermediate ends, which are themselves the means to still further ends. These issues are so important to curricular planning and management that we will look at the horizontal model in two ways, first in terms of function, and then in terms of structure.

3.3. The "Physiology" of Horizontal Systems (Function)

While the construction of systems in this model is often limited by available resources, systems are usually conceived teleologically, in terms of outcomes and implicit impact, and these should reflect the initial conceptual input ("software"), i.e., the medical school's mission, goals, and objectives. In this way, outputs achieve what was planned at the input stage, and the circle is complete. It cannot be emphasized too strongly that the system is designed for an educational purpose, and activities (instruction and assessments) are aligned to achieve that purpose. This is similar to a physiologic system designed to maintain, for instance, short-term results (blood pressure and cardiac output) sufficient to achieve the desired outcome (perfuse vital organs). Assessments and measurements monitor these desired outputs and short-term outcomes to provide feedback into the activities. In the horizontal model for education, feedback mechanisms follow each assessment to provide a correction (more instruction) for any output or short-term outcome (teacher assessment or test performance) that falls below the expected standard.

In medical education it is understood[11,12] and even required[13,14] that students be given feedback on their assessment-based performance. Therefore the system would provide the resources needed for assessment and feedback, such as time for observing students and training in how to observe, time for feedback and training in how to give effective feedback. For the individual student, the sequence of instruction and assessment is designed to fit with the curricular goals that anticipate the desired outcome. Feedback is the system's method of adjusting instruction to result in continually improved performance by each student.

At the program level, the sequence parallels what the system does for the individual student. Arranging assessment data in a "pre-during-post" model for evaluation of education programs[15] provides a linear (horizontal) sequence over time, and sees the system elements in terms of the desired goals. "Post"-curriculum outcome data become dependent variables, with process data from the "during" curriculum phase, and "pre"-instruction input data becoming co-variants. The purpose of this system is fundamentally program evaluation, that is, to relate outputs to inputs in ways that allow us to attribute success to the curriculum, rather than to the quality of the students we have admitted to medical school; processes to gather assessment data systematically for relating success to processes, also reveals the feedback loops that support quality improvement.

3.4. The "Anatomy" of Horizontal Systems (Structure)

To help educators describe, or perhaps confront, the resources needed for an effective system, it seems useful to review the horizontal system in terms of its requirements.

3.4.1. Inputs

As noted above, inputs for an assessment system (see Table 3.2) include both "hardware" and "software" (the ideas underlying assessments, sets of test questions, and the processes to score them).

- *"Hardware"*: books, seminar rooms, simulation centers, faculty who will function as observers, computers for online examinations, printed syllabi, SPs, simulators, and/or video cameras.
- *"Software"*: More fundamental to the assessment of a student's progress are the underlying ideas and assumptions that affect how we structure curriculum and assessment to achieve the right outcomes.

In this sense "software" includes the concepts and beliefs, which are the "mental models" that encompass goals and expectations for students, such as the ACGME competency framework,[16] the CanMEDS physician roles,[17] the RIME framework,[15] entrustable professional activities (EPAs),[15] and "milestones"[18] (see Chapter 2). Further, since processes and outcomes are expected to improve with scholarship and systematic studies, educational research becomes an essential "input" into the process of student assessment.[1] These intangible concepts are *critical* elements of any list of inputs, outputs, and desired outcomes; they express and organize the use of resources (materials[19]) and processes (mechanisms) to achieve intended educational outcomes (formal causes) for the sake of societal impact (teleologic causes). In an effective system, institutional leaders provide the resources and time needed to be sure that these are all aligned and sufficient.

Mental models that underlie the assessment process,[20] include: (1) expectations for students and the timeline on which they are to be achieved, whether these are expressed in analytic, synthetic, or developmental models[19] (see Chapter 2); and (2) the degree of proficiency to be achieved in each area of competency; in other words, the standard to be achieved within the criterion (see Chapter 2) and the sampling needed to establish that the standard has been met.[21]

3.4.2. Activities/Processes

Processes are the "means" (mechanisms) to an "end" (desired outcomes and impact). These processes include design, implementation, and evaluation of instructional methods and assessments for student learning and faculty development, as well as process for their oversight.

Communication and Conversation: Primary among these processes is a series of conversations (whether spoken or by electronic media) that calibrate the performance of students and teachers, and of academic directors (course and clerkship directors) and academic executives (chairs and deans), and for which the system must provide time and training.[9,22] These communicate horizontally over time (for instance providing feedback after assessment) and vertically between the "levels" of the system. The latter will be discussed later in the chapter.

An essential system *process* is to communicate the mental model for evaluation to the teachers, so that the evaluation or assessment rubric is applied consistently across students, across locations, and across time (see Chapter 8). Teachers must be trained in the frame of reference being used for assessment, and in the dimensions of performance for the facets of the framework;[20,23] in other words, teachers must be fully conversant with the competency framework being used for their learners. They must be able to visualize for themselves and their residents what success would look like, for instance, in the domain of systems-based practice for a final year resident.

It is now recognized at the GME level that the institutional system must provide protected time for program directors to fulfill their responsibilities.[24] Faculty development for program directors has been provided by ACGME and by specialty organizations. At the level of the clerkship directors, ACE, which sponsors this book, has recommended that the system provide time, training, and academic progression for clerkship directors that will enable them to fulfill their responsibilities; i.e., that any expectations "of" clerkship directors must be supported by expectations "for" what we provide them.[22]

Logically prior to the process of communication with assessors (faculty development and calibration of teachers), however, is the process whereby assessments are planned and resources allocated. Planning is typically done at several levels of the institution - the faculty as individuals, in courses, or in departments, or at the school level (dean's office and executive curriculum committees). This process should be, of course, iterative. It has to be done not just before the assessment program is deployed, but in an ongoing fashion to reevaluate based on the success of the program, changing requirements from regulatory and accreditation agencies, and more current scholarship in education and assessment. In other words, program evaluation must provide within the system for a system of evaluating the program.[25]

3.4.3. Outputs

There are a wide variety of "process measurements" available to document whether or not the planned activities of the curriculum and of the assessment of students have actually taken place. Many of the chapters in Section Three of this *Handbook* deal with methods for the assessment of individual students, which can be used in the aggregate for program evaluation. For a clerkship rotation these are the "outputs," and they belong with the "planned work" phase of the logic outcomes model[9] described above (Figure 3.1), rather than with "desired result." These outputs could include the number of patients seen on a clinical rotation, the number of problems seen on a single clinical rotation or for the entire clerkship year, faculty contact hours, attendance at conferences, use of training simulators, etc. An indication of efficacy within the curricular system then might be whether the number of diagnoses seen by students during a clerkship correlated with outcomes such as National Board of Medical Examiners (NBME) subject examination scores.

3.4.4. Outcomes

Naming "outcomes" of interest depends on the phase in the curriculum[16] since what is an outcome of one phase may be the baseline for another. For convenience we can describe these as immediate (short-term), intermediate, and long-term outcomes. For the pre-clerkship period immediate outcomes for training typically include written examinations of basic science and basic principles of clinical medicine (see Chapters 15 and 18) and proficiency in "bedside" clinical skills (see Chapters 9 and 16), and longer term outcomes would include performance in the clinical workplace during the clerkship year (see Chapters 8, 9, and 13).

Immediate outcomes for the pre-clerkship period become baseline parameters[16] for the clerkship period (see Chapter 5). The short-term "outcomes" for the clerkship period could include the success with which they accomplished their histories and physicals, scores on an NBME subject examination, or on an end-of-clerkship, end-of-clerkship-year, or end-of-year OSCE. The "intermediate" outcomes would include assessments of function in the post-clerkship period, such as performance level in the final year of medical school, e.g., whether in a subinternship the student had progressed beyond consistent "reporter-interpreter" to consistent manager (see Chapter 6); performance in directly observed clinical tasks, e.g., interviewing a patient or discussing the management plan (see Chapter 9); or performance in a pre-internship assessment of clinical skills (see Chapters 6, 16, and 17).

3.4.5. Impact

To the basic triad of input-process-outcome we may add the desired, ultimate *impact* of the curriculum on patient care during residency training or beyond. This allows us to incorporate the fourth level of the Kirkpatrick hierarchy "(impact)"[25] into the system. Impacts may be long-term when educational epidemiology has matured. In the meantime, sustained post-instruction improvement in trainees' skills may be seen as a surrogate for improvement in patient care outcomes.[26] A visual representation of this sequence is presented above in Figure 3.1.

3.5. Conversation at Interfaces Between Vertical Elements of the System

At this point we can review the undergraduate educational system as a process of oversights and governance, between "levels" in the system, and transition to "vertical" systems. The emphasis now is on the design and control of the system, rather than how it produces a "product" over time. At the operational level, a medical education system may be simplified as a series of relationships between people and groups.

Clerkship Director

Teacher

Student

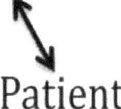

Patient

Figure 3.2.
Two-Way Communications
in the Instructional Process

At the "50,000 foot level," the medical education system also includes the regulatory and accreditation bodies which influence - if not dictate - a school's expectations for student achievement, and this encompassing system includes society at large, which is a prominent stakeholder on education, through support for medical education and through payments to the medical practitioners who are our teachers. These stakeholders and the societal and financial pressures on our students are the "strong forces" which can overwhelm the weaker forces of education theory and practice. These are illustrated in Figure 3.3.

Terms and vocabulary for communication between the levels of our educational systems are less well agreed upon than those for the horizontal structural elements. We are still, as an educational community, working out our terms. The recent and almost simultaneous introduction of the terms "milestones" and EPAs as assessment methods of a trainee's competence, for which regulatory bodies wish programs to observe, measure, and report has not been without confusion, and still requires work after several years.[27]

Biologic models for systems emphasize both function (physiologic communication) and structure (bodily organs). While a medical school typically has administrative departments (structural elements) that are less easy to modify, added value and process improvement are usually obtained by improving the communication between the "fixed" elements.[28] At the very least, a system of communicating goals and, once obtained, outcomes are accepted responsibilities of the system and its leaders. But shared mental models required for harmonization across the elements of the system require a common vocabulary of terms, and our own American system has required adjustments to the six "competencies" to move them "out of the realm of the abstract" and to make them "meaningful."[29,30] We could argue that a simpler vocabulary may be more effective in communication than the elaborate constructs written by educators,[18] in the same way that the body uses small molecules (molecular weight 150) as neurotransmitters, rather than immunoglobulins (molecular weight 150,000) for rapid effective communication.

Figure 3.3. Levels of the forward communication in a vertical model for medical education. The textured arrows indicate strong societal forces.

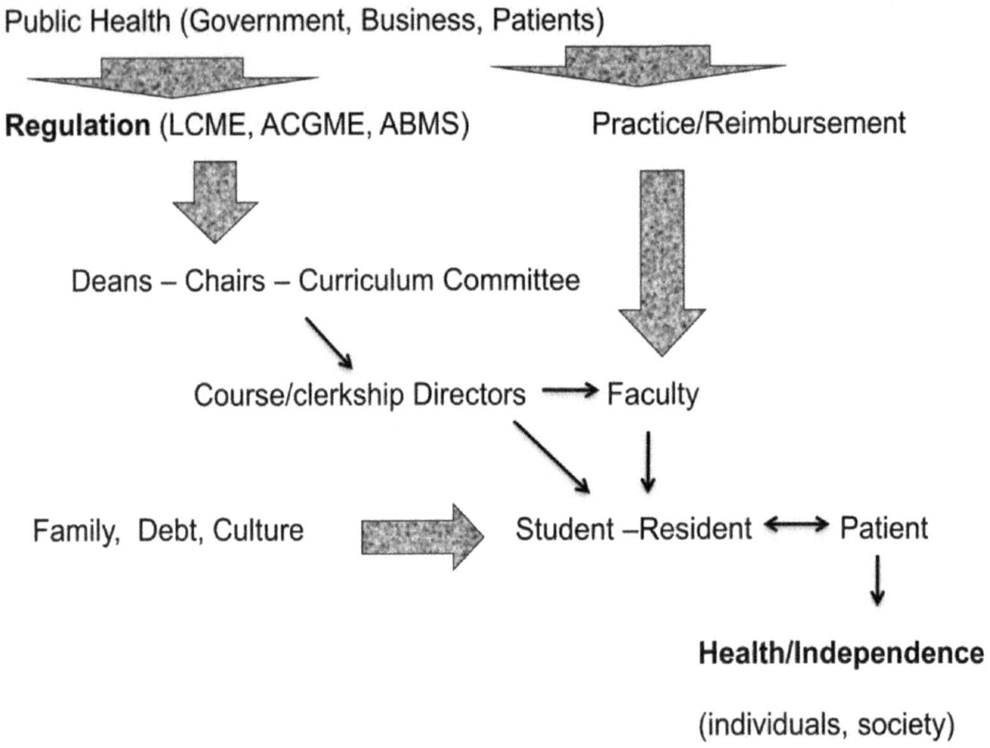

Public Health (Government, Business, Patients)

Regulation (LCME, ACGME, ABMS)　　Practice/Reimbursement

Deans – Chairs – Curriculum Committee

Course/clerkship Directors → Faculty

Family, Debt, Culture　　Student –Resident ↔ Patient

Health/Independence

(individuals, society)

One assumption of this chapter, and in fact of this text, is that a system should achieve accuracy and consistency of assessment across students, and that this depends on a commonality of expectations for students; i.e., a shared mental model.[19] The purposes of a particular assessment method and how this fits into the larger competency framework that is used (see Chapter 1) are critical "inputs" into the system, but their efficacy/utility depends on whether they are used to structure a teacher's observation about students, and whether this use is consistent within teachers over time, and across teachers in a curriculum. The system, in this case, the departmental chair or the medical school dean, must provide the time and training to make this possible.[9]

While we use the term "levels," it should not be taken to mean a hierarchy of importance, or acceptance of a top-down approach. Indeed, it is those "lowest" on the educational hierarchy - the students and their teachers - whose work the system is designed to support.

Figure 3.4. Conversations for System Integration. The three boxes with solid borders illustrate the departmental conversations that support setting goals, consistent evaluation of and feedback for students

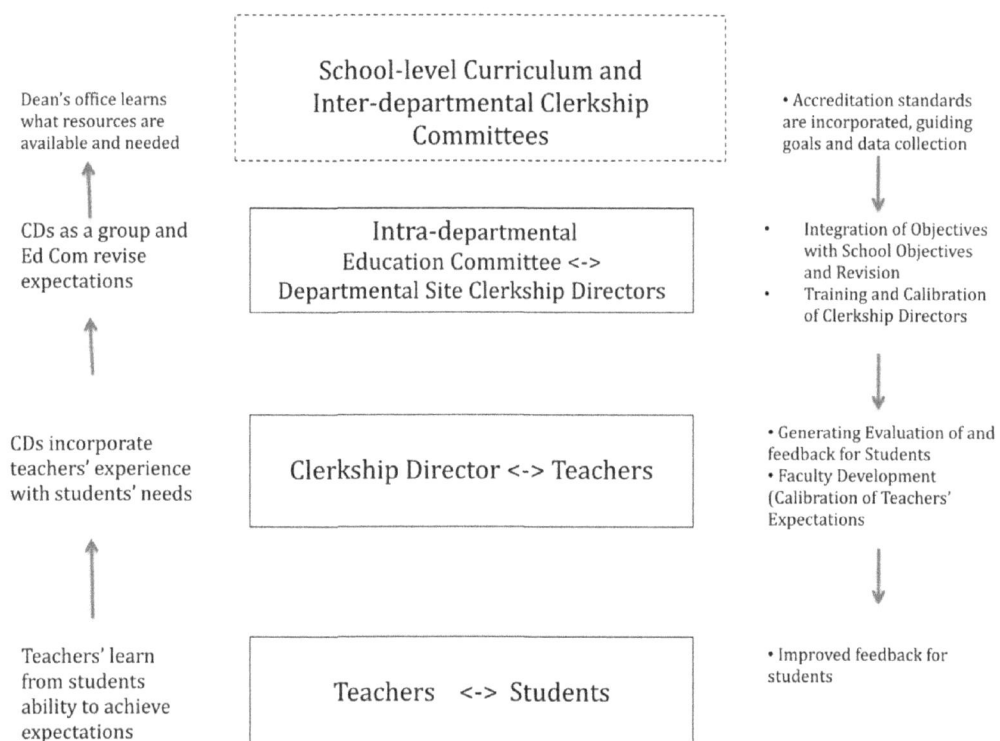

Illustrated in Figure 3.4 is how departmental resources are used in the clinical setting to structure a series for conversation between the principle players in the group: between students and their clinical supervisors, between those supervisors and the clerkship directors at each clerkship site, and between those site clerkship directors and the overall clerkship director, and other departmental leaders such as pre-clerkship clinical skills course directors, subinternship directors, the vice chair for education, the GME program director and the chair of medicine. Such an education committee can provide oversight in achieving the desired consistency in summative evaluation and grading.[31,40] In the U.S., the ACGME now mandates that the compendium of assessments of residents be reviewed by a "competency committee" that will determine whether the resident has achieved the expected level of performance.[33]

As distinguished from "communication" in which the department indicates to clerkship directors, students, and teachers the expectations of the school or accreditation body, "conversation" implies an openness to adjustment of the mental model underlying assessment.[34] The case has been made for face-to-face conversations as enhancing assessment and feedback in the workplace (see Chapter 8); and the benefits of spoken communication

- as opposed to obtaining written assessments from teachers - have been demonstrated. The phrase, "Low tech is good tech," has become an axiom in our own institution.

Whatever the mode of communication, the goal is increased effectiveness through system harmony, and this allows influence of teachers and students to emerge in a setting where control and authority cannot be assumed. In fact, in the complex system of medical education, Mennin has argued that openness, frequent non-linear interactions and abundant short-loop feedback may be essential.[35] Further, it models the willingness of the system to correct itself and be open to adjustment and even criticism; this is consistent with the accepted principles of quality improvement[36] and professionalism.[37,38]

How a specific assessment method is to be used - for instance whether formative or summative, or whether it is "high stakes" for the student - will determine the degree of reproducibility (reliability) that is desired, and this in turn will determine the resources (time and effort) that must be applied. Assessment in the clinical setting is more accurate when resources are committed to calibrating teachers[39,40] (see Chapter 8), going beyond the easy convenience of providing the teacher with an evaluation form (on a sheet of paper or as an e-mail attachment). As has been discussed elsewhere,[18] the "secondary effects" of assessment frameworks mean that frameworks that are more elaborate and less intuitive require more resources to achieve consistency. Those at the nominal top of the education system, certainly chairs and deans, and perhaps even the accreditation bodies, should be sure that resources for the deployment of new assessment methods and for faculty development are provided.

3.6. Cultural Assumptions in a Shifting Environment

Our educational systems exist within large institutions (our academic health centers) and often under the aegis of national accreditation bodies. Different models for systems exist throughout society, and each has assumptions, often tacit, about how the purposes of an institution are accomplished. The input-process-product model described above reflects a model in which outputs are thought to be directly related to the processes and inputs provided. It is not surprising that this would be useful in manufacturing automobiles to achieve consistency in the product across hundreds of thousands of units produced at several plants. In what Schein has described as the "executive culture,"[32] the overall responsibility and control for the processes are at the highest level, the "CEO." It is at this highest level that the value in the institution is assumed to be created. In the "operator culture,"[38] the value is created by those who are on the front lines, doing the work; and until recently it has been physicians, researchers, and teachers who have been seen as creating the value in a university or medical school.

The importance of these business terms to this discussion is that the need to demonstrate the medical profession's commitment to society, and to seeing medical education as a "public good," has led to an increasing demand for consistency in medical education; consistency not just in learners' experiences (such as in LCME requirements in number of diagnoses per students in clerkships) but in the assessment of "competencies" and in a national implementation of "milestones" by specialty[32,33] (see Chapter 2).

Application of the manufacturing or engineering model to medical education has been controversial among some medical educators, but for our purposes it is achieving an essential goal, by focussing on how an enterprise looks at itself as a system; and in aligning the system with an ultimate (teleologic) goal - to guarantee a consistent outcome for society. In the case of undergraduate medical education, this guarantee is to produce a graduate who is ready for supervised practice with a medical degree; i.e., a "license to commit medicine."[41]

We may see the recently increased stipulations for medical schools and academic teaching hospitals as an engineering approach, solving a "complicated" problem in which inputs, processes, and outputs are - or can be - well known, and measured. This has not yet been established, and clerkship directors usually see curricula as a solving a "complex" problem of trying to produce a competent graduate while the practice and regulatory landscapes are always shifting. In other words, the applicable body of knowledge, the available technology, and relationships and reimbursements are subject to frequent change.

Hopefully, studies exploring whether and how these newer models of accountability will be funded and will advance our understanding of how educational systems work. In the meantime, demonstrating our profession's commitment to serve our society is a prime value. It is becoming generally agreed that the medical school graduates of the coming decades should understand their environment and culture as complex, requiring not just content expertise (mastery of certain basic competencies) but also adaptive expertise in which the basics are applied in the unanticipated contexts presented by individual patients.[35]

In any case, the multi-level system of conversations recommended here goes beyond simple "communication" in which expectations are conveyed and observations of competence documented, but is a series of "conversations" in which there is openness to the changing needs of stakeholders, and an expectation that the system will adapt as needed.

3.7. Summary Points

Each student assessment within courses and clerkships should be aligned at the institutional level with expectations of students and for faculty, and the system should provide the resources needed to allow this to happen.

We expect that the reliability and calibration of assessments will be sufficient for how their results are to be used. Departments and schools must provide the needed resources for such assessments and for the network that allows information to be fed back into the curriculum.

Prospective and deliberate data collection about outcomes of interest (i.e., related to curricular goals) is now generally accepted; trying to correlate these outcomes with data for documentation of processes and for inputs and resources may allow clearer understanding of what contributes to results.

Two-way transfer of information at curricular interfaces improves student performance, and may gather real-time feedback from teachers, which will foster ongoing renovation of the curriculum. In addition to transferring quantified assessment data, we recommend the use of the low-tech solution (face-to-face conversation) whenever feasible.

References

1. McGaghie WC, Issenberg SB, Cohen ER, et al. Translational educational research: A necessity for effective health-care improvement. Chest 2012;142(5):1097-1103.
2. Rechtin E. Systems Architecting of Organizations: Why Eagles Can't Swim. Boca Raton, FL: CRC Press, 1999: 4.
3. W.K. Kellogg Foundation Logic Model Development Guide. <www.wkkf.org/resource-directory/resource/2006/02/wk-kellogg-foundation-logic-model-development-guide>. Accessed February 7, 2015.
4. Schuster B, Pangaro LN. Understanding systems of education: What to expect of, and for, each faculty member. In: Pangaro LN, ed. Leadership Careers in Medical Education. Philadelphia: American College of Physicians Press, 2010: 51-72.
5. Mennin S. Complexity and health professions education: A basic glossary. J Eval Clin Pract 2010;16(4):838-840.
6. Gage NL. Hard Gains in the Soft Sciences: The Case of Pedagogy. Bloomington, IN: Phi Delta Kappa International, 1985.
7. Donabedian A. The quality of care: How can it be assessed? JAMA 1988;260(12): 1743-1748.
8. Adapted from: Health Resources and Services Administration. Quality Improvement. <www.hrsa.gov/quality/toolbox/methodology/qualityimprovement/>. Accessed February 7, 2015.
9. Armstrong EG, Barsion SJ. Using an outcomes-logic-model approach to evaluate a faculty development program for medical educators. Acad Med 2006;81(5):483-488.
10. Donabedian A. Evaluating the quality of medical care. Milbank Q 2005;83(4):691-729.
11. Ericsson KA. An expert-performance perspective of research on medical expertise: The study of clinical performance. Med Educ 2007;41(12):1124-1130.

12. Veloski J, Boex JR, Grasberger MJ, et al. Systematic review of the literature on assessment, feedback and physicians' clinical performance: BEME guide no. 7. Med Teach 2006;28(2):117-128.
13. LCME. Functions and Structure of a Medical School. June 2013. <www.lcme.org/publications/functions.pdf>. Accessed May 17, 2015.
14. Barzansky B, Hunt D, Busing N. Evaluation for program and school accreditation. In: McGaghie WC, ed. International Best Practices for Evaluation in the Health Professions. London: Radcliffe, 2013: 329-340.
15. Durning SJ, Hemmer PA, Pangaro LN. The structure of program evaluation: An approach for evaluating a course, clerkship, or components of a residency training program. Teach Learn Med 2007;19(3):308-318.
16. ACGME Core Competencies. 1999. <www.mcw.edu/MedicalSchool/EducationalServices/GraduateMedicalEducation/ACGMECoreCompetencies.htm>. Accessed July 21, 2012; not reachable April 6, 2015, but see <www.gahec.org/CME/Liasions/0)ACGME Core Competencies Definitions.htm>, accessed April 6, 2015.
17. Frank JR, ed. The Royal College of Physicians and Surgeons of Canada. The CanMEDS 2005 Physician Competency Framework. <fhs.mcmaster.ca/pathres/resident_resources/documents/CanMEDS2005_e.pdf>. Accessed February 7, 2015.
18. Pangaro LN, ten Cate O. Frameworks for learner assessment in medicine: AMEE guide no. 78. Med Teach. 2013;35(6):e1197-e1210.
19. Aristotle. Physics, 194a33-195b30. In: McKeon R, ed. The Basic Works of Aristotle. New York: Modern Library, 2001: 240-242.
20. Pangaro LN, Holmboe ES. Evaluation forms and formal rating scales. In: Holmboe ES, Hawkins RE, eds. Practical Guide to the Evaluation of Clinical Competence. Philadelphia: Mosby, 2008: 24-41.
21. van der Vleuten CPM, Schuwirth LW. Assessing professional competence: From methods to programmes. Med Educ 2005;39(3):309-317.
22. Pangaro LN, Bachicha J, Brodkey A, et al. Expectations of and for clerkship directors: A collaborative Statement from the Alliance for Clinical Education. Teach Learn Med 2003;15(3):217-222.
23. Kogan JR, Conforti LN, Iobst WF, Holmboe ES. Reconceptualizing variable rater assessments as both an educational and clinical care problem. Acad Med 2014;89(5):721-727.
24. ACGME Program Requirements for Graduate Medical Education in Internal Medicine. <www.acgme.org/acgmeweb/Portals/0/PFAssets/2013-PR-FAQ-PIF/140_internal_medicine_07012013.pdf>. Accessed February 7, 2015.
25. Aretz HT. Some thoughts about creating healthcare professionals that match what societies need. Med Teach 2011;33(8):608-613.
26. Wayne DB, Siddall VJ, Butter J, et al. A longitudinal study of internal medicine residents' retention of advanced cardiac life support skills. Acad Med 2006;81(10 Suppl):S9-S12.
27. Englander R, Carraccio C. From theory to practice: Making entrustable professional activities come to life in the context of milestones. Acad Med 2014;89(10):1321-1323.
28. Armstrong EG, Mackey M, Spear SJ. Medical education as a process management problem. Acad Med. 2004;79(8):721-728.
29. Green ML, Aagaard EM, Caverzagie KJ, et al. Charting the road to competence: Developmental milestones for internal medicine residency training. J Grad Med Educ 2009;1(1):5-20.

30. Nasca TJ, Philibert I, Brigham T, Flynn TC. The next GME accreditation system: Rationale and benefits. N Engl J Med 2012;366(11):1051-1056.
31. Durning SJ, Pangaro LN, Denton GD, et al. Intersite consistency as a measurement of programmatic evaluation in a medicine clerkship with multiple, geographically separated sites. Acad Med. 2003;78(10 Suppl):S36-S38.
32. Schein EH. Three cultures of management: The key to organizational learning. Sloan Mgmt Rev 1996;38(1):9-20.
33. Frequently Asked Questions: Clinical Competency Committee and Program Evaluation Committee. Common Program Requirements. ACGME. <www.acgme.org/acgmeweb/Portals/0/PDFs/FAQ/CCC_PEC_FAQs.pdf>. Accessed February 7, 2015.
34. Dubberly H, Pangaro P. What is conversation and how can we design for it? Interactions 2009;16(4):22-28. Also available as: What is conversation? How can we design for effective conversation? <www.dubberly.com/articles/what-is-conversation.html>. Accessed February 9, 2015.
35. Mennin S. Self-organisation, integration and curriculum in the complex world of medical education. Med Educ 2010;44(1):20-30.
36. Berwick D. The science of improvement. JAMA 2008;299(10):1182-1184.
37. Colbert CY, Ogden PE, Ownby AR, Bowe C. Systems-based practice in graduate medical education: Systems thinking as the missing foundational construct. Teach Learn Med 2011;23(2):179-185.
38. Bowe CM, Lahey L, Armstrong E, Kegan R. Questioning the "big assumptions": Part II: Recognizing organizational contradictions that impede institutional change. Med Educ 2003;37(8):723-733.
39. Hemmer PA, Pangaro LN. Using formal evaluation sessions for case-based faculty development during clinical clerkships. Acad Med 2000;75(12):1216-1221.
40. Gaglione MM, Moores L, Pangaro LN, Hemmer PA. Does group discussion of student clerkship performance at an education committee affect an individual committee member's decisions? Acad Med 2005;80(10 Suppl):S55-S58.
41. Joy RJ. Personal communication.

Chapter 4
Sharing Student Performance Information Across Courses and Clerkships*

Lynn M. Cleary, M.D.

Many important clerkship director student evaluation responsibilities occur across or outside singular clerkship boundaries. Examples include participation in interdisciplinary assessments, such as integrated clinical skills examinations, clinical progress testing, comprehensive clinical science examinations, or sharing information about student performance in previous clerkships with other clerkship directors. The latter is sometimes called "forward feeding" of student performance information.[1-3] This chapter describes the pros and cons of prospectively sharing student performance information, describes models of how it can be done, and offers a recommendation that schools commit to developing policies and procedures about information sharing as part of a robust, integrated student assessment program (see Chapter 3).

Assessment of medical student performance must change along with the evolution of curricular structures and principles.[4] Competency-based curricula, measurement of milestones, and core entrustable professional activities[5] are being integrated into undergraduate medical education. Longitudinal integrated clerkships require teaching and assessment across multiple disciplines.[6] Research evaluating longitudinal integrated clerkships has demonstrated contextual and developmental advantages when these models are implemented. The majority of clerkship directors' efforts in student performance evaluation are conducted within the clerkship for which they are responsible.[7] Each medical school must implement and manage an effective student assessment program to measure these important, integrated, and competency-based outcomes.[8]

4.1. Advantages for Sharing Information about Individual Students

There are theoretical advantages and disadvantages to sharing information prospectively about student performance, but little research or data to support decisions about its use. A majority of clerkship directors indicated from a recent survey that there are benefits to students when information about performance is shared.[9] They also report a professional obligation to protect the public and the patients whom their graduates will treat. The major disadvantage of sharing performance information is the potential to introduce bias in assessment. Most schools have limited policies about sharing student performance information. However, even in schools where there is no policy, informal discussions about student performance occur regularly.

Arguments supporting forward feeding of performance information[1] include: (1) personalized mentoring, (2) increased detection across clerkships, and (3) fulfilling social responsibility that expectations have been met.

4.1.1. Personalized Mentoring

Early knowledge of weak skill areas within a student will foster personalized mentoring and early opportunities for improvement. Sometimes it takes multiple observations by faculty and residents before a clerkship director is informed about inadequate student skills or problem behavior. There is little time to provide feedback, focussed instruction, and reassessment to a weak student if the clerkship director does not learn about problems until late in the clerkship. This is particularly true in short clerkships, because the average duration of most block clerkships has been reduced recently. Therefore, one cannot approach the performance record for each student in each clerkship as a *tabula rasa*.

Therefore, the benefits to students include the opportunity to receive early and specific evidence-based feedback and guidance, especially about skill areas needing improvement. Students can also be placed with a highly skilled teacher who can coach them appropriately.

4.1.2. Increased Detection Across Clerkships

Sharing performance evaluations across clerkships reduces the likelihood that students with deficiencies in knowledge, skill, or attitude will "fly under the radar" and advance to the post-clerkship phase before problems are recognized. Without early identification of students with substandard performance, they may be passed along to successive clerkships. Anecdotally, clerkship directors are often troubled to hear at end-of-year student promotion committee meetings that problems they saw in an early clerkship also occurred in several others. These clerkship directors have then collectively failed to recognize a consistent weakness until they talked together. Failure to evaluate students rigorously and communicate formative outcomes may result in incompetent students passing all clerkships yet having inadequate skills.

4.1.3. Fulfilling Social Responsibility that Expectations Have Been Met

Clerkship directors and medical schools have a responsibility to the public and to the future patients whom each student will serve. Identifying and remediating inadequate performance is a responsibility that clerkship directors take seriously, and reflects their sense of responsibility to the patients for whom the learners will eventually provide care. The doctoral degree granted by each medical school to each graduating student testifies that the graduate has the skills needed to enter the next phase of medical training.[10] Sharing information about performance in core skills across all clerkships provides confidence that the student has met a robust minimum standard of performance, especially in clinical skills.[11] New residents are responsible for important and complex patient care activities, often without appropriate supervision. Implicit and explicit expectations for competence on entrance to residency must inform assessment at the undergraduate level. This underscores the need for robust and cross-disciplinary collaboration to ensure minimum competence, which benefits society as well as students.

4.2. Disadvantages of Sharing Information about Students

Arguments against forward feeding of performance information[2] include: (1) bias in subsequent evaluations, (2) increased student anxiety, and (3) issues with futility and privacy.

4.2.1. Bias in Subsequent Evaluations

The most significant disadvantage of sharing performance information across clerkships is the possibility that communication about past performance may bias subsequent evaluations. There is also concern that this may become a self-fulfilling prophecy and negatively affect later student performance (the observer-expectancy effect) if the shared information is unfavorable. By contrast, this would not be a disadvantage if favorable information were fed forward (the Pygmalion effect). Students should receive multiple, unbiased assessments of their clinical skills performance.

The risk of introducing bias can be reduced by limiting knowledge of prior performance only to clerkship directors. Faculty and residents who do the actual teaching and assessments need not know about students' previous performances.

4.2.2. Increased Student Anxiety

Another potential disadvantage is that students who are not performing well often try to stay out of the limelight. These students may find it intimidating if a clerkship director or supervising faculty were to engage them directly in conversations about how to address deficits previously noted. Students may feel they are under focussed or even unfair scrutiny. Making feedback on clerkship evaluations the norm, rather than the exception, may mitigate this.

There is little research on what students think about sharing information across courses or clerkships. Clerkship directors report anecdotally that students mistrust it, fearing bias. Literature about the student experience in clerkships indicates that many students struggle with frequent changes in clerkship site and with turnover among supervising residents and attendings. Medical students have more trust in longitudinal, workplace-based assessments and feedback from faculty with whom they work over time. This is an area ripe for additional study.

4.2.3. Futility and Privacy

Scholars question whether medical schools can remediate underlying problems of poor integrative skills, unprofessional behavior, lack of insight, and inability to receive feedback effectively and modify behavior. There is little research in this area. Resources must be available to clerkship directors, including faculty time, counseling services, diagnostic evaluation, and advising support. Concern has been expressed about whether sharing performance information is compliant with the Family Educational Rights and Privacy Act (FERPA) (see Chapter 21).[12] Confusion can be avoided by developing clear institutional policies about the rationale and methods for sharing performance information as part of an integrated, longitudinal assessment model (see Chapter 21).

4.3. Policies and Procedures

Each medical school should develop policies and procedures about sharing student performance information among course and clerkship directors. These policies should be communicated with students and faculty regularly, at least at the beginning of each academic year, and be available online and in a printed student and faculty handbook. Policies should identify the purpose, methods, and limits of sharing information, including who should participate in information-sharing based on their academic roles. Developing a well-articulated policy will help to avoid misunderstandings or accusations of wrongdoing that can arise when information is shared informally.

Many schools have established systematic, explicit methods of identifying students with performance problems early, so that timely remediation can be accomplished. This is usually undertaken by a standing committee of course or clerkship directors (e.g., formally in a promotions committee, or informally in an early identification committee of clerkship directors) on a regular (e.g., monthly or post-clerkship block) basis. It includes systematic review of students with performance problems. Assessment data from each clerkship office and from the registrar's office may include qualitative, descriptive, or narrative information, as well as scores on multiple choice question exams, standardized patient assessments, or other quantitative measures. If the school keeps assessment data on individual skills across clerkships, a computer program can be used to identify students at a threshold of concern. For example, it is common to have a uniform evaluation to assess core competencies across clerkships, which may include data gathering (history, physical exam), interpersonal communications, medical communications (oral presentations, written notes), ability to work as team members, professional behavior, critical analysis, and problem-solving skills. These can be entered into a master database and used to identify skill deficits. Spreadsheets are useful, but dialogue is equally or more important. Incidents of unprofessional behavior may be recorded, and discussions about these events are often critical to identify infrequent but significant problems with professionalism.

These methods would ideally be used for all students along the performance spectrum, from struggling students to those who are clearly proficient, providing opportunities for each individual to work on areas that need improvement. This is time-consuming. Most efforts focus on students whose performance raises the greatest concern. These are the medical students with borderline or inadequate performance, where more is at stake if low achievement is not detected and addressed. Improvement is needed for the sake of not only the students but also the future patients whom they will serve and treat.

4.4. Summary and Recommendations

We know from survey studies that a majority of clerkship directors support the idea of sharing student performance information across clerkships.[9] Most clerkship directors believe that the benefits of this practice outweigh potential risks and biases. These problems can be limited by institutional policies and procedures developed with input from clerkship directors, the curriculum dean, registrar, and institutional counsel. Such a process is recommended as part of a thorough, collaborative, robust, multi-sampling approach that takes advantage of ongoing clinical performance assessments to develop a cumulative record about competence measures. Steps must be taken to avoid bias. It is an important institutional commitment requiring dean's office level of support to help clerkship directors with their responsibility to evaluate and support all students, particularly those with marginal or substandard performance.

References

* The foundation material was published previously in the chapter on medical student evaluation in the *ACE Guidebook for Clerkship Directors* - fourth edition - North Syracuse, NY: Gegensatz Press, 2012.
1. Cleary L. "Forward feeding" about students' progress: The case for longitudinal, progressive, and shared assessment of medical students. Acad Med. 2008;83(9):800.

2. Cox SM. "Forward feeding" about students' progress: Information on struggling medical students should not be shared among clerkship directors or with students' current teachers. Acad Med. 2008;83(9):801.
3. Pangaro LN. "Forward feeding" about students' progress: More information will enable better policy. Acad Med. 2008;83(9):802-803.
4. Cooke M, Irby DM, O'Brien BC. Educating Physicians: A Call for Reform of Medical School and Residency. Stanford, CA: The Carnegie Foundation for the Advancement of Teaching; San Francisco: Jossey-Bass, 2010.
5. AAMC. Core Entrustable Professional Activities for Entering Residency. 2014. <members.aamc.org/eweb/upload/Core%20EPA%20Curriculum%20Dev%20Guide.pdf>. Accessed May 8, 2015.
6. Bates J, Konklin J, Suddards C, et al. Student perceptions of assessment and feedback in longitudinal integrated clerkships. Med Educ 2013;47(4):362-374.
7. Hemmer PA, Durning SJ, Papp KK. What are the discussion topics and usefulness of clerkship directors' meetings within medical schools? A report from the CDIM 2007 National Survey. Acad Med 2010;85(12):1855-1861.
8. Armstrong EG, Mackey M, Spear SJ. Medical education as a process management problem. Acad Med. 2004;79(8):721-728.
9. Frellsen SL, Baker EA, Papp KK, Durning SJ. Medical school policies regarding struggling medical students during the internal medicine clerkships: Results of a national survey. Acad Med. 2008;83(9):876-881.
10. Raymond MR, Mee J, King A, et al. What new residents do during their initial months of training. Acad Med 2011;86(10 Suppl):S59-S62.
11. Angus S, Vu TR, Halvorsen AJ, et al. What skills should new internal medicine interns have in July? A national survey of internal medicine residency program directors. Acad Med 2014;89(3):432-435.
12. Family Educational Rights and Privacy Act (FERPA). <www2.ed.gov/policy/gen/guid/fpco/ferpa/index.html>. Accessed February 7, 2015.

Chapter 5
Using Pre-Clerkship Variables to Identify High-Risk Students

Jeffrey S. LaRochelle, M.D., M.P.H.
Gerald D. Denton, M.D., M.P.H.

Pre-clerkship observations may be used to identify students at risk for poor clerkship outcomes. These may include faculty observations, the results of structured, quantified assessments, or summative grades. This chapter will focus on the observations and evaluations themselves, rather than on any prior summative grades (see Table 5).

Table 5. Pre-Clerkship Observations about Performance of Individual Students

Pre-Clerkship Observations	Quantified (see definitions above in Chapter 2)	Descriptive
Pre-Matriculation Data	Undergraduate GPA and MCAT scores	Medical school admission interviews
Basic Science Course Work	Performance on course or module-based basic science tests: faculty written, subject, or customized examinations from the NBME (National Board of Medical Examiners)	Incidents reflecting unprofessional behavior Faculty observations of performance in small group discussions
Doctoring and Clinical Reasoning Courses	Observations from OSCE or other simulation of clinical skills	Faculty observations of performance in clinical reasoning-type courses
Preceptorships		Faculty observation from clinical practice settings
Cumulative Standardized Examinations	Standardized test scores (e.g., USMLE Step 1 or the NBME Comprehensive Basic Science Self-Assessment)	

This chapter will review the predictive power of some commonly available measurements and then discuss ways this information might be used to identify at-risk students. We know that test performance predicts test performance, and prior measures of knowledge predict a student's ability to acquire factual knowledge during later clerkships.[1-4] However, competence in clinical skills, professionalism, data interpretation, and problem solving are also critical to successful clerkship outcomes. Few data are currently available to support the ability of pre-clerkship variables to predict deficits in skill and attitude domains. Most of the advice in this section is informed by published educational literature, but some recommendations stem from the authors' experience and judgment. Since more medical schools now begin the clinical clerkships prior to the beginning of the third academic year, we will use the term "pre-clerkship," rather than "first" or "second year." Consideration of the benefits and risks of using prior observations, as well as institutional policy for their use to inform subsequent student guidance or assessment, is also discussed in Chapter 4.

5.1. The Use of Pre-Matriculation Data

5.1.1. Undergraduate Grade Point Average

A strong positive correlation between undergraduate GPA and subsequent measures of knowledge has been reported consistently.[3,4] Undergraduate GPA is one of the strongest predictors of future academic performance in medical school.[4] Low science and non-science undergraduate GPA has a strong correlation with NBME subject exam failure with high specificity. However, undergraduate GPA does not predict clinical performance.[4] This supports the common observation that clinical skills and professionalism do not track consistently with acquired knowledge. A strong knowledge base does not protect a student from deficits in other areas. Since the correlation between undergraduate GPA and NBME failure is only 50%-60% sensitive, clerkship directors may have difficulty predicting poor performance using this information.[3]

5.1.2. MCAT

Many studies demonstrate the predictive validity of MCAT scores for academic performance in medical school and on future standardized tests, including licensure examinations and NBME subject examinations.[3,5,6] Like undergraduate GPA, MCAT scores predict early medical school academic performance with some variability. Meta-analyses that employ regression models using MCAT scores to explain pre-clerkship and clerkship grades demonstrate predictive variability coefficients (*r-values*) of 0.39 and 0.46, although some studies indicate *r-values* as high as 0.59 for pre-clerkship grades.[5-7] MCAT scores have also been shown to predict USMLE scores for Steps 1, 2, and 3 with *r-values* of 0.70, 0.60, and 0.62, respectively.[5-7] Previous research has shown that the MCAT predictive validity is limited to the total score. Subtest scores and the former writing sample do not explain significant variance in traditional measures of academic performance; e.g., medical school grades, standardized test performance.[7] The former writing sample did not contribute to these traditional measurements of performance but did correlate with other clerkship outcomes, including global clinical competence, data gathering, and communication skills.[8] Additionally, total MCAT scores are inversely correlated with academic difficulty defined by delayed graduation, early withdrawal, or early dismissal from medical school.[5,6]

More recent studies demonstrate that total MCAT scores are able to predict which students will progress through medical school unimpeded, as defined by completion of training within five years and first time passing of USMLE Step 1, Step 2 Clinical Knowledge (CK) and Step 2 Clinical Skills (CS).[9] However, some medical students still struggle academically despite high MCAT scores, while others excel academically despite low MCAT scores. This indicates that other factors must be considered when predicting medical student performance.[6] In 2015, a new version of the MCAT will be launched that will focus more on problem solving, critical analysis, and reasoning skills as foundation competencies for future physicians. In addition, the revised MCAT will include an assessment of the psychological and social foundations of behavior in an attempt to address the social and behavioral determinants of health.[10] A focus on these concepts may further predict student performance in the clinical setting, but this will need to be studied closely.

5.1.3. Admission Committee Interviews

Comments from medical school admission interviews, reference letters, personal essays, and other narrative sources can be a rich source of pre-clerkship information.[11-13] The interview process is not standardized between institutions and sometimes not even within the same institution.[13] Several studies demonstrate a large proportion of variance related to the interviewer experience. This suggests that the interview process has limited value in predicting future medical school success.[14,15] However, use of a structured interview focussing on such non-cognitive factors as maturity, interpersonal skills, motivation, and personal achievement can predict clinical performance better than undergraduate GPA or MCAT scores.[11,12]

The next generation of structured interviews is a series of observed encounters, putting applicants into several scenarios to assess their non-cognitive skills. One approach involves three scenarios termed "medical judgment vignettes" that focus on morality, altruism, and dutifulness.[16] The medical judgment vignettes produced high interrater reliability. Total scores from matriculating applicants on these vignettes also explained a significant amount of the variance in history and physical exam skills, professionalism, problem solving, and motivation (21%, 30%, 38%, and 20%, respectively) as measured by clinical preceptors at the end of the clerkship year.[16,17] Therefore, as the earliest observation by a school's own faculty, a well designed interview process can identify students who may subsequently have difficulty in clinical skills and non-cognitive domains. Of course, candidates with negative comments are less likely to be admitted to medical school and observations about successful applicants are not regularly provided to clerkship directors to allow structured assistance of identified weaknesses. Additionally, recent work on the use of emotional intelligence scores measured at the time of applicant interviews and at matriculation did not reliably predict future performance in medical school.[18]

Admissions committees and educators should work together to develop a structured process to identify candidates who will best fit the mission of the institution. Given the current body of evidence, interventions based on comments from admission committee interviews may not yield improved clinical performance. A meta-analysis of twenty studies looking at a variety of admission interviews (predominantly loosely or moderately structured) found that the admission interview was a weak predictor of academic ($r = 0.06$) or clinical ($r = 0.17$) performance.[19] More research is needed on the use of highly structured admission interviews to determine their true potential for predicting student performance.

5.2. Use of Pre-Clerkship Performance

5.2.1. Pre-Clerkship Performance

Similar to the predictive validity of undergraduate GPA, pre-clerkship GPA can predict future clerkship performance.[20] However, the poor sensitivity of this measure means that pre-clerkship GPA may not be practically useful to identify at-risk students.[21] There is evidence to suggest a correlation between pre-clerkship GPA using numerical grades and clerkship performance measured by both exams and clinical competence; i.e., students with lower pre-clinical GPAs were more likely to have delayed graduation or fail USMLE Step 1.[22] Non-numerical grading formats may not be as meaningful to clerkship directors, due to a lack of predictive validity originating from narrow scale bandwidth; i.e., four-point (A-B-C-D) or Pass/Fail vs. 100-point scales.[22] In addition to overall pre-clerkship GPA, performance on individual written exams can predict performance on future written exams in the clerkship years and may identify at-risk students who need early remediation.[23]

Student educational portfolios are a new source of information for clerkship directors. Portfolios may guide educational interventions tailored to student needs indicated by their portfolio strengths, weaknesses, and omissions.[24] However, recent studies demonstrate that portfolios are often poorly completed or not used by trainees at all, and there are often discrepancies between the trainee's self-reflections and the faculty assessments of the trainee.[25] Given variability in student portfolios, caution should be applied when using this information to predict future performance. Although there is value in trainee self-reflection, future research is necessary to understand better the potential use of this information.

5.2.2. USMLE Step 1

Several reports have correlated USMLE Step 1 scores with NBME subject exam scores for the clinical clerkships. Failure on the first attempt at USMLE

Step 1 predicts students at risk for poor scores on clerkship final examinations.[3,21] In addition, USMLE Step 1 scores correlate with composite clinical evaluations at the end of clerkships.[26] Although failure of USMLE Step 1 places students at increased risk for failure of clerkship exams, this did not predict poor clinical performance measured by faculty and resident evaluations.[26] Unfortunately, many medical schools have policies that do not allow clerkship directors access to USMLE scores (personal communication, CDIM). Additionally, the NBME does not provide a separate score for Step 1 clinical skills questions, which might be valuable information for clerkship directors.[27]

5.2.3. Pre-Clerkship Clinical Skills and Clinical Reasoning Performance

Mastery of fundamental skills learned during pre-clerkship introduction to clinical medicine (ICM) clinical skills and clinical reasoning courses is essential to successful student practice and mastery during clerkships and beyond. While there is a paucity of literature supporting the predictive validity of ICM courses, students who perform at a substandard level in an ICM course may be at higher risk of a failing internal medicine clerkship grade.[28] Although multiple choice testing in an ICM course demonstrates a weak correlation with clerkship outcomes,[29] there is significant variability not only in the goals of pre-clerkship courses but also in how students are assessed.[30] A common form of assessment at the end of pre-clerkship training is the OSCE, which may predict future clinical clerkship performance.[23,31] In fact, performance on a pre-clerkship, three-station OSCE may be able to identify students at risk of failing a future clerkship OSCE.[32] In this study, students falling below the 20% rank for their class on the pre-clerkship OSCE had an odds ratio of 21.09 for failure of the clerkship OSCE with a sensitivity and specificity of 0.77 and 0.86, respectively.[32] In addition, a combination of clinical skills and clinical reasoning outcomes may collectively provide stronger predictive value for future performance in the clerkship years. Regardless, improved standardization of pre-clerkship clinical skills goals via better dialogue between clerkship directors and ICM directors would likely improve predictive validity of these courses.

5.2.4. Clerkship "Pretests"

A test given on the first day of a clerkship ("pretest") can identify students at risk of poor performance measured by faculty evaluations and scores on the NBME subject exam.[33] This study of a 100-question, faculty-written multiple choice format examination also found significant overlap between other pre-clerkship predictors (i.e., pre-clerkship GPA, USMLE Step 1 scores) of student performance and the pretest, even though these predictors measure different student skills. Since pre-clerkship GPA and USMLE Step 1 scores may not be accessible to clerkship directors, a clerkship pretest offers a reasonable alternative while providing the same predictive power as the USMLE Step 1 and pre-clerkship GPA to identify at-risk students. Additionally, a pretest may provide better sensitivity in identifying at-risk students than the USMLE Step 1 exam.[34]

5.2.5. Incidents Reflecting Professionalism

Professionalism deficiencies during medical school have been significantly associated with subsequent adverse licensure actions among graduates, while traditional cognitive markers, such as grades and test scores, are not predictive of future unprofessional behavior.[35] Irresponsibility and diminished capacity for self improvement were identified as significantly important for predicting future unprofessional behavior.[36] Such deficiencies may be corrected by early remediation, but this has not been clearly established. Other intangible qualities of character and professionalism may predict clerkship performance, but little hard data supports their predictive validity or even how to measure them reliably. Traits including punctuality, reliability, work ethic, knowledge of one's limits, ability to get along with others, and situation awareness are well-recognized characteristics of successful professionals that, when present, would logically be associated with enhanced clerkship outcomes.

A recent study developed a conscientiousness index (CI) as a tool for quantifying behaviors associated with attendance, timely submission of work, voluntary participation in educational activities, and other quantifiable events during medical school.[37] This research found that the CI correlated with preceptor evaluations of a student's professionalism which indicates there may be a valid and feasible method for objectively measuring professional behavior among medical students.[37] More work is needed to determine the predictive validity of such a tool and to determine if unprofessional behaviors can be changed once they are identified. In the physician charter for professionalism, the American Board of Internal Medicine (ABIM) spells out a compelling need to reaffirm professionalism as the basis of medicine's societal contract.[38]

The need to assess and monitor the professional development of medical students is apparent in this era of renewed emphasis on basic principles of professional behavior. A recent study found that medical knowledge, clinical reasoning, and professionalism issues were the most common deficits found in learners referred to a remediation program, with most learners having deficits in multiple domains and professionalism issues being more prevalent at higher levels of training.[39] Wider implementation of longitudinal professionalism assessment and tracking in conjunction with information on medical knowledge and clinical reasoning would be useful to clerkship directors, and such systems should be implemented.

5.3. Use of Baseline Information

5.3.1. Avoiding Bias

Medical school officials and students express concern that future teachers and clerkship directors could be biased by prior knowledge of student performance that profiles students as academically weak. Data on the predictive validity of various pre-clerkship prognostic measures are accumulating. However, little is known about how to use this pre-clerkship information to improve clerkship performance. Students who struggle in the pre-clinical years may wish to start their clinical rotations with a clean slate. Fairness dictates that clerkship directors should use baseline information to address previously identified deficits and improve student performance, and to avoid prejudging students (see Chapter 4).

5.3.2. Confidentiality and Disclosure

Proper use of baseline information includes protection of student confidentiality. Concerns about confidentiality and fairness may prevent medical school officials from sharing pre-matriculation and pre-clerkship information with clerkship directors. If pre-clerkship information is used, disclosure outlining the nature of its use, and policies governing dissemination of prior academic data, are important to reassure students that the process is unbiased and respects their privacy.

5.3.3. Protecting Future Patients, Discovering Important Patterns

Students participating in clinical clerkships have important roles in patient care as first-line reporters and patient confidants. Any system of evaluation should take into consideration safe and effective patient care. While there may be reluctance to "poison the well" by sharing potentially adverse information about an individual student, sharing information between course and clerkship directors is justifiable when done in the service of patient safety. Deficits in clinical competence should be tracked longitudinally because, when seen together, isolated clerkship incidents may reveal a pattern of weakness in the student spanning from the pre-clerkship period to or across clerkships. An approach that balances student rights articulated through the office of student affairs with the rights of future patients, articulated by faculty through an advisory committee or a student promotions committee, should be entrusted with longitudinally tracking deficits in student performance.

5.4. Summary

Prior assessments of student knowledge and prior faculty observations of professional behavior, clinical skills, and non-cognitive performance are part of every medical student's record. These data could be valuable to clerkship directors to facilitate early interventions. There is increasing evidence about the predictive validity of pre-clerkship information. However, no single measure can predict student clerkship success or failure. There is less evidence about accurate identification of students at risk for failure. However, an argument can be made to use a broad spectrum of pre-clerkship measurements looking for patterns of behavior or areas of consistent weakness. Collaboration across disciplines and further study may lead to development of useful prediction models to identify at-risk students with adequate sensitivity and specificity to justify early intervention.

References

1. Glew RH, Ripkey DR, Swanson DB. Relationship between students' performances on the NBME Comprehensive Basic Science Examination and the USMLE Step 1: A longitudinal investigation at one school. Acad Med. 1997;72(12):1097-1102.
2. Holtman MC, et al. Using basic science subject tests to identify students at risk for failing Step 1. Acad Med. 2001;76(10 Suppl):S48-S51.
3. Constance E, et al. Coaching students who fail and identifying students at risk for failing the National Board of Medical Examiners medicine subject test. Acad Med. 1994;69(10 Suppl):S69-S71.
4. Salvatori P. Reliability and validity of admissions tools used to select students for the health professions. Adv Health Sci Educ Theory Pract. 2001;6(2):159-175.
5. Mitchell KJ. Traditional predictors of performance in medical school. Acad Med. 1990;65(3):149-158.
6. Julian ER. Validity of the Medical College Admission Test for predicting medical school performance. Acad Med. 2005;80(10):910-917.
7. Donnon T, Paolucci EO, Violato C. The predictive validity of the MCAT for medical school performance and medical board licensing examinations: A meta-analysis of the published research. Acad Med. 2007;82(1):100-106.
8. Hojat M, et al. A validity study of the writing sample section of the Medical College Admission Test. Acad Med. 2000;75(10 Suppl):S25-S27.
9. Dunleavy DM, Kroopnick MH, Dowd KW, et al. The predictive validity of the MCAT exam in relation to academic performance through medical school: A national cohort study of 2001-2004 matriculants. Acad Med 2013;88(5):666-671.
10. Kirch DG, Mitchell K, Ast C. The new 2015 MCAT: Testing competencies. JAMA 2013;310(21):2243-2244.
11. Murden R, et al. Academic and personal predictors of clinical success in medical school. J Med Educ 1978;53(9):711-719.
12. Meredith KE, Dunlap MR, Baker HH. Subjective and objective admissions factors as predictors of clinical clerkship performance. J Med Educ. 1982;57(10 Pt 1): 743-751.
13. Johnson EK, Edwards JC, Current practices in admission interviews at U.S. medical schools. Acad Med. 1991;66(7):408-412.
14. Harasym PH, et al. Reliability and validity of interviewers' judgments of medical school candidates. Acad Med. 1996;71(1 Suppl):S40-S42.
15. DeVaul RA, et al. Medical school performance of initially rejected students. JAMA. 1987;257(1):47-51.
16. Donnon T, Paolucci EO. A generalizability study of the medical judgment

vignettes interview to assess students' noncognitive attributes for medical school. BMC Med Educ. 2008;8:58.
17. Donnon T, Paolucci EO, Violato C. A predictive validity study of medical judgment vignettes to assess students' noncognitive attributes: A 3-year prospective longitudinal study. Med Teach 2009;31(4):e148-e155.
18. Humphrey-Murto S, Leddy JJ, Wood TJ, et al. Does emotional intelligence at medical school admission predict future academic performance? Acad Med. 2014;89(4):638-643.
19. Goho J, Blackman A. The effectiveness of academic admission interviews: An exploratory meta-analysis. Med Teach 2006;28(4):335-340.
20. Roop SA, Pangaro LN. Effect of clinical teaching on student performance during a medicine clerkship. Am J Med 2001;110(3):205-209.
21. Armstrong A, Dahl C, Haffner W. Predictors of performance on the National Board of Medical Examiners obstetrics and gynecology subject examination. Obstet Gynecol 1998;91(6):1021-1022.
22. Gonnella JS, Erdmann JB, Hojat M. An empirical study of the predictive validity of number grades in medical school using 3 decades of longitudinal data: Implications for a grading system. Med Educ 2004;38(4):425-434.
23. Wilkinson TJ, Frampton CM. Comprehensive undergraduate medical assessments improve prediction of clinical performance. Med Educ 2004;38(10):1111-1116.
24. Buckley S, Coleman J, Davison I, et al. The educational effects of portfolios on undergraduate student learning: A best evidence medical education (BEME) systematic review: BEME guide no. 11. Med Teach 2009;31(4):282-298.
25. Goodyear HM, Bindal T, Wall D. How useful are structured electronic portfolio templates to encourage reflective practice? Med Teach 2013;35(1):71-73.
26. Myles T, Galvez-Myles R. USMLE Step 1 and 2 scores correlate with family medicine clinical and examination scores. Fam Med 2003;35(7):510-513.
27. Omori DM, Wong RY, Antonelli MA, Hemmer PA. Introduction to clinical medicine: A time for consensus and integration. Am J Med 2005;118(2):189-194.
28. Poremba J. Using second year student performance in clinical skills courses to predict substandard clerkship outcome. Unpublished data, 2004.
29. Peitzman SJ, Nieman LZ, Gracely EJ. Comparison of "fact-recall" with "higher-order" questions in multiple-choice examinations as predictors of clinical performance of medical students. Acad Med 1990;65(9 Suppl):S59-S60.
30. LaRochelle J, Gilliland W, Torre D, et al. Readdressing the need for consensus in preclinical education. Mil Med 2009;174(10):1081-1087.
31. Cleland JA, Milne A, Sinclair H, et al. Cohort study on predicting grades: Is performance on early MBChB assessments predictive of later undergraduate grades? Med Educ 2008;42(7):676-683.
32. Klamen DL, Borgia PT. Can students' scores on preclerkship clinical performance examinations predict that they will fail a senior clinical performance examination? Acad Med 2011;86(4):516-520.
33. Denton GD, Durning SJ, Wimmer AP, et al. Is a faculty developed pretest equivalent to pre-third year GPA or USMLE Step 1 as a predictor of third-year internal medicine clerkship outcomes? Teach Learn Med 2004;16(4):329-332.
34. Hemmer PA, Grau T, Pangaro LN. Assessing the effectiveness of combining evaluation methods for the early identification of students with inadequate knowledge during a clerkship. Med Teach 2001;23(6):580-584.
35. Papadakis MA, Hodgson CS, Teherani A, Kohatsu ND. Unprofessional behavior in medical school is associated with subsequent disciplinary action by a state medical board. Acad Med 2004;79(3):244-249.

36. Papadakis MA, Teherani A, Banach MA, et al. Disciplinary action by medical boards and prior behavior in medical school. N Engl J Med 2005;353(25):2673-2682.
37. McLachlan JC, Finn G, Macnaughton J. The conscientiousness index: A novel tool to explore students' professionalism. Acad Med 2009;84(5):559-565.
38. ABIM Foundation, ACP-ASIM Foundation, European Federation of Internal Medicine. Medical professionalism in the new millennium: A physician charter. 2002. <www.abimfoundation.org/~/media/Foundation/Professionalism/Physician%20Charter.ashx?la=en> and <www.abimfoundation.org/Professionalism/Physician-Charter.aspx>. Accessed May 2, 2015.
39. Guerrasio J, Garrity MJ, Aagaard EM. Learner deficits and academic outcomes of medical students, residents, fellows, and attending physicians referred to a remediation program, 2006-2012. Acad Med 2014;89(2):352-358.

Chapter 6
Assessment in the Post-Clerkship Year

Meenakshy K. Aiyer, M.B.B.S.
Matthew Joseph Mischler, M.D.

6.1. Post-Clerkship Period: The Final Phase of Medical School

The post-clerkship period is defined as the time from completion of mandatory core clerkships until graduation from medical school. Assessments during this period that focus on preparedness for residency and attainment of institutional graduation competencies can help address the challenges described in the literature regarding students' preparedness for internship.[1-3] For many years the final year of medical school has not been subject to the attention and consistency expected in clerkships, and fourth-year challenges are formidable.[4] As we discuss below, the experience of many students in the post-clerkship phase is variable, and although they achieve what they need for graduation, they do not always achieve preparedness for residency. Bridging medical school to internship with post-clerkship assessments is a commitment to the concept of the "continuum of medical education."

Recently there has been a call for innovation across medical education, with standardization of learning outcomes and individualization of curriculum to meet learners' unique requirements.[4] The post-clerkship period is ideal for fostering the fundamental values of the medical profession in learners, and also for providing time to demonstrate competence prior to graduation. Unfortunately, variability and lack of clarity in curricula and structure during this period have led to controversy regarding the utility of this phase of training.[5-8] However, recent studies see this time as an opportunity for students to explore and finalize their career choices, and to prepare effectively for residency.[9] Program directors in several disciplines have defined competencies needed by incoming interns, while expressing concern about large gaps in interns' knowledge and skills at the start of residency.[2,3] Recently the AAMC has proposed thirteen entrustable professional activities (EPAs) which interns should be able to perform on the first day of their residency, regardless of their discipline.[10] To achieve these EPAs, and to ensure that students are prepared for residency, formal assessment and feedback during the post-clerkship period would be critical.

The post-clerkship period has usually included electives, intensive care unit (ICU) rotations, advanced clinical responsibilities in the form of subinternships (four to eight weeks of intern-level responsibility under direct supervision) and audition rotations.[5,11] As students transition from minimal expectations as reliable "reporters" in their clerkships to "interpreters" or "managers" (see Chapters 5 and 20), increased responsibility, coupled with appropriate assessments, will ensure progression through these experiences.

6.2. Purposes of Post-Clerkship Assessment

6.2.1. Assessment of Graduation Competence

This period represents the final opportunity for schools to ensure that students have satisfied the "graduation competencies" that are linked to the school's institutional mission. Students are required to participate in standardized assessments, such as the USMLE Step 2 CK and Step 2 CS or the COMLEX (Comprehensive Osteopathic Medical Licensing Examination of the United States), during their fourth year. While these tests do not address the unique and specific mission of each individual medical school, they may help to establish national benchmarks by ensuring the presence of core knowledge and some data-gathering skills in each student, regardless of their residency. We should be aware that the generally used national assessments of graduation competence have not tested management skills; this has been left to each school.

6.2.2. Assess Preparedness for Residency

Students must achieve according to guidelines set out by their educational institutions in order to graduate. However, the experience of many students in the post-clerkship phase is variable, and, as noted above, although they achieve what they need to graduate, they do not always achieve preparedness for residency.[12,13] Program directors have expressed concerns over the lack of preparedness of interns at the start of residency.[2] This has led program directors and subinternship directors to define skills expected of new interns.[3] In addition, the recently defined entrustable professional activities (EPAs), suggested for all graduating students, should help to facilitate transition to internship, equipping students to deal with difficult clinical and social situations, while providing safe, quality care.[13,14]

6.2.3. Document Learner Experiences

The educational experiences of students in the post-clerkship period may vary in the level of responsibility expected, relevant to their residency fields, and possibly in their educational effectiveness. Upon graduation, new interns assume heavier workloads than what they had experienced as students.[13] The ED-2 requirements of the LCME oblige institutions to define the patient conditions, appropriate clinical settings for education, and the level of responsibility that students will experience while on clinical rotations.[15] However, there is no uniform process needed to define these parameters during the post-clerkship period.[5] This period can provide opportunity to define, document, and assess higher level responsibilities, such as order writing, advanced care planning, facilitating transitions of care, and higher level communication in the health care system.

6.2.4. Feedback for Personal and Professional Development

Significant elective time allows students to individualize learning. Goals and objectives for each rotation can be aligned with institutional goals, particularly as they pertain to a specific field. However, aligning goals and objectives of each rotation with the learner's own goals is a more arduous task, since specific goals vary for each learner, and altering an educational experience for each individual would be resource-intensive. As a support for personal growth, formative feedback - based on direct observation of performance - can help to build the self-efficacy of the students, and facilitate their growth through the focus, guidance, and contextual and objective information provided by that feedback.[16] Also, portfolios, discussed below, are one method to document students' progress toward their individual goals.[17]

Table 6. Clerkship Assessments Compared to Post Clerkship Assessments

	Clerkship Assessment	Post Clerkship Assessment
Goals	Meet the goals and objectives of the individual clerkship	Preparedness for residency; learner self-efficacy of skills
Miller's Level of Assessment	"Knows how" to "shows how"	"Shows how" to "does"
Type of Assessment	Summative and Formative: used for providing a grade at the end of the clerkship	Formative with feedback: continued development of knowledge, skills, and attitudes
Assessment Tools	Established tools with validity evidence (subject examinations and end-of-clerkship OSCEs)	Need for development of new assessment tools, or application of existing tools to this phase of education
Skills Development (Dreyfus Model)	Novice to Advanced Beginner	Competent for supervised practice
Areas of Focus	Grades for the clerkships which certify mastery of specialty-specific learning objectives	Personal and professional growth; self-preparedness and verification of EPAs
Potential Sources of Feedback	Various faculty across many services; clerkship directors	Specified OSCE faculty; specialty-focussed in some cases; "close" mentor
Career-Relatedness	Can help to inform decision making in the student	Can help to increase self-efficacy, especially post-match, confirmatory for chosen specialty or to identify areas for the student to fine tune for internship

6.3. Post-Clerkship Assessments vs. Clerkship Assessments

Approaches to clerkship and post-clerkship assessments are outlined in Table 6. For the most part, the pre-clerkship and clerkship phases of the curriculum ensure "standardization" across students; i.e., that each student has met certain basic expectations in knowledge, skills, and professionalism to function at a basic level. While these expectations may include EPAs, to be certified in the period before graduation, the principle of "individualization" broadens the assessment strategy to include ongoing personal development.

6.4. General Principles for Assessment in the Post-Clerkship Period

Here are principles derived from literature and reflected in the prior chapters of this *Handbook*.

- Assessment methods should be broad in scope (covering a broad range of competencies, such as those of the ACGME) and diverse in methods (including both workplace assessments and final examinations). The range of available post-clerkship experiences requires a diverse range of assessments performed in a variety of learning environments.
- Performance assessment methods such as direct observation in the clinical setting and OSCEs should focus on higher levels of function, using frameworks such as Miller's pyramid of "shows how" / "does," or "reporter" / "interpreter" / "manager" in the RIME framework (see Chapter 8).
- Low stakes vs. high stakes: A series of low-stakes, formative assessments provide opportunities for learners to process content and enhance developing knowledge, skills, and attitudes. High-stakes assessments can ensure that the knowledge, skills, and attitudes needed for graduation and/or residency competency are in place.
- Departmental vs. centralized process: Assessments made at the departmental level should focus on the competency of each learner with an agreed-upon set of skills related to the field of choice. A centralized process should ensure that each student's departmental assessments are congruent with the career choice for an agreed-upon set of knowledge, skills, and attitudes that should exist regardless of the field.
- The domains for assessments during the fourth year of training can be categorized into:
  - Assessments of core institutional graduation competencies/skills.
  - Assessments of critical competencies that help assess readiness for internship.
  - EPAs used as a conceptual framework to refocus the assessment of "competency," and guide formative and summative assessment. The RIME model may help to provide a road map to begin to implement EPAs into post-clerkship assessments. The use of the RIME model for learner assessment combined with the use of EPAs in the post-clerkship period could be a powerful assessment tool as we move

toward "standardization and individualized learning objectives."[4,18]
- Creation and assessment of individualized learning plans to foster professional development, accountability and self-directed learning.
- Validity and reliability considerations should be evaluated when developing assessment tools. The current medical literature shows a gap in such tools for post-clerkship assessment, making the development of new tools crucial to proper assessment.
- Assessments need to be tailored to the needs of the individual institution, with emphasis on cost and feasibility.

6.5. Specific Post-Clerkship Assessments Approaches

6.5.1. Entrustable Professional Activities (EPAs)

The ACGME has introduced milestones as an integral concept of resident evaluation.[19] Recognizing the continuum of medical education and the challenges with learner transitions, the AAMC has defined, for students, thirteen EPAs as "tasks or responsibilities to be entrusted to the unsupervised execution by a trainee once he or she has attained sufficient specific competence."[20] An EPA is a construct that synthesizes multiple competencies, and includes specialized functions/skills that should be observable and measurable to gain entrustment.[18,20] Utilizing the EPAs as a framework for assessment provides faculty an objective lens through which the learner can be observed. Various approaches to the development and implementation of an EPA have been described, including selection, practice location, barriers, functions, identifying and developing assessment tools, and defining criteria for advancement through EPAs.[21] Faculty and learner engagement and development through an iterative process is critical to effective implementation. In addition, given the varied nature of post-clerkship rotations, content and process-specific activities will characterize each rotation.[22] For example, "recognize a patient requiring emergent care and initiate evaluation and management" could occur during an ICU or emergency medicine rotation, while process activities such as "discuss patient preferences for advanced care planning" may occur across many rotations. Operationalizing EPAs for assessment is in its infancy, but holds promise for the post-clerkship period.

6.5.2. Assessment During Subinternships

The subinternship has been an integral part of most medical school fourth year curricula.[11] The majority of program directors expect that students complete a required subinternship in their residency field prior to graduation.[2] The internal medicine subinternship task force has defined the core competencies and discussed assessment methods to evaluate learners during subinternship.[23] Other subinternship experiences may not be required in the curriculum, but can be weighted in students' overall assessment based on their residency choice. These assessments could be summative or formative and are applicable across clinical specialties. The workplace assessment methods described in Chapter 8 for calibrating faculty observations are also very useful for subinterns, and we recommend that providing the time needed for these would be worthwhile.

6.5.3. Direct Observational Assessment

Direct observation of a student performing a clinical task with formative feedback has been well described as a method for students to receive feedback during their rotations, involving psychomotor skills, communication skills, and other aspects of patient care.[26,27] Time and personnel are major barriers to implementation, and faculty development is critical to its success. The mini clinical evaluation exercise (mini-CEX) is a well-defined assessment tool, adaptable to many clinical environments, and provides an objective guide to give highly useful formative feedback with direct observation of the learner. These observations can occur across varied clinical settings, and can be used to provide direct feedback on any facet of clinical care, including procedures, communication skills, to history and physical exam, and clinical reasoning.[28,29] The evaluator needs to have a clear sense of the assessment goal in regard to the skill being assessed, particularly as the learner moves through the RIME construct. The lack of a gold standard and the wide variation in evaluation without a structured format are limitations of direct observation, but it is an immensely powerful tool when performed by a skilled educator.[26]

6.5.4. Objective Structured Clinical Exam (OSCE)

OSCEs are a well established method of assessing a learners' further progress in skills gained during the core clerkships.[24] This includes not only the acquisition and evaluation of data, but the ability to communicate the data through communication with patients, families, and health care providers in delivering bad news, disclosing medical errors, and calling consults.[12] An OSCE provides a controlled environment with a reproducible clinical scenario that can be used to assess various clinical skills. A multi-station OSCE that focusses on different types of skills (Figure 6) such as writing discharge orders or admit orders, calling consults or primary care providers, patient handoffs, dealing with nurse calls, or discussing adverse events with patients allows for better sampling of these skills and decreases threats to validity. These skills are process-specific and can be applied to any subinternship.

The lack of validated instruments and resources needed to run an OSCE pose a challenge to implementation. The OSCE should be constructed with consideration given to the optimal number of learners and stations, clarity regarding the domains assessed, and interrater reliability of the assessors.[25] The domains assessed during an OSCE should reflect institutional goals, and/or be aligned with the EPAs.

Figure 6. Sample Multi-Station OSCE for Subinternships

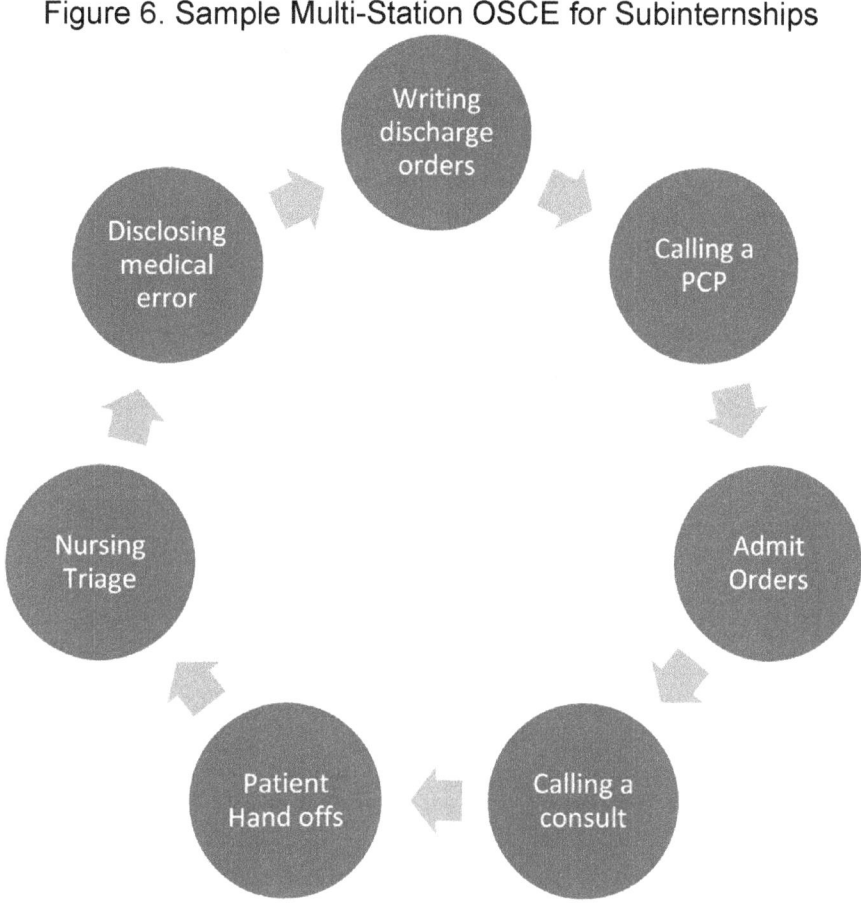

6.5.5. Other Simulation-Based Assessments

Simulation-based assessments apply significantly to providing formative and summative evaluation in the post-clerkship period, ranging from simple task-based stations, to complex skills development such as managing a critically ill patient, running a code, or dealing with a conflict (see Chapter 17).

6.5.6. Assessment Portfolios

Assessment portfolios are models of educational development that allow learners to record, tabulate, reflect on, and process key events in their professional development. These portfolios serve as compilations of personal and professional growth, and provide powerful longitudinal assessment tools for both students and evaluators.[17] They have been implemented as summative assessment tools, and have been shown to improve student and faculty reflective practice.[30] Successful implementation requires benchmarks and frame of reference training to raters of portfolios, and venues to discuss scores and reach consensus. Although studies using portfolios have not always been shown to correlate with other assessment outcomes, consideration should be given to triangulating this assessment with other methods.

6.5.7. Intern Preparedness Course, "Capstone" or "Boot Camps"

Intern preparedness courses, sometimes called "capstone" or "boot camp" courses, are instructional rather than assessments, and are designed to be a culmination of all four years of medical school curriculum near the end of undergraduate training. These courses are being implemented during the post-clerkship period in some schools in an effort to better prepare students for residency. They vary in content and structure, ranging from a two-day to a four-week experience, offered as an independent elective or a culmination of a longitudinal course. Many "boot camps" began to develop the skills of students going into surgical specialties in a short, high-yield course just prior to graduation.[31] These courses have evolved to embrace other disciplines and skill sets, and some schools now require them as part of the fourth year curriculum for all students.[2] The content taught in these courses varies widely, but may be broadly classified into advanced communication skills, transitions of care, and professionalism, coupled with or contrasted to discipline-specific skills, such as laparoscopy or suturing for future surgical interns. Given the paucity of information on the optimal method of assessment of competence in these areas, a "capstone" course may provide a method by which, not only to impart, but also to assess many of these skills.[32]

Studies have shown both increased self-confidence and improved skills in students who have participated in these courses prior to graduation.[34-37,42] The environment of such courses is low stress, usually free of patient ethics concerns, and provides deliberate practice time for students. The content can be adjusted to fit the overall longitudinal content of each individual learning institution. Teamwork and interprofessional learning can be taught and assessed using simulations. OSCE stations, direct observation during simulated exercises, global rating scales, portfolios can all be utilized during these courses. However, the lack of widely validated and available assessment instruments limits the assessment of impact of these courses on clinical performance after medical school and will be a topic for future research. As more capstone and intern preparedness courses are implemented, the tools with which to assess their effectiveness will undoubtedly emerge for wider applicability.

6.6. Post-Clerkship Electives

The post-clerkship period of medical school typically provides elective time to medical students who have previously followed a fairly rigid schedule.[9,11] "Elective" courses are generally described as courses that students select of their own choosing in any field, any time, at any institution locally or globally. "Selective" courses are choices that students have to make between various clinical options outlined by their institutions. Recommended rotations have included subinternships in students' future fields of choice or in internal medicine (IM) and rotations in IM or pediatric subspecialties, critical care medicine, emergency medicine, and ambulatory medicine.[2] During elective rotations, ongoing assessment can be challenging, as students may be rotating outside their fields of residency choice, may have had a brief prior exposure, or are rotating with teachers not considered "core faculty."

Some institutions have utilized elective reports as an assessment tool to provide a detailed record of the student electives, and to hold students accountable for choosing high-quality, well sequenced electives.[38]

6.6.1. Assessment in Electives

Combinations of the various assessment tools discussed above can be considered for use during electives, with direct observation being the simplest to achieve. We would recommend considering an assessment portfolio that accompanies the student during elective time. With the recently proposed EPAs, an assessment portfolio will allow the elective to enhance the student's clinical knowledge, while allowing the preceptor the ability to tailor the elective to areas of development still required for the student's progression. Rather than considering electives to be grade-free rotations, we would also recommend that there be explicit, minimum requirements to be met during elective courses, such as those tailored to the student's residency choice; i.e., a student about to enter internal medicine may have different learning objectives on a surgical subspecialty rotation, than a student entering a surgical specialty. Reflective essays at the end of the electives to illustrate personal development, coupled with global rating scales are some examples of assessments that have also been described.[39]

6.6.2. Audition Electives

Students participate in electives at another institution either to enhance their opportunities for residency; i.e., they are "auditioning," or to experience another clinical setting. This poses interesting challenges for assessments, since they are usually completed by the host institution, rather than by the student's own school. Furthermore, lack of standardized expectations and role clarity impacts the validity and reliability of such assessments.

6.6.3. Longitudinal Course Assessments

These represent assessments of tracks or pathways that may have begun during the pre-clerkship phase, but culminate in a capstone project or experience in the post-clerkship phase. Topics such as research, humanities, quality improvement, and service-oriented curricula lend themselves to a longitudinal track. Assessment portfolios, reflective portfolios, and oral examinations are previously used assessment methods.[40,41]

6.6.4. Future Directions

The post-clerkship period prior to graduation should be extensively utilized to ensure preparedness for graduation, as well as for the start of graduate medical education. However, significant variability in the structure and quality of the educational experience of this period leaves many areas for future research to identify the best methods for post-clerkship instruction.

- Should the starting point of a "milestones meeting" at the beginning of the first postgraduate year be a hard look at a compendium of M4 assessments or an M4 portfolio?
- Can and should schools have uniformly higher expectations in the final year of medical school?
- In an era of ACGME milestones and the NAS, should program directors review a summary of a capstone product from an M4 who has spent considerable time developing scholarly work?
- How do we implement the EPAs broadly, standardizing minimum expectations of all graduate medical students, regardless of their chosen residencies?
- Can we learn from traditional Ph.D. programs with their thesis/dissertation model, where learners are expected to produce a synthesis of their learning?
- What is the role of forward feeding from the clerkship period? (See Chapter 4.)
- Is the "interview trail" of audition electives trumping curriculum in the final phase of medical school? With so much time and effort dedicated to job searching, are assessment efforts diminished?

6.7. Conclusions

Assessment in the post-clerkship period is important for students' continued professional development, assurance of a class's readiness to graduate, and of an individual's preparedness for residency. It is a critical element in evaluating learners as they progress through their medical education, and the post-clerkship phase is invaluable for refining and inculcating learners with the tools needed to be successful physicians. However, significant work needs to be done in this phase, not only in creating validated assessment tools, but also critically addressing some of the issues related to learner transitions and medical education continuum.

References

1. Lypson ML, Frohna JG, Gruppen LD, Woolliscroft JO. Assessing residents' competencies at baseline: Identifying the gaps. Acad Med 2004;79(6):564-570.
2. Lyss-Lerman P, Teherani A, Aagaard E, et al. What training is needed in the fourth

year of medical school? Views of residency program directors. Acad Med 2009;84(7):823-829.
3. Angus S, Vu TR, Halvorsen AJ, et al. What skills should new internal medicine interns have in July? A national survey of internal medicine residency program directors. Acad Med 2014;89(3):432-435.
4. Cooke M, Irby DM, O'Brien BC. Educating Physicians: A Call for Reform of Medical School and Residency. Stanford, CA: The Carnegie Foundation for the Advancement of Teaching; San Francisco: Jossey-Bass, 2010.
5. Walling A, Merando A. The fourth year of medical education: A literature review. Acad Med 2010;85(11):1698-1704.
6. Kanter SL. How to win an argument about the senior year of medical school. Acad Med 2009;84(7):815-816.
7. Chang LL, Grayson MS, Patrick PA, Sivak SL. Incorporating the fourth year of medical school into an internal medicine residency: Effect of an accelerated program on performance outcomes and career choice. Teach Learn Med 2004;16(4):361-364.
8. Petrany SM, Crespo R. The accelerated residency program: The Marshall University family practice 9-year experience. Fam Med 2002;34(9):669-672.
9. Wolf SJ, Lockspeiser TM, Gong J, Guiton G. Students' perspectives on the fourth year of medical school: A mixed-methods analysis. Acad Med 2014;89(4):602-607.
10. AAMC. Core Entrustable Professional Activities for Entering Residency: Curriculum Developers' Guide. Washington DC: AAMC, 2014.
11. Aiyer MK, Vu TR, Ledford C, et al. The subinternship curriculum in internal medicine: A national survey of clerkship directors. Teach Learn Med 2008;20(2):151-156.
12. Mischler M, Miller G, Aldag J, Aiyer MK. Last chance to observe: Assessing residency preparedness following the 4th-year subinternship. Teach Learn Med 2013;25(3):242-248.
13. Raymond MR, Mee J, King A, et al. What new residents do during their initial months of training. Acad Med 2011;86(10 Suppl):S59-S62.
14. Teo AR, Harleman E, O'Sullivan PS, Maa J. The key role of a transition course in preparing medical students for internship. Acad Med 2011;86(7):860-865.
15. LCME. ED-2. <www.lcme.org/connections/connections_2013-2014/ED-2_2013-2014.htm>. Accessed February 7, 2015.
16. Reiser RA, Gagné RM. Characteristics of media selection models. Review of Educational Research. 1982;52(4):499-512.
17. Buckley S, Coleman J, Davison I, et al. The educational effects of portfolios on undergraduate student learning: A best evidence medical education (BEME) systematic review: BEME guide no. 11. Med Teach 2009;31(4):282-298.
18. Pangaro LN, ten Cate O. Frameworks for learner assessment in medicine: AMEE guide no. 78. Med Teach. 2013;35(6):e1197-e1210.
19. ACGME. <www.acgme.org/acgmeweb/>. Accessed February 10, 2015.
20. ten Cate O. Nuts and bolts of entrustable professional activities. J Grad Med Educ 2013;5(1):157-158.
21. Aylward M, Nixon J, Gladding S. An entrustable professional activity (EPA) for handoffs as a model for EPA assessment development. Acad Med 2014;89(10): 1335-1340.
22. Warm EJ, Mathis BR, Held JD, et al. Entrustment and mapping of observable practice activities for resident assessment. J Gen Intern Med 2014;29(8):1177-1182.
23. Alliance for Academic Internal Medicine. AAIM Connect. CDIM Subinternship Curriculum and Training Problems. <connect.im.org/p/cm/ld/fid=661>. Accessed February 10, 2015.
24. Stillman PL, Regan MB, Swanson DB, et al. An assessment of the clinical skills

of fourth-year students at four New England medical schools. Acad Med 1990; 65(5):320-326.
25. Downing SM, Yudkowsky R, eds. Assessment in Health Professions Education. New York: Routledge, 2009.
26. Kogan JR, Holmboe ES, Hauer KE. Tools for direct observation and assessment of clinical skills of medical trainees: A systematic review. JAMA 2009;302(12):1316-1326.
27. Jelovsek JE, Kow N, Diwadkar GB. Tools for the direct observation and assessment of psychomotor skills in medical trainees: A systematic review. Med Educ 2013;47(7):650-673.
28. Kessler CS, Kalapurayil PS, Yudkowsky R, Schwartz A. Validity evidence for a new checklist evaluating consultations, the 5Cs model. Acad Med 2012;87(10):1408-1412.
29. Farnan JM, Paro JA, Rodriguez RM, et al. Hand-off education and evaluation: Piloting the observed simulated hand-off experience (OSHE). J Gen Intern Med 2010;25(2):129-134.
30. Davis MH, Friedman Ben-David M, Harden RM, et al. Portfolio assessment in medical students' final examinations. Med Teach 2001;23(4):357-366.
31. Okusanya OT, Kornfield ZN, Reinke CE, et al. The effect and durability of a pregraduation boot camp on the confidence of senior medical student entering surgical residencies. J Surg Educ 2012;69(4):536-543.
32. Mery CM, Greenberg JA, Patel A, Jaik NP. Teaching and assessing the ACGME competencies in surgical residency. Bull Am Coll Surg 2008;93(7):39-47.
33. Krajewski A, Filippa D, Staff I, et al. Implementation of an intern boot camp curriculum to address clinical competencies under the new Accreditation Council for Graduate Medical Education supervision requirements and duty hour restrictions. JAMA Surg 2013;148(8):727-732.
34. Esterl RM Jr, Henzi DL, Cohn SM. Senior medical student "boot camp" can result in increased self-confidence before starting surgery internships. Curr Surg 2006; 63(4):264-268.
35. Brunt LM, Halpin VJ, Klingensmith ME, et al. Accelerated skills preparation and assessment for senior medical students entering surgical internship. J Am Coll Surg 2008;206(5):897-904; discussion: 904-907.
36. Klingensmith ME, Brunt LM. Focused surgical skills training for senior medical students and interns. Surg Clin North Am 2010;90(3):505-518.
37. Antonoff MB, Swanson JA, Green CA, et al. The significant impact of a competency-based preparatory course for senior medical students entering surgical residency. Acad Med 2012;87(3):308-319.
38. University of Cambridge School of Clinical Medicine. Assessment Methods. <www.medschl.cam.ac.uk/education/courses/standard/assessment-methods/>. Accessed February 8, 2015.
39. Lumb A, Murdoch-Eaton D. Electives in undergraduate medical education: AMEE guide no. 88. Med Teach 2014;36(7):557-572.
40. University of Iowa Carver College of Medicine. M.D. Program. Humanities Distinction Track. <www.medicine.uiowa.edu/md/humanities/>. Accessed February 9, 2015.
41. Vanderbilt University School of Medicine. Vanderbilt Program in Interprofessional Learning. <medschool.vanderbilt.edu/vpil/>. Accessed February 8, 2015.
42. Cohen ER, Barsuk JH, Moazed F, et al. Making July safer: Simulation-based mastery learning during intern boot camp. Acad Med 2013;88(2):233-239.
43. Wayne DB, Cohen ER, Singer BD, et al. Progress toward improving medical school graduates' skills via a "boot camp" curriculum. Simul Healthc 2014;9(1):33-39.
44. Wilcox JE, Raval Z, Patel AB, et al. Imperfect beginnings: Incoming residents vary in their ability to interpret basic electrocardiogram findings. J Hosp Med 2014;9(3):197-198.

Section Two

Chapter 7
Introduction to Section Two: Integrating Assessment Methods with Blueprints*

Louis N. Pangaro, M.D.

This chapter provides an overview of how those managing academic programs integrate a variety of assessment methods with a group of domains (or dimensions) of competence. Its purpose is to help course and clerkship directors to place the assessment methods listed by William McGaghie in Chapter 1, and discussed in detail in the chapters following this one, into a well-structured plan of assessment.

Assessment methods should be suitable for purposes closely related to the institutional or departmental goals for the curriculum, in such a way that will eventually allow a judgment to be made about the readiness of the trainee for the next level of training.[1] In the case of a medical student, this would be readiness for supervised practice in the first postgraduate year (internship). For a resident it would be readiness for unsupervised practice in one's specialty, if competence has been demonstrated. The methods reviewed in this section of the *Handbook* are essential for formative evaluation, and may also be incorporated into grading.

In Chapter 3 the focus was on how the flow of information within an educational system could (a) result in knowledge about how the system was working, and (b) be sufficient to allow improvements in the system. This chapter introduces Section Two and its focus is on how blueprints may facilitate alignment of methods reviewed with dimensions of performance. Blueprinting in the design of individual written examinations is discussed in Chapter 19.

Chapters 8 through 11 deal with available assessment methods that allow formative assessment that will be linked to feedback in the workplace. They are means whereby we assess the progress of students toward readiness for GME in several dimensions of competence to form a multi-method assessment plan.[2,3]

7.1. "Dimension-by-Method" Blueprints

One common assessment blueprint is a "dimension-x-method" blueprint, which provides a synoptic view of the assessment plan; "synoptic" meaning seeing the components together at one time. In such a blueprint the various dimensions of interest would be displayed in the left column, and the available methods (detailed in Chapter 1) in the top row (see Table 7.1).

Table 7.1. Performance "Dimension by Assessment Method" Blueprint (modified from Klass[2] and used with permission).

The Xes indicate how generally useful each assessment method is for the dimension of performance: X = marginal contribution to evidence; XX = significant contribution but not large or efficient; XXX = significant contribution; XXXX = independently sufficient for decision making (not used in this table because no current method of assessment is considered sufficient in itself).

ACGME Competencies	CanMED Roles	Descriptive Workplace Evaluations	Direct Observation Protocols, Mini-CEX	Observing Procedures	Clinical Reasoning, Computer Case Simulations	Professionalism Assessments (360°) and Peers	Multiple-Choice Tests, Written Examinations	Standardized Patients and OSCEs	Portfolio †
		Chapter 8	Chapter 9 Chapter 18	Chapter 10 Chapter 18	Chapter 11	Chapter 12	Chapter 15 Chapter 16	Chapter 17	Chapter 12
Medical Knowledge	Medical Expert, Scholar	xx	xx	x	xx	xx	xxx	x	x
Interpersonal and Communication Skills	Communicator, Collaborator	xx	xx	xx	x	xxx	x	xxx	x
Professionalism	Professional, Collaborator, Health Advocate	xxx	x	xx	x	xx	x	x	xx
Patient Care	Manager, Health Advocate, Medical Expert	xxx	xxx	xxx	xx	xx	xx	xx	xxx
System-Based Practice	Manager, Health Advocate, Collaborator	xx	x	x	x	xxx	x	x	x
Practice-Based Learning	Medical Expert, Scholar	x	x	x	x	x	x	x	xxx

The dimensions of performance in the left column could be the ACGME competencies,[4] the CanMEDS roles,[5] or any other analytic framework in which competence was refracted into different dimensions of performance to be looked at separately. Typically these dimensions are an expansion of the knowledge-skills-attitudes (KSA)[6] or attitudes-skills-knowledge (ASK) model.

In Chapter 8, Drs. Rodriguez and Hemmer discuss the principles and processes of descriptive evaluations and clinical performance evaluations in the workplace. This remains one of the most important problems in clinical education, as such evaluations often have the greatest weight in grading, but too often are the most questionable.[7] Chapter 8 provides guidance for reliably collecting and synthesizing teachers' observations over a clerkship.

The methods of assessment displayed in the top row of the blueprint could also include the direct observation of students' clinical skills, for which Dr. Holmboe in Chapter 9 provides practical and evidence-based guidance in students' encounters with patients. The top row could also include methods for evaluating medical procedures in transfer to the bedside, discussed by Drs. Barsuk and Szmuilowicz in Chapter 10; methods for assessing clinical reasoning, the topic of Drs. Durning, Rencic, and Schuwirth in Chapter 11; and methods for meaningfully evaluating students' attitudes and professional relationships, covered by Drs. Anderson and Kuczewski in Chapter 12.

The blueprint's top row of assessment methods may also include the structured, quantified, *in vitro* methods, to be addressed in Section Three, including multiple choice tests (Chapters 15 and 16), standardized observations of clinical skills with SPs (Chapter 17) and with other forms of simulation (Chapter 18). See Chapter 19 for a sample blueprint of an OSCE in a surgical clerkship.

Assessments in a synthetic framework[6] look at functions that require the student to combine the necessary knowledge, skills and attitudes in order to solve the problem at hand. In fact, the student would be expected to determine what the problem at hand is; what skills are needed to assist this patient; and then to bring these to bear with the appropriate level of proficiency and economy. This depends on a synthetic approach to a student's function, in which competence is the ability to bring to each situation all that the patient requires - and little in excess.[8]

In such an approach, the left column of the blueprint might specify *the setting* in which proficiency must be demonstrated, such as inpatient ward, outpatient clinic, consultative service, emergency room, disaster relief, etc. (see Table 7.2.) These settings help define the context in which a student or resident must demonstrate clinical decision making.[9] The horizontal row across the top of the blueprint could include dimensions of the problem such as organ system, "unknown" (problem in search of a diagnosis) vs. "known" (diagnosis in search of a treatment), solo vs. team-based, single problem vs. complex), and so forth.

Table 7.2. Setting-by-Problem Blueprint (after Klass[2])

	Problem Content (pulmonary, skin, etc)	**Problem Type** "Unknown" vs. "Known"
Settings		
inpatient ward		
outpatient clinic		
long term care facility		
consultative service		
emergency room		
disaster relief		

7.2. Developmental Approaches

When the goal is to plan assessments to document progressively higher levels of performance, then the left column usually represents expected levels of performance as described in Table 7.3. Developmental frameworks are more holistic, (seeing function as a whole, rather than as discrete aspects of knowledge, skill, or attitude), and knowledge-skills-attitudes are not assessed discretely.

In using milestones, the diagram constructed in advance by the clerkship director or program director sets expectations that the learner should be able to achieve at specific points in time. The horizontal row across the top now includes specific times, and the grid blocks are completed with words describing what is expected.

Table 7.3. Developmental Models and Their Terms for Progress

Model	Terms for Progress
Dreyfus[10]	Novice - Advanced Beginner - Competent - Proficient - Expert - Master
RIME[8]	Reporter - Interpreter - Manager - Educator
Milestones[11]	Deficient - Adequate - Ready for Practice - Aspirational
EPAs[12]	Not Ready to Try - Supervised - Unsupervised

In a developmental representation of progress the horizontal (Y) axis of the blueprint - or rather in this case diagram (Figure 7.1) reflects the year of training. The cells of such a table would include the behavioral descriptors of success for each level (milestones).

Figure 7.1. Progress through the years of medical education from UME to GME until independent practice, based on when RIME (reporter-interpreter-manager-educator) levels are introduced, repeated, and when proficiency is expected. When in independent practice, the physician has mastery of all RIME roles, which are often in a patient encounter at the same time. Key: I = introduced in the curriculum; R = repetition, practice; P = sufficient proficiency for the next level of practice; M = mastery in practice

Medical School Year into GME

	I	II	III	IV	PGY1	PGY2/3	Practice
EDUCATOR	I		R	R	R	P	M
MANAGER				I	R	P	M
INTERPRETER		I	R	P			M
REPORTER	I	R	P				M

Finally, it should be emphasized that developmental models expect not only increasing proficiency in doing a procedure, but increased consistency in repeating the procedure, or across cases and clinical problems. This can be represented in Figure 7.2 using the RIME model in which average consistency rises over time (from left to right) but the variability in performance decreases. We would say that by the time one is ready for independent practice at the end of residency, one should be at the "manager"/"educator" level for *all* core problems in one's specialty. Being at the "reporter"/"interpreter" level for a patient with congestive heart failure would be a "red flag" for an internal medicine resident, whereas being at the R-I level for a patient with acromegaly would not.

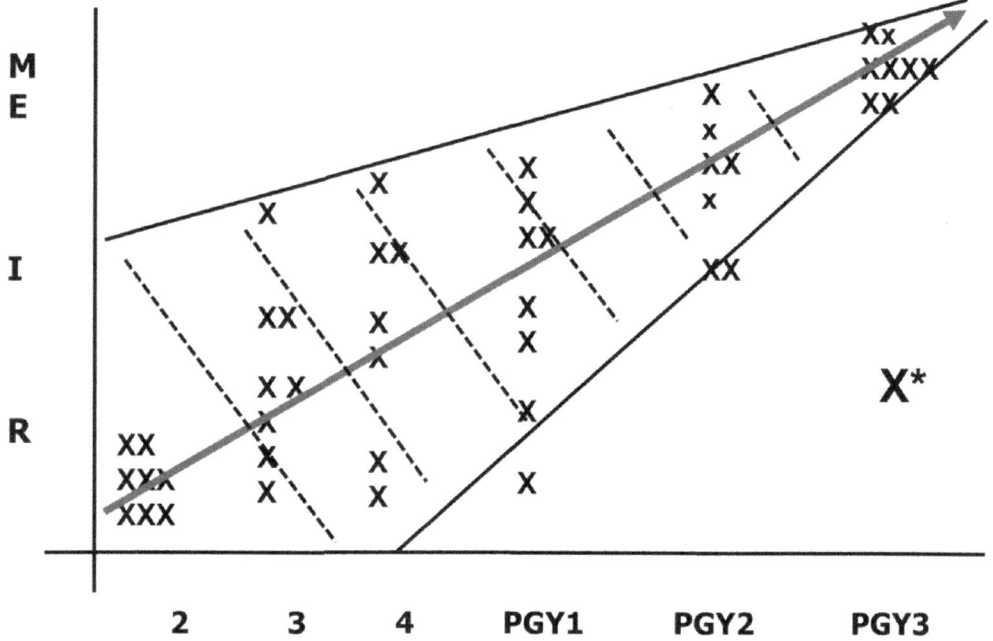

Figure 7.2. A representation of expected increases in levels of skill and consistency across problems with time in developmental models (not empirical data). The asterisk indicates a possible "red flag," as described in the text.

Table 7.4. (after Green[11]). How RIME terms and milestone phrasing align expectations for time in the residency program

	6 months	12 Months	18 months	24 months
RIME Term	REPORTER	INTERPRETER	MANAGER	EDUCATOR
Milestone phrasing	Acquire accurate and relevant history from the patient	Synthesize all data to define each patient's clinical problem	With supervision manage patients with common clinical disorders	Develop a system to track, pursue and reflect on clinical question

In the final chapter of this section, Drs. Leggio and Albritton discuss feedback as a critical step for us to get right in the whole educational system. While there is no single correct blueprint or single correct approach (analytic, synthetic, developmental) for course or clerkship directors to use in planning assessments, we must relate guidance for students to how our observations and assessment methods reflect their progress toward independence.

References

* The opinions herein are the author's own, and do not represent those of the Uniformed Services University or the Department of Defense.
1. van der Vleuten CPM, Schuwirth LW, Driessen EW, et al. A model for programmatic assessment fit for purpose. Med Teach 2012;34(3):205-214.
2. Klass DJ. Developing a system for evaluation of learners. In: Pangaro LN, ed. Leadership Careers in Medical Education. Philadelphia: American College of Physicians Press, 2010: 151-178.
3. Hawkins RE, Holmboe ES. Constructing an evaluation system for an educational program. In: Holmboe ES, Hawkins RE, eds. Practical Guide to the Evaluation of Clinical Competence. Philadelphia: Mosby, 2008: 216-237.
4. ACGME Core Competencies. 1999. <www.mcw.edu/MedicalSchool/EducationalServices/GraduateMedicalEducation/ACGMECoreCompetencies.htm>. Accessed July 21, 2012; not reachable April 6, 2015, but see <www.gahec.org/CME/Liasions/0)ACGME Core Competencies Definitions.htm>, accessed April 6, 2015.
5. Frank JR, ed. The Royal College of Physicians and Surgeons of Canada. The CanMEDS 2005 Physician Competency Framework. <fhs.mcmaster.ca/pathres/resident_resources/documents/CanMEDS2005_e.pdf>. Accessed February 7, 2015.
6. Pangaro LN, ten Cate O. Frameworks for learner assessment in medicine: AMEE guide no. 78. Med Teach. 2013;35(6):e1197-e1210.
7. Williams RG, Klamen DA, McGaghie WC. Cognitive, social, and environmental sources of bias in clinical performance ratings. Teach Learn Med 2003;15(4): 270-292.
8. Pangaro LN. Investing in descriptive evaluation: A vision for the future of assessment. Med Teach 2000;22(5):478-481.
9. Durning SJ, Artino AR Jr, Pangaro LN, et al. Perspective: Redefining context in the clinical encounter: Implications for research and training in medical education. Acad Med 2010;85(5):894-901.
10. Carraccio CL, Benson BJ, Nixon LJ, Derstine PL. From the educational bench to the clinical bedside: Translating the Dreyfus developmental model to the learning of clinical skills. Acad Med 2008;83(8):761-767.
11. Green ML, Aagaard EM, Caverzagie KJ, et al. Charting the road to competence: Developmental milestones for internal medicine residency training. J Grad Med Educ 2009;1(1):5-20.
12. ten Cate O, Scheele F, Competency-based postgraduate training: Can we bridge the gap between theory and clinical practice? Acad Med 2007;82(6):542-547.

Chapter 8
Descriptive Evaluations and Clinical Performance Evaluations in the Workplace

Rechell G. Rodriguez, M.D.
Paul A. Hemmer, M.D., M.P.H.

8.1. The Purpose of Descriptive Evaluations*

Descriptive evaluation is the term applied to the words instructors use in assessing students' demonstrated competency across the domains of knowledge, skills and attitudes; it is usually based on their observations of students over a given period of time (a clinical rotation). It is called "descriptive" to contrast with "quantified" evaluations that use numbers or rating scales (see Chapter 2). Teachers' words should provide evidence of a student's strengths and weaknesses, give examples of achievement or deficiencies, and serve as the basis for direct, meaningful feedback to the student and for recommending advancement or remediation. Some have described this as "clinical performance appraisal."[1]

8.1.1. Workplace-Based Assessment

Descriptive evaluation is typically embedded within the clinical work environment: ambulatory or inpatient care, etc. As such, descriptive evaluation draws on actions, activities, observation, and reflection in the workplace, and thus can be considered part of workplace-based assessment.[2] It should draw from many of the observations made as part of workplace-based assessment; e.g., mini-CEX,[3] case based discussions, clinical encounter cards,[4,5] and multisource feedback. These assessments can and should result in feedback to trainees about their current level of achievement, and how they can take their "next step."[2] Assessments based on actual performance in the clinical arena may be regarded as "authentic," as opposed to performance under controlled conditions.[6] Using an analogy to the clinical setting we sometimes refer to this as *in vivo* rather than *in vitro*.

8.1.2. Characteristics of Descriptive Evaluation

Descriptive evaluation is often, erroneously, referred to as "subjective" evaluation.[7,8] This may have been encouraged by psychometrics and behavioral science, which may label narrative judgments as unreliable and "soft." As a result faculty may be urged to focus on methods that yield "objective" assessments,"[9] and reflecting the bias in favor of that which is expressed in numbers rather than in words.[10] However, Eisner has asserted that expert judgment is likely the superior approach to evaluating competence in fields in which science and art are mixed[11] and, more recently, Govaerts has asserted that, from the constructivist-interpretivist viewpoint, the traditional notions of reliability and validity related to quantitative psychometric-based evaluation of assessment practices have limited usefulness in the evaluation of socially situated performance interpretations or clinical work settings.[12] Additionally, with the rise of team-based health care, the assessment of competence is shifting focus from individuals to collaborative care.[13] Ringsted *et al.*, cited by Hodges, wrote: "In the assessment of physicians it must be acknowledged that physicians often work in teams and systems, rendering it impossible to attribute quality of practice to a single person."[13] The importance of narrative information has been reasserted in recent years with competency and role-based frameworks for assessing trainee performance. Specifically, "the assessment of such general competencies will increasingly be based on qualitative, descriptive and narrative information rather than on, or in addition to, quantitative, numerical data."[14] Hanson *et al.* have asserted that narrative descriptions should replace grades and numerical ratings for clinical performance in medical education.[15] "Performance assessment is a judgment and decision making process, in which rating outcomes are influenced by interactions between individuals and the social context in which assessment occurs."[12]

8.1.2.a. Descriptive ("Subjective") and Quantified ("Objective")

The term "subjective" is potentially detrimental to the evaluation process, in that students and faculty often infer that a "subjective" assessment method is inferior to an "objective" (or quantifiable) method. One must bear in mind that "objectivity does not necessarily result from the strategies of objectification (strategies to reduce measurement error), and the application of these strategies may have undesirable consequences."[16] The critical issue is not that judgments about what is observed vary from evaluator to evaluator, but that these judgments may be lost when translated into numbers on a scale.[15] In fact, the challenge of descriptive evaluation is to make it as rigorous as possible "without trivializing the content for 'objectivity' reasons."[14] "Descriptive" more accurately defines this type of evaluation - conveying one's ideas, thoughts, observations, and a synthesized judgment with words.

Descriptive evaluation is one component of an overall system of evaluation that also frequently incorporates quantifiable examinations of knowledge and/or skills evaluation.[17-19] Descriptive evaluation is unique because it involves all aspects of the evaluation system, including evaluators, students, content of evaluation, and learning environment.[12,20] Additionally, it can be utilized to assess competencies not easily measured by knowledge or skills examinations, such as responsibility, integrity, compassion, maturity, professionalism and collaboration, and the application of knowledge in the clinical problem-solving of direct patient care.[12,20]

Evaluation methods within and across clerkships are rapidly evolving, including a greater emphasis on frameworks for descriptive evaluation and direct observation of learners. Clerkship directors place great emphasis on instructors' comments in determining grades.[17] Studies of required internal medicine clerkships in the U.S. and Canada demonstrated that clinical instructors' evaluations account for 40%-60% (range, 0%-100%) of students' final clerkship grades.[17] Given the reliance on descriptive evaluations in the grading process, clerkship directors must strive for narratives of performance that are dependable, trustworthy, and have sources of evidence that support their validity.

Furthermore, the evaluations should be based on as many direct clinical observations of the students as feasible, describe students' performance according to uniform criteria established by the clerkship faculty, and cite specific examples of behavior and performance.[1,21-23] Evaluators should make precise, behaviorally based comments that cite strengths and weaknesses, thereby providing meaningful feedback to the students. As a result, the evaluations would help clerkship directors and faculty teaching in the clerkship to discern and tailor interventions for those students who are superior, average, or marginal, as well as those who are failing.[12,21,24,25]

Studies of instructors' ratings have shown a remarkable similarity in the elements that instructors emphasize. Typically, these elements include the students' interpersonal skills in dealing with colleagues and patients, their professional attitudes and behaviors, as well as their ability to apply knowledge and solve clinical problems.[18,21,26,27] Instructors at various levels of training and experience may place greater emphasis on different factors. Residents may value a student's procedural skills, work ethic, and motivation to help the team; attending physicians place greater value on a student's knowledge and reasoning skills.[28,29] Peers provide another perspective: Fellow medical students value personal attributes, team contributions, and cognitive abilities when evaluating their student colleagues.[30] These studies are based primarily on instructors' annotations to a rating scale, and not on their narrative comments. Despite their limitations, these studies demonstrate that instructors' evaluations of students assess the breadth of competency: knowledge and its application, problem-solving skills, and professional qualities.

8.1.2.b. Professionalism in Descriptive Evaluation

Many faculty believe that assessing qualities of professionalism may be the most important aspect of evaluating medical students[31] (see Chapter 13). There may be no better evaluation method to assess professional qualities than faculty and residents who observe performance on a daily basis. In fact, faculty ratings and comments form the centerpiece of an evaluation process focussing on professionalism,[32] and such comments made by teachers about students may identify those at risk of future unprofessional conduct.[33,34]

Table 8.1. Problems Encountered in the Evaluation of Medical Students During the Clinical Years (adapted from Tonesk and Buchanan[20])
% = percent of those surveyed who rated problem as "serious."

Clerkship Directors	%	Instructors	%
1. Faculty members' unwillingness to record negative evaluations	40.4	1. Inadequate guidelines for handling problem students	36.7
2. Lack of early warning system regarding problem students	43.6	2. Lack of information about problems students bring with them into the rotation	34.8
3. Breakdown in transmission of information across rotations and clerkships	43.5	3. Faculty members' unwillingness to record negative evaluations	34.5
4. Lack of training of evaluators	35.1	4. Failure to act on negative evaluations	36.6
5. Tardy submission of required evaluations	27.2	5. Lack of training of evaluators	25.8
6. Criteria of evaluation insufficiently defined	29.2	6. Reversal or dilution of negative evaluations	25.1
7. Inadequate guidelines regarding repeaters	32.2	7. Criteria of evaluation insufficiently defined	22.6
8. Reversal or dilution of negative evaluations	25.6	8. Delays in feedback to students	21.9
9. No follow-up of effectiveness of remediation	23.3	9. Role as evaluator not clearly defined	15.3
10. Lack of agreement among evaluators	16.9	10. Insufficient communication with clerkship or site coordinator	15.3
11. Failure to act on negative evaluations	26.4	11. Tardy submission of required evaluations	14.3
12. Lack of integration of information about the student from various sources	12.5	12. Insufficient opportunity to observe students directly	18.2
13. Delays in feedback to students	14.1	13. Excessive reliance on residents for information about students	14.3
14. Lack of integration of information about the student over time	15.1	14. Inadequate evaluation form	12.9
15. Inadequate guidelines regarding temporary or conditional grades	17.2		
16. Lack of correspondence between grades and narrative evaluation	16.5		
17. Inadequate evaluation form	12.8		
18. Inappropriateness of remedy applied to problems identified in students	14.5		
19. Underutilization of existing counseling system	9.4		
20. Excessive reliance on residents for information about students	11.3		
21. Paucity of counseling options	8.8		
22. Insufficient support from administration for the evaluative process	9.6		

8.2. Limitations of Descriptive Evaluation

Some studies of written comments by evaluators have concluded that these comments often were general or non-specific ("a pleasure to work with"),[35] lacked specific examples of performance, and, in general, did not meet minimal standards for what would be considered effective feedback.[35,36] Some proposed reasons for this are: time constraints in busy clinical environments, reluctance to provide feedback that may have negative impacts on learners, poor feedback role modeling, and ineffective or absent training on how to provide effective feedback.[37]

8.2.1. Teacher Reluctance to Record Negative Observations

Instructors may be unwilling to *record* negative comments, but this does not necessarily mean that instructors are not willing to *identify* at-risk students (see Table 8.1).[9,24,38] Reasons for this reluctance include fear of legal action, lack of administrative support for unpopular decisions, an unwillingness to be involved in follow through on difficult cases, fear that receiving poor teacher evaluations may affect future academic promotion, or "passing the buck" to other evaluators.[20] Also, instructors may feel their role as teacher and mentor may be in conflict with that as evaluator, or they may have difficulty with delivering "bad news."

Surveys regarding grade inflation showed that 82% of respondents believed that faculty were reluctant to provide low evaluations because of students' expectations of higher grades, fear of legal action, student "hassle," belief that students with strong work ethic should not fail, or that assigning higher grades may entice students to their own specialty.[39,40] Forty-three percent of the clerkship directors surveyed in one study felt that we are unable to identify incompetent students.[39] These issues persist.[41]

Faculty should be aware of several facts: First, the courts have consistently upheld the judgment of faculty in cases in which students have not met standards[32,42] (see Chapter 21). Second, the "halo effect" continues strongly to influence an instructor's evaluation.[43] Third, students' expectations, sense of entitlement, or tenacity in challenging grades appear to have undue influence on instructors.[44] Given the reluctance to offer a "negative" evaluation, there is likely substantial merit if even only one instructor states or records a negative comment.[33,45,46] Finally, any limitations in what teachers are willing to document are as true of numerical ratings as they are of descriptive comments.

8.2.2. Reliability of Descriptive Evaluation[47,48]

Studies of instructors' ratings of students' written case reports, as well as ratings of videotaped encounters of trainees interviewing, examining, or presenting a patient have shown low intrarater and interrater reliability.[49-51] Although some of the low reliability may be due to instructors focussing on different aspects of student performance, standardized rating scales only modestly improved reliability.[28,29,51,52]

Other studies suggest that instructors' clinical evaluations can achieve sufficient reliability for "high-stakes" academic decisions. Using a standardized descriptive clerkship evaluation form, faculty have achieved a reliability of 0.8 for assigning clerkship grades, when at least seven observations of student performance were available. A reliability of 0.8 has also been achieved when evaluating surgical residents at least eight times, with no improvement in the reliability when more rating scales were added to the evaluation form.[22] Time during the academic year, clerkship site, and academic level of the rater had little effect on the ratings. In another study, the students' scores seemed to depend on the instructor to whom they were assigned and the clinical context in which the rating was performed.[53] Yet another demonstrated that experts were more likely than novice instructors to pay attention to the situation-specific cues in the context of the assessment, as well as to provide more interpretations of what they observed, rather than strictly literal descriptions.[54]

8.3. Rating Scales

Use of global rating scales has demonstrated a modest increase in interrater reliability.[28,29,51,52,55] This higher degree of interrater reliability may be due to a number of actions designed to achieve that reliability: definition of the parameters rated; instructors who had direct, prolonged observation of relatively few students; ratings which were assigned after consensus among all supervisors; and training the raters to use the evaluation forms. In another study,[56] physician ratings of 120 videotaped medical student encounters also demonstrated good interrater reliability (mean 0.85). The high level of agreement was also felt to be due to collaboration on the rating scales that were used in the study. These studies highlight the roles of rater training, creating consensus among teachers about which elements are to be evaluated, and how to go about doing so. More recently, Ginsburg et al. reported interrater reliabilities across three attending (supervising) physicians' rankings of evaluation form written comments of up to 0.83. They concluded that experienced faculty have a shared understanding and conceptualization of residents' performance in real-world settings. Their study echoes recent calls to rely on the wisdom and expertise of assessors.[57]

While high reliability coefficients are desirable, lack of agreement among instructors' evaluations is not necessarily undesirable. Different instructors may focus on different domains, and some may witness performance that not all observe. In aggregate, the ratings should provide a more comprehensive picture of a student's performance.[22,28,29] Ultimately, the clerkship director must decide whether areas of disagreement among instructors are desirable or undesirable.

8.4. Validity[47]

The evidence for the validity of descriptive evaluations has been questioned in studies that have centered on the predictive, concurrent, content, and face validity of descriptive evaluations (recognizing that validity may be most appropriately viewed globally as construct validity, with predictive, concurrent, and content being sources of evidence).[58] Overall competence has been better predicted than professional behavior during residency. Students with good communication skills were more likely to receive higher overall competence ratings.[59] Students who had deficiencies identified by teachers during an internal medicine clerkship were thirteen times more likely to receive low ratings or comments from internship directors.[60] As previously noted, comments and ratings that identify unprofessional behavior of medical students highlight individuals who are at risk of continued unprofessional behavior.[33,34]

Studies have also raised concerns about the concurrent validity of instructors' evaluations, evidenced by low correlation between instructors' end-of-clerkship evaluations and students' performance on knowledge and/or skills examinations.[8,61-65] This low correlation with quantified examinations may not be unexpected. In addition to students' knowledge, instructors' evaluations assess clinical skills and attitudes, thereby assessing characteristics beyond the scope of knowledge or skills examinations. Different types of evaluations measure different characteristics.[61,62,64,66-68]

Content and face validity have also been questioned. Instructors' ratings of videotaped case presentations seemed to depend on the "likeability" of the student, and, as noted, judgments about competency reflected students' communication skills.[49,67] Assessment of one trait (e.g., knowledge) on an evaluation form correlated with assessment of other traits (clinical skills, personal characteristics).[64] Residents have been shown to give higher ratings to students than those given by faculty. Resident evaluations have shown better internal consistency than faculty; adding resident evaluations to those of faculty improves their dependability.[65] Rating forms tailored to a specific task, such as the mini-CEX, have content validity, and faculty can be trained to observe and record accurately.[69,70]

Other factors may affect reliability and validity: a teacher's sense of personal failure if one's student does not improve; a desire to be liked; evaluations that lack specific, behaviorally based comments; substitution of a grade for comments; differing expectations among instructors; limited student-instructor encounter time; lack of a trusting relationship between teacher and learner; failure to observe student performance directly; the interest of raters in the process of evaluation; the types of interactions (such as attending rounds vs. work rounds); and differences in the training environment.[66,71-73] Length of observation may also be a factor. In a surgery clerkship, faculty's descriptive evaluations of knowledge after four-week rotations or longitudinal small-group interactions were better correlated with subject examination scores than after two-week electives.[63] It is becoming increasingly common for teaching faculty to attend on inpatient wards for one or two-week intervals rather than four weeks; there is need for further research on this area. Perceived lack of rewards for teaching may also impact instructors' willingness to participate effectively in the evaluation process. The introduction of longitudinal integrated clerkships (LICs) facilitates student/preceptor(s) continuity for extended periods of time from six months to one year. There is evidence that preceptors and students perceive evaluation in an LIC more favorably than evaluation on block clerkships.[74] Further research is needed on the reliability and validity of LIC evaluations.

Many of the above cited factors highlight that raters themselves are a source of error in the evaluation process.[75] Lack of experience, exposure, or training on the assessment tools used by faculty, especially if in electronic formats, may result in inaccurate or incomplete evaluations.[76] If faculty base their evaluations not on established criteria but on some other factor(s), rater error will increase and this can affect the evaluation process.[58,77] Rater training (see below) and other statistical adjustments can counter rater error,[75] but a clerkship director must be aware of the presence of rater error.

8.5. Improving Descriptive Evaluation

General interventions to improve instructors' evaluations include developing and reinforcing clear performance guidelines, improving communication among faculty members, and offering faculty development regarding evaluation skills.[24,65,78,79] Reliability may be improved by using additional raters, investigating sources of disagreement among evaluators, or statistical methods such as generalizability theory that seek to uncover sources of variation in the evaluation process.[14,48,75,80] Using a computerized evaluation form may improve the timeliness of evaluations as well as the number and quality of comments.[72,81,82] However, there is some recent evidence of delay in completion of online work-based assessments, which affects timeliness of feedback. There is the possibility that faculty training and converting to better technologies such as smart phone and tablet applications will improve this in the future.[76] Relying on instructors for evaluation but not grading may improve the quality of instructors' comments. Feedback to instructors on their evaluation or grading patterns may help to improve future evaluations.[23,35]

Adding behaviorally based descriptors ("anchors") in each evaluation category for each level of performance enhances the reliability of instructors' evaluations, a benefit lost when the descriptors were subsequently withdrawn.[27] Behavioral descriptors on an evaluation form may contribute to instructors making more detailed written comments.[83] Sixteen recommendations to improve clinical performance ratings and these are summarized in Table 8.2. It takes time for the process of descriptive evaluation to be effective, and it needs to be interactive between the clerkship director (or site director) and the teachers. Additionally, administrative resources are needed for transcription of descriptive comments into a narrative format.

Table 8.2. Recommendations for Improvement in Clinical Performance Assessment (Descriptive Evaluation) (adapted from Williams, Klamen, and McGaghie[21])

Recommendation	Example
Broad, Systematic Sampling	Plan multiple observations (may be brief), multiple settings, includes simulations; ideally, 7-10 ratings
Observation by Multiple Raters	Addresses "idiosyncrasies" of single raters
Keep Rating Instruments Short	For progress decisions (grades): 5-10 items plus global rating; when feedback is goal, make form specific to event rated
Separate Appraisal for Teaching, Learning, and Feedback from Appraisal for Promotion	Feedback should be immediate, not saved for written comments on end of rotation rating form
Encourage Prompt Recording	Record observations during the clerkship, as they occur
Supplement Formal Observation with Unobtrusive Observation	Use nurse and patient observations
Consider Making Promotion and Grading Decisions via Group Review	Broadens base of knowledge, perspectives; more likely to make "tough" decisions
Supplement Traditional Clinical Performance Ratings with Standardized Clinical Encounters and Skills Training and Assessment Protocols	Allows all members of group to have clinical skills assessed in standard manner; comparisons to peers and gold standards possible
Educate Raters	Familiarize raters with forms; Provide frame of reference training
Provide Time for Rating	Gather raters together to accomplish ratings (e.g., evaluation sessions)
Encourage Raters to Observe and Rate Specific Performances	Use of mini-CEX form (from American Board of Internal Medicine)
Use No More than Seven Quality Rating Categories	Discourage two-level rating (e.g., 1-3 unsatisfactory, 4-6 satisfactory)
Establish the Meaning of Ratings	Use consistent rating form; did forms help identify excellent or poor performers (e.g., those asked to leave program); provide descriptors
Give Raters Feedback about Stringency and Leniency	Let them know how they compare to others
Learn from Other Professions	Aviation, clergy, military; team performance
Acknowledge the Limits of Ratings	Insufficient by themselves to assess clinical competence

8.6. The RIME Framework

In the early 1990s at the Uniformed Services University of the Health Sciences (USUHS), Pangaro implemented a framework for the descriptive evaluation of medical students designed to assess and foster their progression from "reporter" to "interpreter" to "manager" to "educator" (RIME),[84,85] a scheme which has been widely adopted among medical schools - and even veterinary schools.

8.6.1. Reporter

Students must: (1) take ownership of the facts about their patients and accurately and independently gather information; (2) use appropriate terminology to clearly communicate their findings, both orally and in writing; (3) interact professionally with patients and staff; and (4) consistently and reliably carry out their responsibilities. Success in this RIME category requires that students have an adequate knowledge base, the basic skills to perform fundamental tasks, and core attributes of honesty, reliability, and commitment. Students who are reporters can answer the "What?" questions about their patients.

8.6.2. Interpreter

Students must: (1) take ownership of explaining their patients' findings, (2) demonstrate ability to identify and prioritize problems independently, and (3) offer three *reasonable* explanations for new problems, generating and defending differential diagnoses. This category requires a greater knowledge base, increased confidence and skill in selecting and applying clinical facts to a specific patient, and the ability to begin to pose clinical questions. Interpreters organize, prioritize, synthesize, and interpret problems. Students who are interpreters can answer the "Why?" questions about their patients.

8.6.3. Manager

Students must be more "proactive," taking ownership of solving their patients' problems, suggesting diagnostic and therapeutic plans that include reasonable diagnostic options and possible therapies. This level takes even greater knowledge, more confidence, and the skill to select interventions for an individual patient. Managers understand their patients' needs and desires and can enter into "relationship-centered care."

8.6.4. Educator

Becoming a manager is an action closely tied to being an educator. Students take ownership for getting to a higher level of expertise, and must identify questions related to their patients that cannot be answered from textbooks; they cite evidence that new or alternative therapies or tests are worthwhile, and share their acquired knowledge with other members of the health care team. Desire and ability to educate one's self and others is intrinsic to being a manager and reflects a desire not only to teach colleagues but also, and most importantly, to help the patient. A manager/educator answers the "How?" questions, for themselves, and their patients. It is not simply a matter of "bringing in articles to the team."

In a curriculum in which the basic "reporter" skills of interviewing, symptom characterization, comprehensive history and physical exam had been introduced in the first year, "passing" a core clerkship (typically in the third year) may require mastery of "reporter" skills and also evidence of some transition toward "interpreter." Acquisition of skills as a consistent, *reasonable* "interpreter" constitutes a higher level of performance. Consistently demonstrating skills at the "manager/educator" level reflects performance beyond expectations for a clerkship student, in other words what might be expected of a fourth-year student or subintern (see Chapter 6).

RIME captures what clinicians do when they interact with patients: observation (reporter), reflection (interpreter), action (manager/educator) and what they write: "subjective/symptoms" and "objective/observations" (reporter), "assessment" (interpreter), "plan" (manager/educator). RIME is "synthetic" - success in each RIME category requires a combination of elements in the traditional analytic framework - knowledge, skills, and attitudes - brought together by the student.[86]

RIME also helps teachers to understand the minimal level of performance below which a trainee cannot fall. For example, accomplished interpretation skills are unacceptable if the student cannot demonstrate the ability to obtain reliably and independently the information from the patient. In this way, it provides a criterion-based framework for evaluating the performance of students.

RIME is applicable in both ambulatory care and inpatient settings, in which it readily becomes part of the terminology that teachers use. In a study assessing the feasibility and acceptability of RIME, Battistone *et al.*[23,84,87,88] found that residents and faculty believed that the new descriptive system was "more valid" than the prior evaluation method. Eighty percent of students found RIME to be "helpful" or "very helpful" with overall student satisfaction. More than half of the students reported they heard the RIME terminology in the feedback from their teachers within the first year of implementation.[23,84,87,88] Students felt such feedback was more useful and helped them identify specifically how to improve.

8.7. Formal Evaluation Sessions

Formal evaluation sessions are meetings held with teachers during a clinical clerkship[90] and can be used to train faculty to use any desired educational framework, such as the ACGME competencies or the CanMEDS framework. There are studies that establish the value of this as a method for training faculty to use the RIME framework.[46,60,87,89,90]

8.7.1. Implementing Evaluation Sessions

The evaluation sessions are formal, planned meetings that are held at the midpoint and the last week of the rotation at each clerkship site. The clerkship director or the onsite coordinator for the clerkship moderates each session, during which, fifteen minutes is devoted to discussing each medical student. All instructors, including residents and faculty, are asked to attend. Each evaluator is asked to describe and assess the student's strengths and/or weaknesses and is allowed to speak uninterrupted. The moderator may ask for clarifications about, or specific examples of, demonstrated knowledge, skills, and attitudes and makes handwritten notes of each teacher's comments. Typically, the most junior evaluator speaks first, and the attending physician last, to encourage the house staff to voice their observations uninfluenced by the comments of the more senior attending physician, who usually has had less time to observe the student. At the end of the comments, the facilitator asks for a recommended summary evaluation and the "next steps" for the student to progress along the RIME framework.

The spoken comments are paraphrased and included in the final narrative summary and can be distinguished from the written comments made by the teacher on their evaluation form. The clerkship director or site directors can also provide faculty development by giving feedback to the teachers through frame of reference training[91] (see Chapter 9). The clerkship director or site director meets with each student the following day to provide feedback by expressing the verbal comments from evaluators and having the student review the evaluation forms with the written comments.

Meeting with ambulatory teachers may require a bit more flexibility than in the inpatient setting, but such sessions are possible in either setting. More than 40% of U.S. internal medicine clerkships currently use some version of face-to-face meetings with teachers *during* the clerkship.[17]

8.7.2. Faculty Development through Evaluation Sessions

Evaluation sessions also create formal opportunities for: (1) defining clerkship objectives and how they can be assessed; (2) defining expectations of and for instructors; (3) facilitating communication among faculty members; and (4) providing faculty development.[20,39,78,89] These sessions must be considered "protected time." In addition, because they take place *during* the clerkship, these sessions meet the students' need for formative evaluation and feedback by identifying and discussing strengths and weaknesses.

Importantly, the sessions facilitate identification of marginally performing students by capitalizing on instructors' willingness to discuss verbally concerns regarding students.[45,46] Evaluation sessions have enhanced predictive validity over traditional evaluation methods for identifying students with marginal funds of knowledge, as well as those students who are likely to have problems during their first postgraduate year of training.[46,60] The sessions improve the detection and description of unprofessional behavior.[45] Using the RIME framework in conjunction with the formal sessions has achieved (1) an internal consistency of descriptive evaluation of student performance similar to that of quantifiable examinations[92] and (2) consistency of evaluation across geographically widely separated clerkship sites.[93]

Evaluation sessions have been implemented at other institutions on various clerkships.[17,87,90,94-96] Residency program directors and local leaders support these sessions by allowing residency lecture time to be used for these sessions, signaling the importance of trainee evaluation and also teachers' professional development.[87,96] Teachers do indeed attend the meetings, with attendance rates ranging from 72% to nearly 100%.[87,96] Some clerkships may have students at such a large number of teaching sites that face-to-face meetings may not be feasible. What seems to be most important is the interaction between the clerkship director and the teachers, which, for some programs, necessitates advanced communication technology to facilitate.

During a 10-12 week clerkship, to complete this evaluation process, a cumulative total of 45-60 minutes per student is invested. This is similar to the time invested in evaluation by clerkship directors who use alternative evaluation and grading methods. The time and resources to administer the evaluation sessions are commensurate with expectations of clerkship directors outlined by the Alliance for Clinical Education and others.[96-98]

8.8. Putting It Together: The Final Narrative of a Student's Clerkship Performance

At the completion of the clerkship, the clerkship director is responsible for synthesizing into a final grade all of the information gathered about a student during the clerkship (see Chapter 20). This will involve creating a narrative of the descriptive evaluations submitted by the teachers from the clerkship or discussed during the formal sessions.

8.9. "Rules" for Clerkship Narratives

There are some general recommendations to follow when creating such a narrative:

- It should reflect the input of anyone who provided a descriptive evaluation.
- It should describe over what period of time each individual teacher worked with and observed the student.
- If teachers make a recommendation about a final evaluation (e.g., Honors, Pass, Fail, A, B, C, level within RIME, etc.), then this should be recorded.
- As much as possible, use the teachers' comments verbatim. There may be circumstances in which it is appropriate to edit a teacher's comments, particularly if the comments reflect a teacher who is not evaluating the student based on established criteria.
- Specific examples are always desirable.
- Be careful about excluding comments that describe concerns; remember, even concerns from a single evaluator may have merit.

Another part of the clerkship narrative should be a summary section written by the clerkship director. The clerkship director should synthesize all of the teacher's comments and the student's examination performance to generate as comprehensive a picture of the student's performance as possible. If the RIME framework is used, summarize where the student currently is in the RIME transitions and cite examples. If the ACGME competency framework is used, summarize what was achieved within the domains that were assessed. If possible, address the student's response to feedback, desire for self-improvement, reliability, and responsibility, and whether the student is fulfilling the promises of duty and expertise that we expect them all to begin to make toward patients. The final paragraph should be complete enough to give a comprehensive picture of the student's performance at the end of the clerkship.

This summary paragraph should not be used to predict the student's future performance, or to recruit a student to a given specialty. It may be best to think of this paragraph as it might be used in a letter of evaluation or in the Medical Student Performance Evaluation (MSPE). When a departmentally based review committee has determined a final grade that is less than Pass, there are other considerations, such as referring to the committee's review of the "entirety" of the student's record (see Chapter 21). Spending time to write this concluding paragraph not only may help with citing areas of performance important to residency program directors, such as aspects of professionalism, but also could improve the specificity and richness of the description by providing specific examples of achievement or deficiency.[99]

8.10. Conclusion

Credible descriptive evaluations of medical students require use of the same expectations for both formative and summative evaluation, and careful calibration of teachers.[84] This takes time, both for the clerkship director and for the teachers.[97] Improving descriptive evaluation can be accomplished if clerkship directors talk with teachers on a regular basis. If faculty or resident time is an issue, then this certainly requires the support of the medical school, the department, and local teaching site leadership. It is unreasonable to assume that, without training and faculty development, instructors will be able to improve evaluation skills or feel support to identify concerns regarding students. Clerkship directors should consider the language in which they ask teachers to evaluate, and whether the terms being used are actually grasped by evaluators and students. Providing descriptive evaluations will enhance the MSPE reports,[100] written by the dean's office, which will help residency program directors to determine qualified candidates from applicants who come from institutions with Honors/Pass/Fail grading systems, which are growing in prevalence.

References

* The foundation material was published previously in the chapter on medical student evaluation in the *ACE Guidebook for Clerkship Directors* - fourth edition - (Gegensatz Press, 2012). This is now expanded and updated to report new developments.
1. Clerkship Directors in Internal Medicine. Evaluating the internal medicine clerkship: A CDIM commentary. Am J Med 1994;97(5):i-vii.
2. Norcini JJ, Burch V. Workplace-based assessment as an educational tool: AMEE guide no. 31. Med Teach 2007;29(9):855-871.
3. Kogan JR, Holmboe ES, Hauer KE. Tools for direct observation and assessment of clinical skills of medical trainees: A systematic review. JAMA 2009;302(12):1316-1326.
4. Bennett AJ, Goldenhar LM, Stanford K. Utilization of a formative evaluation card in a psychiatry clerkship. Acad Psychiatry. 2006;30(4):319-324.
5. Richards ML, Paukert JL, Downing SM, Bordage G. Reliability and usefulness of clinical encounter cards for a third-year surgical clerkship. J Surg Res 2007; 140(1):139-148.
6. Pangaro LN. Investing in descriptive evaluation: A vision for the future of assessment. Med Teach 2000;22(5):478-481.
7. Awad SS, Liscum KR, Aoki N, et al. Does the subjective evaluation of medical student surgical knowledge correlate with written and oral exam performance? J Surg Res 2002;104(1):36-39.
8. Marienfeld RD, Reid JC. Subjective vs. objective evaluation of clinical clerks. N Engl J Med 1980;302(18):1036-1037.
9. Tonesk X. The Evaluation of Clerks: Perceptions of Clinical Faculty. A Summary of Issues and Proposed Actions. Washington, DC: AAMC, 1983.
10. Simpson MA. Medical student evaluation in the absence of examinations. Med Educ. 1976;10(1):22-26.
11. Eisner EW. The Educational Imagination. New York: MacMillan, 1979.

12. Govaerts MJ, van der Vleuten CPM, Schuwirth LW, Muijtjens AM. Broadening perspectives on clinical performance assessment: Rethinking the nature of in-training assessment. Adv Health Sci Educ Theory Pract 2007;12(2):239-260.
13. Hodges B. Assessment in the post-psychometric era: Learning to love the subjective and collective. Med Teach 2013;35(7):564-568.
14. van der Vleuten CPM, Schuwirth LW. Assessing professional competence: From methods to programmes. Med Educ 2005;39(3):309-317.
15. Hanson JL, Rosenberg AA, Lane JL. Narrative descriptions should replace grades and numerical ratings for clinical performance in medical education in the United States. Front Psychol 2013;4:668.
16. Norman GR, van der Vleuten CPM, De Graaff E. Pitfalls in the pursuit of objectivity: Issues of validity, efficiency and acceptability. Med Educ 1991;25(2):119-126.
17. Hemmer PA, Papp KK, Mechaber AJ, Durning SJ. Evaluation, grading, and use of the RIME vocabulary on internal medicine clerkships: Results of a national survey and comparison to other clinical clerkships. Teach Learn Med 2008;20(2):118-126.
18. Hunt DD. Functional and dysfunctional characteristics of the prevailing model of clinical evaluation systems in North American medical schools. Acad Med 1992;67(4):254-259.
19. Tonesk X. AAMC program to promote improved evaluation of students during clinical education. J Med Educ 1986;61(9 Pt 2):83-88.
20. Tonesk X, Buchanan RG. An AAMC pilot study by 10 medical schools of clinical evaluation of students. J Med Educ 1987;62(9):707-718.
21. Williams RG, Klamen DA, McGaghie WC. Cognitive, social, and environmental sources of bias in clinical performance ratings. Teach Learn Med 2003;15(4):270-292.
22. Williams RG, Verhulst S, Colliver JA, Dunnington GL. Assuring the reliability of resident performance appraisals: More items or more observations? Surgery 2005;137(2):141-147.
23. Holmboe ES. Faculty and the observation of trainees' clinical skills: Problems and opportunities. Acad Med 2004;79(1):16-22.
24. Tonesk X. Clinical judgment of faculties in the evaluation of clerks. J Med Educ 1983;58(3):213-214.
25. Williams RG, Dunnington GL, Klamen DL. Forecasting residents' performance - partly cloudy. Acad Med 2005;80(5):415-422.
26. Grim DR, Miller MD. Criteria for evaluating performance of third-year medical students. Fam Med 1993;25(6):388-390.
27. Maxim BR, Dielman TE. Dimensionality, internal consistency and interrater reliability of clinical performance ratings. Med Educ 1987;21(2):130-137.
28. Metheny WP. Limitations of physician ratings in the assessment of student clinical performance in an obstetrics and gynecology clerkship. Obstet Gynecol 1991;78(1):136-141.
29. Stillman RM. Pitfalls in evaluating the surgical student. Surgery 1984;96(1):92-96.
30. Levine RE, Kelly PA, Karakoc T, Haidet P. Peer evaluation in a clinical clerkship: Students' attitudes, experiences, and correlations with traditional assessments. Acad Psychiatry 2007;31(1):19-24.
31. Arnold L. Assessing professional behavior: Yesterday, today, and tomorrow. Acad Med 2002;77(6):502-515.
32. Papadakis MA, Loeser H, Healy K. Early detection and evaluation of professionalism deficiencies in medical students: One school's approach. Acad Med 2001;76(11):1100-1106.

33. Papadakis MA, Hodgson CS, Teherani A, Kohatsu ND. Unprofessional behavior in medical school is associated with subsequent disciplinary action by a state medical board. Acad Med 2004;79(3):244-249.
34. Papadakis MA, Teherani A, Banach MA, et al. Disciplinary action by medical boards and prior behavior in medical school. N Engl J Med 2005;353(25):2673-2682.
35. Lye PS, Biernat KA, Bragg DS, Simpson DE. A pleasure to work with: An analysis of written comments on student evaluations. Ambul Pediatr 2001;1(3):128-131.
36. Braend AM, Gran SF, Frich JC, Lindbaek M. Medical students' clinical performance in general practice: Triangulating assessments from patients, teachers and students. Med Teach 2010;32(4):333-339.
37. Canavan C, Holtman MC, Richmond M, Katsufrakis PJ. The quality of written comments on professional behaviors in a developmental multisource feedback program. Acad Med 2010;85(10 Suppl):S106-S109.
38. Teherani A, Hodgson CS, Banach M, Papadakis MA. Domains of unprofessional behavior during medical school associated with future disciplinary action by a state medical board. Acad Med 2005;80(10 Suppl):S17-S20.
39. Speer AJ, Solomon DJ, Fincher RM. Grade inflation in internal medicine clerkships: Results of a national survey. Teach Learn Med 2000;12(3):112-116.
40. Cacamese SM, Elnicki M, Speer AJ. Grade inflation and the internal medicine subinternship: A national survey of clerkship directors. Teach Learn Med 2007; 19(4):343-346.
41. Permutt ZD, DeFer TM, Fazio S. Grade Inflation in the Internal Medicine Clerkship: A National Survey. Abstract presented at the annual meeting of the Clerkship Directors in Internal Medicine, San Antonio, TX, October 14-17, 2010.
42. Irby DM, Milam S. The legal context for evaluating and dismissing medical students and residents. Acad Med 1989;64(11):639-643.
43. Gough HG, Hall WB, Harris RE. Evaluation of performance in medical training. J Med Educ 1964;39(7):679-692.
44. Dubovsky SL. Coping with entitlement in medical education. N Engl J Med 1986;315(26):1672-1674.
45. Hemmer PA, Hawkins R, Jackson JL, Pangaro LN. Assessing how well three evaluation methods detect deficiencies in medical students' professionalism in two settings of an internal medicine clerkship. Acad Med. 2000;75(2):167-173.
46. Hemmer PA, Pangaro LN. The effectiveness of formal evaluation sessions during clinical clerkships in better identifying students with marginal funds of knowledge. Acad Med 1997;72(7):641-643.
47. Cook DA, Beckman TJ. Current concepts in validity and reliability for psychometric instruments: Theory and application. Am J Med 2006;119(2):166.e7-e16.
48. Downing SM. Reliability: On the reproducibility of assessment data. Med Educ 2004;38(9):1006-1012.
49. Kalet A, Earp JA, Kowlowitz V. How well do faculty evaluate the interviewing skills of medical students? J Gen Intern Med 1992;7(5):499-505.
50. McLeod PJ. Faculty assessments of case reports of medical students. J Med Educ 1987;62(8):673-677.
51. Noel GL, Herbers JE Jr, Caplow MP, et al. How well do internal medicine faculty members evaluate the clinical skills of residents? Ann Intern Med 1992;117(9): 757-765.
52. Pangaro LN, Holmboe ES. Evaluation forms and formal rating scales. In: Holmboe ES, Hawkins RE, eds. Practical Guide to the Evaluation of Clinical Competence. Philadelphia: Mosby, 2008: 24-41.

53. Kreiter CD, Ferguson K, Lee WC, et al. A generalizability study of a new standardized rating form used to evaluate students' clinical clerkship performances. Acad Med 1998;73(12):1294-1298.
54. Govaerts MJ, Schuwirth LW, van der Vleuten CPM, Muijtjens AM. Workplace-based assessment: Effects of rater expertise. Adv Health Sci Educ Theory Pract 2011;16(2):151-165.
55. Keynan A, Friedman M, Benbassat J. Reliability of global rating scales in the assessment of clinical competence of medical students. Med Educ 1987;21(6): 477-481.
56. MacRae HM, Vu NV, Graham B, et al. Comparing checklists and databases with physicians' ratings as measures of students' history and physical-examination skills. Acad Med 1995;70(4):313-317.
57. Ginsburg S, Gold W, Cavalcanti RB, et al. Competencies "plus": The nature of written comments on internal medicine residents' evaluation forms. Acad Med 2011;86(10 Suppl):S30-S34.
58. Downing SM, Haladyna TM. Validity threats: Overcoming interference with proposed interpretations of assessment data. Med Educ 2004;38(3):327-333.
59. Dawson-Saunders B, Paiva RE. The validity of clerkship performance evaluations. Med Educ 1986;20(3):240-245.
60. Lavin B, Pangaro LN. Internship ratings as a validity outcome measure for an evaluation system to identify inadequate clerkship performance. Acad Med 1998; 73(9):998-1002.
61. Campos-Outcalt D, Witzke DB, Fulginiti JV. Correlations of family medicine clerkship evaluations with scores on standard measures of academic achievement. Fam Med 1994;26(2):85-88.
62. Case SM, Ripkey DR, Swanson DB. The relationship between clinical science performance in 20 medical schools and performance on Step 2 of the USMLE licensing examination. 1994-95 Validity Study Group for USMLE Step 1 and 2 Pass/Fail Standards. Acad Med 1996;71(1 Suppl):S31-S33.
63. Farrell TM, Kohn GP, Owen SM, et al. Low correlation between subjective and objective measures of knowledge on surgery clerkships. J Am Coll Surg 2010; 210(5):680-683; discussion: 683-685.
64. Hull AL, Hodder S, Berger B, et al. Validity of three clinical performance assessments of internal medicine clerks. Acad Med 1995;70(6):517-522.
65. Littlefield JH, Harrington JT, Anthracite NE, Garman RE. A description and four-year analysis of a clinical clerkship evaluation system. J Med Educ 1981;56(4): 334-340.
66. Greenberg LW, Getson PR. Assessing student performance on a pediatric clerkship. Arch Pediatr Adolesc Med 1996;150(11):1209-1212.
67. Lawrence PF, Nelson EW, Cockayne TW. Assessment of medical student fund of knowledge in surgery. Surgery 1985;97(6):745-749.
68. Stenchever MA, O'Toole B, Irby D. Evaluating student performance in an obstetrics and gynecology clerkship. Am J Obstet Gynecol 1979;134(3):235-237.
69. Holmboe ES, Hawkins RE, Huot SJ. Effects of training in direct observation of medical residents' clinical competence: A randomized trial. Ann Intern Med. 2004;140(11):874-881.
70. Holmboe ES, Huot S, Chung J. Construct validity of the miniclinical evaluation exercise (miniCEX). Acad Med 2003;78(8):826-830.
71. Carline JD, Paauw DS, Thiede KW, Ramsey PG. Factors affecting the reliability of ratings of students' clinical skills in a medicine clerkship. J Gen Intern Med 1992;7(5):506-510.

72. Ten Eyck RP, Maclean TA. Improving the quality of emergency medicine rotation/clerkship evaluations. Am J Emerg Med 1994;12(1):113-117.
73. Weaver CS, Humbert AJ, Besinger BR, et al. A more explicit grading scale decreases grade inflation in a clinical clerkship. Acad Emerg Med 2007;14(3):283-286.
74. Mazotti L, O'Brien B, Tong L, Hauer KE. Perceptions of evaluations in longitudinal versus traditional clerkships. Med Educ 2011;45(5):464-470.
75. Downing SM. Threats to the validity of clinical teaching assessments: What about rater error? Med Educ 2005;39(4):353-355.
76. Basu I, Parvizi S, Chin K. The perception of online work-based assessments. Clin Teach 2013;10(2):73-77.
77. McLaughlin K, Vitale G, Coderre S, et al. Clerkship evaluation: What are we measuring? Med Teach 2009;31(2):e36-e39.
78. Stemmler EJ. Promoting improved evaluation of students during clinical education: A complex management task. J Med Educ 1986;61(9 Pt 2):75-81.
79. Norcini JJ, Holmboe ES, Hawkins RE. Evaluation challenges in the era of outcomes-based education. In: Holmboe ES, Hawkins RE, eds. Practical Guide to the Evaluation of Clinical Competence. Philadelphia: Mosby, 2008: 1-9.
80. Kreiter CD, Ferguson K, Lee WC, et al. A generalizability study of a new standardized rating form used to evaluate students' clinical clerkship performances. Acad Med 1998;73(12):1294-1298.
81. Bennett AJ, Arnold LM. Use of a computerized evaluation system in a psychiatry clerkship. Acad Psychiatry 2004;28(3):197-203.
82. Duque G. Web-based evaluation of medical clerkships: A new approach to immediacy and efficacy of feedback and assessment. Med Teach 2003;25(5):510-514.
83. Ainsworth MA, Speer AJ, Solomon DJ. A clinical evaluation form to improve faculty critique of students. Acad Med 1995;70(5):445.
84. Pangaro LN. A new vocabulary and other innovations for improving descriptive in-training evaluations. Acad Med. Nov 1999;74(11):1203-1207.
85. Pangaro LN. Investing in descriptive evaluation: A vision for the future of assessment. Med Teach 2000;22(5):478-481.
86. Pangaro LN, ten Cate O. Frameworks for learner assessment in medicine: AMEE guide no. 78. Med Teach 2013;35(6):e1197-e1210.
87. Battistone MJ, Milne C, Sande MA, et al. The feasibility and acceptability of implementing formal evaluation sessions and using descriptive vocabulary to assess student performance on a clinical clerkship. Teach Learn Med 2002;14(1):5-10.
88. Battistone MJ, Pendleton B, Milne C, et al. Global descriptive evaluations are more responsive than global numeric ratings in detecting students' progress during the inpatient portion of an internal medicine clerkship. Acad Med 2001;76(10 Suppl):S105-S107.
89. Hemmer PA, Pangaro LN. Using formal evaluation sessions for case-based faculty development during clinical clerkships. Acad Med 2000;75(12):1216-1221.
90. Noel GL. A system for evaluating and counseling marginal students during clinical clerkships. J Med Educ 1987;62(4):353-355.
91. Pangaro LN, Holmboe ES. Evaluation forms and formal rating scales. In: Holmboe ES, Hawkins RE, eds. Practical Guide to the Evaluation of Clinical Competence. Philadelphia: Mosby, 2008: 24-41.
92. Roop SA, Pangaro LN. Effect of clinical teaching on student performance during a medicine clerkship. Am J Med. 2001;110(3):205-209.

93. Durning SJ, Pangaro LN, Denton GD, et al. Intersite consistency as a measurement of programmatic evaluation in a medicine clerkship with multiple, geographically separated sites. Acad Med. 2003;78(10 Suppl):S36-S38.
94. Albritton TA, Fincher RM, Work JA. Group evaluation of student performance in a clerkship. Acad Med 1996;71(5):551-552.
95. Metheny WP, Espey EL, Bienstock J, et al. To the point: Medical education reviews evaluation in context: Assessing learners, teachers, and training programs. Am J Obstet Gynecol 2005;192(1):34-37.
96. Ogburn T, Espey E. The R-I-M-E method for evaluation of medical students on an obstetrics and gynecology clerkship. Am J Obstet Gynecol. Sep 2003;189(3):666-669.
97. Pangaro LN, Bachicha J, Brodkey A, et al. Expectations of and for clerkship directors: A collaborative statement from the Alliance for Clinical Education. Teach Learn Med 2003;15(3):217-222.
98. Pangaro LN. Expectations of and for the medicine clerkship director. Am J Med 1998;105(5):363-365.
99. Shea JA, O'Grady E, Wagner BR, et al. Professionalism in clerkships: An analysis of MSPE commentary. Acad Med 2008;83(10 Suppl):S1-S4.
100. AAMC. A Guide to the Preparation of the Medical Student Performance Evaluation. 2002. <www.aamc.org/download/64496/data/mspeguide.pdf>. Accessed February 7, 2015.

Chapter 9
Direct Observation of Students' Clinical Skills

Eric Holmboe, M.D.

Despite tremendous advances in medical technology, the clinical skills of interviewing, physical examination, and informed decision making and counseling remain essential to the successful care of patients. The AAMC strongly endorses the evaluation of students in these clinical skills.[1] The Institute of Medicine has placed *patient-centered care* at the heart of its five core competencies for all physicians.[2] Substantial research exists on the importance of strong communication skills and quality of care for patients.[3,4] Faculty observation of students performing medical interviews, physical examinations, or informed decision making/counseling is still essential for the reliable and valid assessment of these skills.

The development of SPs to evaluate clinical skills has been a major advance in the assessment of students.[5-9] However, standardized patients should be optimally applied in clinical skills teaching and assessment as a supplement to similar activities in the real clinical setting; they cannot replace the observation of students by faculty on an ongoing basis with actual patients.[10-13] This direct observation is the focus of this chapter.

Accurate assessment of performance with actual patients by faculty constitutes the essential ingredient needed for effective feedback to help students develop strong clinical skills.[14-16] Lack of high-quality assessment and feedback makes it very difficult for students to reach their full potential. Unfortunately many faculty are not sufficiently prepared to observe accurately and provide effective corrective feedback about these clinical skills. In this chapter we will first explore problems in students' clinical skills and the challenges faced by faculty performing direct observation. We will then outline some practical methods to improve faculty observation skills along with useful tools that faculty can use when performing observations.

9.1. Reasons for and Challenges of Direct Observation

Numerous studies have documented serious deficiencies in medical interviewing and counseling that have persisted over time. In the views of some, history taking skills may have actually declined.[17-22] More importantly, research has demonstrated positive associations between good communication skills and improved patient outcomes.[3,23,24] Errors are also common in physical examination skills.[25-31] For example, deficiencies in auscultatory skills among trainees were noted over 40 years ago,[27,28] and poor cardiac and pulmonary physical exam skills continue to plague U.S. students and residents today.[29-31]

These findings are relevant because we know that, despite advances in technology, accurate data collection during medical interviews and physical exams remains the most potent diagnostic tool available to physicians.[32-35] Two important past studies showed that the medical interview alone produced the correct diagnosis in nearly 80% of patients presenting to an ambulatory care clinic with previously undiagnosed conditions.[32,34] Bordage noted that errors in data collection are one of the principal factors in diagnostic errors committed by physicians.[36] More recently, Graber found that while systems factors were important in adverse events experienced by hospitalized patients, errors in data collection and synthesis of clinical information were also major factors.[37] Overuse of potentially dangerous tests and procedures is also partly the result of inadequate clinical skills. Ensuring that students and residents acquire strong clinical skills can therefore be part of the solution to improve the quality of care and reduce the alarming rise in health care costs. The Choosing Wisely and High Value Care initiatives highlight the importance of strong clinical skills in avoiding unnecessary and potentially harmful care for patients.[38,39] Without accurate evaluation of clinical skills, which must be accomplished by direct observation, improvement in the clinical skills of physicians is unlikely.[40-42]

9.2. Lack of Direct Observation by Faculty

Perhaps the biggest problem in the evaluation of clinical skills is simply getting faculty to observe students. One of the most prominent physician-scientists and educators of the twentieth century, the late George Engel, strongly advocated direct observation of the history and physical examination skills of trainees about forty years ago.[43,44] Dr. Engel commented in a 1976 editorial: "Evidently it is not deemed necessary to assay students' (and residents) clinical performance once they have entered the clinical years. Nor do clinical instructors more than occasionally show how they themselves elicit and check the reliability of clinical data. To a degree that is often at variance with their own professed scientific standards, attending staff all too often accept and use as the basis for discussion, if not recommendations, findings reported by students and house staff without ever evaluating the reporter's mastery of the clinical methods utilized or the reliability of the data obtained."[44]

Sadly, little may have changed since Engel wrote this passage. The AAMC found that, among 97 medical schools it visited between 1993 and 1998, faculty rarely observed student interactions with patients, noting that the majority of a student's evaluation was based on faculty and resident recollections of student presentation skills and knowledge.[45] In a more recent study, Lypson and colleagues found medical school graduates about to start an internal medicine internship lacked many of the basic skills believed to be necessary to begin internship safely and effectively.[17] In a 2004 AAMC report, Corbett and Whitcomb found that less than 15% of both U.S. and Canadian medical schools had a formal clinical skills curriculum during the clinical years of medical school.[46] It is yet unclear whether the institution of the USMLE Step 2 CS exam has produced any improvements, but, despite the pressure from this licensing requirement, the AAMC Graduate Questionnaire still finds a substantial proportion of students reporting that they were never or rarely observed by faculty.[47] In my time at the ABIM we still found that over 30% of PGY-2 and 3 residents were never directly observed or assessed during the entire year (personal communication).

9.3. Quality of Faculty Observation

Although several studies show that four to seven observations produces sufficient reliability in the evaluation of clinical skills for "Pass/Fail" determinations, less is known about the validity and accuracy of faculty rating.[48] Noel and Herbers, in two important studies of the ABIM's traditional "long case" clinical evaluation exercise (CEX), found substantial deficiencies in the accuracy of faculty ratings.[49,50] They demonstrated that faculty failed to detect up to 68% of errors committed by a resident scripted to depict marginal performance on a training video. Use of specific checklists prompting faculty to look for certain skills increased accuracy of error detection nearly twofold, but the checklist did not produce more accurate overall ratings of competence. Nearly 70% of faculty still rated a resident depicting marginal performance as satisfactory or superior overall.

Kalet examined the reliability and validity of faculty observation skills using videos of student performance on an OSCE designed to evaluate interviewing skills.[51] She found that faculty were inconsistent in identifying the use of open-ended questions and empathy, and that the positive predictive value of faculty ratings for "adequate" interviewing skills was only 12%. Another study found that faculty could not reliably evaluate 32% of the physical exam skills assessed, and had the most difficulty with examination of the head, neck, and abdomen.[52] One potential reason for the inaccuracy of faculty ratings may relate to the clinical skills of the faculty.[33] Kogan and colleagues found that one of the more important factors in faculty ratings on the mini-CEX was the faculty's own clinical skills. Faculty with more complete history and physical exam skills, as well as more effective communication skills, appropriately rated resident clinical skills more stringently.[53]

More recently several important studies have begun to uncover some of the specific factors that affect the quality of faculty assessment through observation. Kogan and colleagues found that variable frames of reference, inference, faculty's own competence, local culture and experiential modifiers all affected faculty direct observation ratings.[53,54] Most concerning was the finding that faculty's primary frame of reference was self, or "how I would do it." Concern arises, insofar as Kogan's studies found variable competence among faculty across all clinical skills.[53] Yeates in the UK found that faculty were affected by often subconscious stereotypes, plus other factors such as recency bias and idiosyncrasy in what they attended to during an observation.[55-57] Govaerts in the Netherlands also found substantial idiosyncrasies among faculty, but noted that more experienced faculty attended to greater detail.[58,59] Finally, Gingerich remarked that not all idiosyncrasy is necessarily bad - leveraging a faculty's idiosyncratic strengths through appropriate sampling might be very helpful toward improving the quality of assessment.[60] Table 9.1 provides a summary of factors that affect faculty ratings.

Table 9.1. Factors that Affect Faculty Ratings and Judgments

1. Frame of reference	a. Self ("how I would do it") b. Level of learner (normative to peer) c. Practicing physicians d. Criterion-based	
2. Inference (about the learner)	a. Skills	i. Knowledge ii. Competence iii. Work ethic
	b. Prior experiences	Familiarity with scenario
	c. Feelings	i. Comfort ii. Confidence iii. Intentions iv. Ownership
	d. Personality	
	e. Culture	
3. Anticipatory feedback	Anticipating reaction to possible feedback at end of observation	
4. Stereotypes		
5. Recency bias	Effects of previous observations on current observation/rating	
6. Rater idiosyncrasy		
7. Faculty/rater experience		

All these studies have greatly deepened our understanding of rater cognition and the factors that affect the quality of ratings. The studies reinforce the importance of appropriate and multiple sampling of performance. Without good sampling strategies and observations performed by multiple observers, learners will not receive enough high-quality feedback. The studies by Yeates, Govaerts, and Gingerich also highlight the limits of rater training and that faculty development cannot replace the need for multiple samples of performance.[55-60] However, it is clear that we still need approaches to help faculty improve their rating and observation skills. After all, we cannot forget that in the middle of the observation is a patient who deserves to experience high-quality care, even in a training setting. With this in mind, let's explore some promising techniques to help faculty improve their observation skills.

9.4. Practical Approaches to Training Faculty

Given the essential role of faculty observation in the evaluation of basic clinical skills, medical schools and residency programs must better prepare faculty for this important task. Recent research in medical education has demonstrated that effective training approaches can improve observation skills. A brief description of each approach and how it applies to faculty development for competency evaluation of medical students is described below.

9.4.1. Behavioral Observation Training (BOT)

Behavioral observation training is focussed on improving the detection, perception, and recall of actual performance.[61] There are two main strategies emphasized in BOT. The first is simply to increase the number of observations, or increased sampling of actual performance. This helps to improve recall of performance and provides multiple opportunities for skill practice in observation by the rater - the "practice makes perfect" principle." The second strategy is to provide some form of observational aide that raters can then use to record observations, sometimes referred to as "behavioral diaries." Studies show that even something as simple as a 3 x 5 inch index card used to record observation notes improves the quality of information provided on evaluation forms. As described below, the mini-CEX form and checklists can serve as an immediate "behavioral diary" to record a rating of an observation.[62]

Observation of clinical skills also requires that faculty "prepare" for the observation. First, faculty should determine the objectives and/or goals of the observation before entering the patient's room with the student. For example, if you plan to perform an observation of a student's physical examination skills, what would be the appropriate components of a physical exam for the patient's chief complaint or medical condition? Positioning is also very important because, as faculty, you want to minimize interference with the student-patient interaction whenever possible. Figure 9.1 demonstrates the principle of triangulation that maximizes the ability of faculty to observe while minimizing interference. Table 9.2 lists some important yet simple rules for performing student observation.

Figure 9.1. Principle of Triangulation

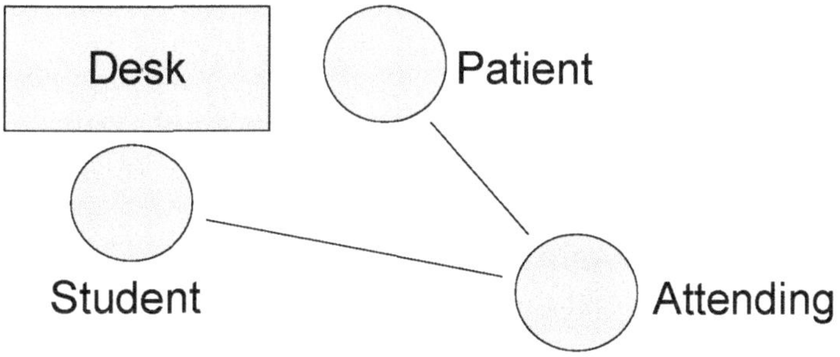

Table 9.2. Five Simple Rules for Observation

Rule	Description
Correct Positioning.	As the rater, try to avoid being in the line of sight of either the patient or trainee, especially when they are communicating. Use the principle of triangulation. However, during physical examinations, be sure you can view the trainee's techniques accurately.
Minimize External Interruptions.	Let your staff know you will be with the resident for 5-10 minutes, avoid taking routine calls, etc.
Avoid Intrusions.	Don't interject or interrupt if at all possible. Once you interject yourself into the trainee-patient interaction, the visit is permanently altered. However, there will be many times at some point in the visit where you need to interject yourself in order to correct misinformation, etc. from the resident.
Be Prepared.	Know before you enter the room what your goals are for the observation session. For example, if a physical exam, have the trainee present the history first; then you will know what the key elements of the PE should be.
Prepare the Trainee *and* the Patient.	Let the trainee know what you plan to do during the observation, including your interaction with the patient. You also need to let the patient know what your role will be and your relationship with the trainee.

9.4.2. Performance Dimension Training (PDT)

This type of training is designed to teach and familiarize the faculty with the appropriate performance dimensions used in their own evaluation systems.[63-65] PDT simply starts with a review of the definitions and criteria for each dimension of performance or competency. The goal should be to define all those criteria and student *behaviors* that constitute a superior performance from the perspective of patient outcomes and should be grounded in the best available evidence for the clinical skill of interest. This technique, by emphasizing a criterion-based approach, helps to ground the observation in what the patient needs and will also help to produce better feedback. The next step in PDT is to give faculty the opportunity to "interact" with the definitions, using videos or actual evaluation examples to improve their understanding of the definitions and criteria. The overarching goal of PDT is to ensure that faculty first understand the definitions and criteria for the competency of interest as a group, so that some degree of consensus is shared among faculty. In other words, PDT helps to create a shared mental model about what constitutes competence in clinical skills.

This will be particularly important as the community continues to evolve to an outcomes-based approach to medical education, as evidenced by the recent proposal of graduation EPAs for medical students.[66] Table 9.3 provides a very straightforward and useful proactive PDT exercise that can be done with faculty to facilitate interaction with competency in clinical skills. We recommend performing PDT exercises in small groups and then having the small groups share their results. Inevitably differences occur among the groups. These differences, however, lead to productive discussions on what constitute the core elements and criteria of competency in counseling or in other clinical skills. Once faculty have shared their criteria for competence with each other, the next step should be to provide best evidence for each clinical skill and to decide what constitutes minimal performance in the context of safe, effective, patient-centered care. This is particularly useful when evidenced-based criteria exist. PDT exercises can be done for two clinical skills over approximately one hour of time. Another approach to PDT is reactive: using actual evaluations or videos of clinical skills, to which faculty can react when performing the PDT exercise.

Table 9.3. Sample Performance Dimension Training and Frame of Reference Exercise

The purpose of this group exercise is to develop specific criteria for a dimension of clinical competency.	
Situation: A student is seeing a patient who has been diagnosed with hypertension and failed a trial of diet and weight loss. The student now needs to start a new medication for this patient. What are the criteria for a superior, highly effective counseling and patient education session? In other words, what criteria will you use to judge the counseling and patient education performance of this student? Once you have defined all the criteria, check off those criteria a student would have to perform in order to receive a satisfactory rating.	
With your group: Define the components/criteria of effective patient counseling and education, based on the attitudes, skills, knowledge (ASK) model. Be sure your criteria are "behavioral" - remember you are developing these elements inthe context of faculty observation.	
Knowledge	What questions and "content" should the student ask the patient?
Skills	How should the interview be conducted? How should questions be asked?
Attitudes	Define behaviors that would signal to an attending that a student was displaying a compassionate, interested, professional attitude.

9.4.3. Frame of Reference Training (FoRT)

This type of training specifically targets accuracy in rating. Table 9.4 describes the complete FoRT process. FoRT is really an extension of PDT, but the main goal of FoRT is establishing the different performance criteria that distinguish *levels* of performance. The main focus of FoRT should be to define three or four levels of performance and again, to ground "satisfactory" or competent performance using the patient's needs as the frame of reference. The PDT exercise should first define the criteria and definitions for a superior performance from the perspective of optimal patient outcomes. The second step of the exercise (Table 9.3) is to define the minimal criteria for a satisfactory performance. These criteria serve as an important anchoring point to define marginal and unsatisfactory performance in Step 3. Once the group defines marginal criteria, then by default any other type of performance is unsatisfactory. This type of exercise is critical to help faculty develop a shared mental model of what constitutes various levels of performance.

Without a shared "frame of reference" faculty tend to use gestalt as they would in their clinical work. The equation below is a helpful way to think about observation and how to choose an appropriate frame of reference. Essentially, the level, or competence, of the trainee must be matched to the appropriate level of supervision to assure that the patient receives high-quality care that is safe, effective and patient-centered as a minimum.

Trainee Performance (a function of level of competence in context) x Appropriate Level of Supervision (a function of attending competence in context) *Must* = Safe, Effective, Patient-Centered Care

Figure 9.2 provides a schematic for faculty development using the three techniques described above.

Figure 9.2. Approaches to Faculty Development (adapted from Peter Katsufrakis and William Iobst, personal communication) Key: PDT = Performance dimension training; BOT = Behavioral observation training; FOR = Frame of reference training

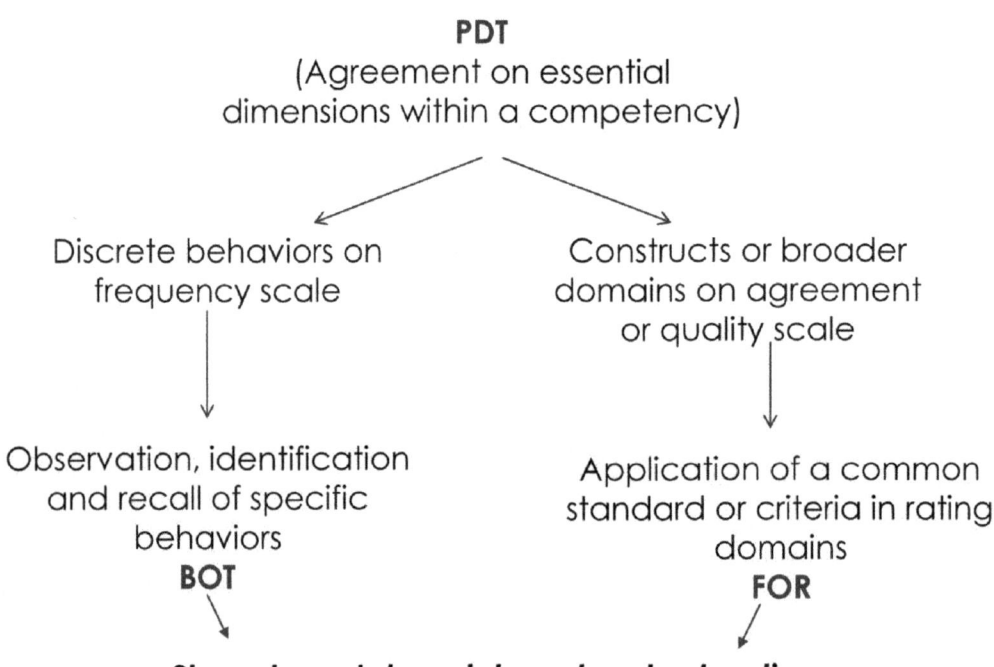

9.5. Direct Observation of Competence (DOC) Training

Direct observation of competence training uses the methods of BOT, PDT, FoRT, and standardized patient training methods to train faculty in observation. There are two versions of DOC training: The "short course" form involves BOT, PDT, and FoRT exercises, using small group discussion and video encounters. The long course version includes a half day of skill practice with standardized residents and patients.[67] To date, one study found that the full day course with the live practice led to meaningful changes in rating behavior that lasted up to eight months; but unfortunately a two-hour workshop version of the training, using only video, did not lead to changes in faculty rating behavior.[68] Observation is a skill that requires training and practice; future work in faculty development will need to test more longitudinal models to allow for ongoing skill practice.

Table 9.4. Steps for Frame of Reference Training

Step	Description of task
1	Performance dimension training (PDT). After an initial group discussion, faculty are given descriptions for each dimension of competence followed by a discussion of what they believe the qualifications are for each dimension.
2	Faculty define what constitutes optimal (the most effective criteria and behaviors) performance from the perspective of optimal patient outcomes (see equation).
3	Next, faculty define and reach consensus on the minimal criteria for satisfactory performance defined as safe, effective, patient-centered care. Once the satisfactory criteria are set, marginal criteria are defined. Everything else by default is unsatisfactory performance.
4	Participants are given clinical vignettes describing critical incidents of performance from unsatisfactory to average to outstanding. (Frame of Reference). For clinical skills, video encounters are the best method.
5	Participants use vignettes to provide ratings on a behaviorally anchored rating scale.
6	Session trainer/facilitator provides feedback on what the "true" ratings should be along with an explanation for each rating.
7	Training session wraps up with an important discussion on the discrepancies between the participants' ratings and the "true" ratings.

9.5.1. Useful Tools to Guide Observation

9.5.1.a. The Mini Clinical Evaluation Exercise (Mini-CEX)

The mini-CEX was originally designed to evaluate residents in a setting reflecting day-to-day practice. Faculty observe a resident performing a *focussed* history, *focussed* physical, or counseling session during routine care experiences on the inpatient wards, intensive care units, outpatient clinics, or the emergency department. However, the mini-CEX has also been used in student clerkships.[69] The mini-CEX facilitates multiple observations over time by different faculty members. This improves both the reliability and validity of the evaluations. This longitudinal nature of the mini-CEX is one of its most important strengths as an evaluation tool and method.

In the first large study of the mini-CEX, Norcini *et al.*[70] reported the results of 388 mini-CEX evaluations for 88 residents at five different residency programs. Over half of the encounters occurred in the inpatient setting. In this initial study, most of the participating residents were in the PGY-1 year, and each resident underwent a mean of 4.4 observations (range 2-10). The authors noted that the standard error for just four mini-CEXs per resident was acceptable enough for Pass/Fail determinations. Trainees reported high satisfaction ratings for the mini-CEX format and, interestingly, there was a modest correlation between faculty satisfaction ratings and resident performance. In a study of the mini-CEX with students, Kogan and colleagues found that nearly 90% of students on a twelve-week medicine clerkship were able to obtain at least nine mini-CEX observations.[50] The reliability coefficient for eight mini-CEXs was 0.77 and the mini-CEX was used in both the inpatient and outpatient clerkship settings.[50] Holmboe and colleagues, using scripted videotapes, found that the mini-CEX evaluation form does possess construct validity.[71]

More recently, Kogan and colleagues in their systematic review of all tools available for direct observation found the mini-CEX was the most studied internationally and possessed the best validity evidence of all the instruments available.[72] This article is also a useful resource to review other available tools that can be used with students, such as the SEGUE communications tool. I recommend the mini-CEX because it is the best studied, with over twenty publications, but the bottom line is that the instrument is only as good as the faculty rater using it.[72] Changes to the rating form itself will, on average, explain only 10% or less of the variance. I strongly encourage programs to choose an existing tool in most circumstances and to spend the majority of their efforts in helping faculty to perform the observation well and to use the instrument or tool effectively.

9.5.1.b. Feedback and the Mini-CEX

An essential component of the mini-CEX, as with any evaluation, is feedback. One study investigated the feedback generated from the mini-CEX observation by audio recording the attending-resident feedback session, with particular focus on interactive feedback.[73] Interactive feedback was defined as any feedback that provided a recommendation plus self-assessment, allowing the learner to react to the feedback, and the development of an action plan. The study showed that 80% of the feedback sessions included at least one recommendation for improvement by the resident, and on average each feedback session contained two recommendations. The majority of recommendations, as might be expected, involved the clinical skills of medical interviewing, physical examination, and counseling. However, despite the large number of recommendations, only eight sessions concluded with a specific action plan from the faculty member on how to carry out the recommendation or to improve.[73] This is a very important aspect of feedback: including an action plan to enable the learner to act on the recommendations provided.

More recently, Kogan and colleagues explored the complexities of feedback associated with direct observation. In this qualitative study, two broad themes were identified in faculty members' descriptions of the feedback process: (1) substantial variability in feedback techniques and (2) how faculty think and feel about delivering feedback. Faculty used multiple approaches in delivering feedback and experienced tensions in balancing positive and negative feedback, in their own perceived self-efficacy for giving good feedback, and in their perceptions of the resident's insight, receptivity, skill, and potential. Faculty also highlighted the importance and challenge of the faculty-resident relationship in the feedback process.[74] In sum, the observation-rating-feedback process is complex, and faculty development is essential to help faculty use assessment methods and tools more effectively.

9.5.1.c. Checklists and Structured Clinical Observation

Checklists targeting specific skills are another tool that can improve the quality of faculty observation. However, since the purpose of faculty direct observation is to assess performance of actual clinical practice, it is not feasible to develop highly detailed checklists for every patient encounter. Some degree of faculty interpretation of behavior and skills will be required when working in actual clinical settings. A number of checklists for assessment of interviewing skills have been developed and tested for reliability. Both the SEGUE and Calgary-Cambridge checklists are useful tools to guide the evaluation of process and general content of medical interviewing.[75,76] Structured clinical observation (SCO) is another observation technique that uses guidelines and observation sheets systematically to assess skills in history taking, physical examination, and information-giving.[77] The value of the SCO approach is the use of narrative and does not require a rating or "grade." Narrative assessment through words is a useful and valid method for formative assessment to help students improve. It is important to recognize that numbers are nothing more than a means to represent a judgment made by the faculty. The observation of faculty and the words used to describe the quality of clinical behaviors are the most important substrate for the student through verbal and written feedback.

9.5.2. Creating an Observation System

There are three simple steps in creating a faculty observation system. First, determine what your faculty are doing in regard to observation. If no observation is occurring, you will probably have to create a "need" for observation. Highlighting the substantial deficiencies in clinical skills among students provides ample evidence that you can use to demonstrate the need to perform observation.[78,79] Second, start small and get the faculty to do some form of observation. Usually what happens is that faculty will notice these deficiencies. Once that happens, it becomes very difficult for your faculty to argue they do not need to observe students, especially from a patient-centered perspective.

The next step is to improve faculty skill in observation. Depending on your educational climate, this can be done concurrently with creating the need for observation. (You may also need to help faculty improve their own clinical skills.) I recommend that you start with performance dimension and behavioral observation training. This is can be done in a series of brief workshops, evaluation sessions, or at faculty meetings. Once your group feels comfortable with the definitions and criteria for the clinical skills competencies, you can then move on to frame of reference training and direct observation of competence training to improve faculty accuracy and ability to distinguish between levels of competence.

9.5.3. Milestones

For a number of reasons, training programs, especially in GME, have struggled to operationalize the general "competencies." One reason has been the lack of a shared understanding of the competencies among educators and of what the developmental trajectories of the competencies should be. In an attempt to address these challenges and to embrace further the outcomes-based philosophy, the specialties have created milestones for each of the six competencies.[80] Milestones have the potential to help guide not only curriculum but also direct observation. Green *et al.* and Nabors *et al.* used the original internal medicine milestones to revise their evaluation forms to help faculty focus on a limited set of behavioral milestones across the competencies that were most relevant for the goals of the specific rotation.[81,82] Moving forward, the milestones can serve as a type of "item bank" to guide assessments through direct observation linked to the goals of the curricular experience.

9.6. Conclusions

The successful practice of medicine requires the effective application of medical interviewing, physical examination, and counseling skills. Studies continue to document significant deficiencies in all three of these clinical skills areas among students. Direct observation by medical faculty remains an essential method to assess core clinical skills with actual patients. Furthermore, faculty are in the best position to assess students' acquisition and refinement of clinical skills and to provide critical feedback longitudinally over time.

References

1. Nutter D, Whitcomb M. The AAMC Project on the Clinical Education of Medical Students. 2007. <www.aamc.org/download/68522/data/clinicalskillsnutter.pdf>. Accessed May 7, 2015.
2. Institute of Medicine. Health Professions Education: A Bridge to Quality. Washington, DC: National Academies Press, 2003.

3. Bernabeo EC, Holmboe ES. Patients, providers, and systems need to acquire a specific set of competencies to achieve truly patient-centered care. Health Affairs 2013;32(2):250-258.
4. Henry SG, Holmboe ES, Frankel RM. Evidence-based competencies for improving communication skills in graduate medical education. A review with suggestions for implementation. Med Teach 2013;35(5):395-403.
5. Richards BF, Rupp R, Zaccaro DJ, et al. Use of a standardized-patient-based clinical performance examination as an outcome measure to evaluate medical school curricula. Acad Med. 1996;71(1 Suppl):S49-S51.
6. Anderson MB, Stillman PL, Wang Y. Growing use of standardized patients in teaching and evaluation in medical education. Teach Learn Med 1994;6(1):15-22.
7. Sloan DA, Donnelly MB, Schwartz RW, Strodel WE. The objective structured clinical examination: The new gold standard for evaluating postgraduate clinical performance. Ann Surg. 1995;222(6):735-742.
8. Stillman PL, Swanson D, Regan MB, et al. Assessment of clinical skills of residents utilizing standardized patients. A follow-up study and recommendations for application. Ann Intern Med. 1991;114(5):393-401.
9. Barrows HS. An overview of the uses of standardized patients for teaching and evaluating clinical skills. Acad Med. 1993;68(6):451-453.
10. van der Vleuten CPM, Swanson DB. Assessment of clinical skills with standardized patients: State of the art. Teach Learn Med 1990;2(2):58-76.
11. Rethans JJ, Sturmans F, Drop R, et al. Does competence of general practitioners predict their performance? Comparison between examination setting and actual practice. BMJ 1991;303:1377-1380.
12. Hodges B, Regehr G, McNaughton N, et al. OSCE checklists do not capture increasing levels of expertise. Acad Med. 1999;74(10):1120-1134.
13. Regehr G, MacRae H, Reznick RK, Szalay D. Comparing the psychometric properties of checklists and global rating scales for assessing performance on an OSCE-format examination. Acad Med 1998;73(9):993-997.
14. Hattie J, Timperley H. The power of feedback. Rev Educ Res 2007;77(1):81-112.
15. Ericsson KA. Deliberate practice and the acquisition and maintenance of expert performance in medicine and related domains. Acad Med 2004;79(10 Suppl):S70-S81.
16. Sargeant J, Armson H, Chesluk B, et al. The processes and dimensions of informed self-assessment: A conceptual model. Acad Med 2010;85(7):1212-1220.
17. Lypson ML, Frohna JG, Gruppen LD, Wolliscroft JO. Assessing residents' competencies at baseline: Identifying the gaps. Acad Med 2004;79(6):564-570.
18. Platt FW, McMath JC. Clinical hypocompetence: The interview. Ann Intern Med 1979;91(6):898-902.
19. Meuleman JR, Caranasos GJ. Evaluating the interview performance of internal medicine interns. Acad Med 1989;64(5):277-279.
20. Beaumier A, Bordage G, Saucier D, Turgeon J. Nature of the clinical difficulties of first-year family medicine residents under direct observation. Can Med Assoc J 1992;146(4):489-497.
21. Sachdeva AK, Loiacono LA, Amiel GE, et al. Variability in the clinical skills of residents entering training programs in surgery. Surgery 1995;118(2):300-309.
22. Pfeiffer C, Madray H, Ardolino A, Willms J. The rise and fall of student's skill in obtaining a medical history. Med Educ 1998;32(3):283-288.
23. Stewart MA, McWhinney IR, Buck CW. The doctor-patient relationship and its effect upon outcome. J R Coll Gen Pract 1979;29(199):77-81.
24. Levinson W, Lesser CS, Epstein RM. Developing physician communication skills for patient-centered care. Health Affairs 2010;29(7):1310-1318.

25. Weiner S, Nathanson M. Physical examination: Frequently observed errors. JAMA 1976;236(7):852-855.
26. Wray NP, Friedland JA. Detection and correction of house staff error in physical diagnosis. JAMA 1983;249(8):1035-1037.
27. Butterworth JS, Reppert EH. Auscultatory acumen in the general medical population. JAMA 1960;174(1):32-34.
28. Raftery EB, Holland WW. Examination of the heart: An investigation into variation. Am J Epidemiol 1967;85(3):438-444.
29. Mangione S, Nieman LZ. Cardiac auscultatory skills of internal medicine and family practice trainees: A comparison of diagnostic proficiency. JAMA 1997;278(9):717-722.
30. Fox RA, Ingham Clark CL, Scotland AD, Dacre JE. A study of pre-registration house officers' clinical skills. Med Educ 2000;34(12):1007-1012.
31. Vukanovic-Criley JM, Criley S, Warde CM, et al. Competency in cardiac examination skills in medical students, trainees, physicians, and faculty: A multicenter study. Arch Intern Med 2006;166(6):610-616.
32. Peterson MC, Holbrook JH, Von Hales D, et al. Contributions of the history, physical examination, and laboratory investigation in making medical diagnoses. West J Med 1992;156(2):163-165.
33. Kirch W, Schaffi C. Misdiagnosis at a university hospital in 4 medical eras: Report on 400 cases. Medicine 1996;75(1):29-40.
34. Hampton JR, Harrison MJ, Mitchell JR, et al. Relative contributions of history-taking, physical examination, and laboratory investigation to diagnosis and management of medical outpatients. BMJ 1975;2(5969):486-489.
35. Bowen JL. Educational strategies to promote clinical diagnostic reasoning. N Engl J Med 2006;355(21):2217-2225.
36. Bordage G. Why did I miss the diagnosis? Some cognitive explanations and educational implications. Acad Med 1999;74(10):S138-S143.
37. Graber ML, Franklin N, Gordon R. Diagnostic error in internal medicine. Arch Intern Med 2005;165(13):1493-1499.
38. American Board of Internal Medicine. Choosing Wisely. <www.choosingwisely.org>. Accessed February 5, 2015.
39. American College of Physicians. High Value Care. <hvc.acponline.org>. Accessed February 7, 2015.
40. Turnbull J, Gray J, MacFadyen J. Improving in-training evaluation programs. J Gen Intern Med 1998;13(5):317-323.
41. Duffy FD. Dialogue: The core clinical skill. Ann Intern Med 1998;128(2):139-141.
42. Johnson BT, Boohan M. Basic clinical skills: Don't leave teaching to the teaching hospitals. Med Educ 2000;34(9):692-699.
43. Engel GL. The deficiencies of the case presentation as a method of clinical teaching: Another approach. N Engl J Med 1971;284(1):20-24.
44. Engel GL. Are medical schools neglecting clinical skills? JAMA 1976;236(7):861-863.
45. Szenas P. The role of faculty observation in assessing students' clinical skills. Contemp Issues Med Educ 1997;1:1-2.
46. Corbett EC, Whitcomb M. The AAMC Project on the Clinical Education of Medical Students: Clinical Skills Education. 2004. <www.aamc.org/download/68526/data/clinicalskillscorbett.pdf>. Accessed May 5, 2015.
47. AAMC. Medical School Graduation Questionnaire (GQ). <www.aamc.org/data/gq/>. Accessed May 5, 2015.
48. Norcini JJ, Blank LL, Duffy FD, Fortna GS. The mini-CEX: A method for assessing clinical skills. Ann Intern Med 2003;138(6):476-481.

49. Noel GL, Herbers JE Jr, Caplow MP, et al. How well do internal medicine faculty members evaluate the clinical skills of residents? Ann Intern Med 1992;117(9): 757-765.
50. Kogan JR, Bellini LM, Shea JA. Feasibility, reliability, and validity of the mini-clinical evaluation exercise (mCEX) in a medicine core clerkship. Acad Med 2003;78(10 Suppl):S33-S35.
51. Kalet A, Earp JA, Kowlowitz V. How well do faculty evaluate the interviewing skills of medical students? J Gen Intern Med 1992;7(5):499-505.
52. Elliot DL, Hickam DH. Evaluation of physical examination skills: Reliability of faculty observers and patient instructors. JAMA 1987;258(23):3405-3408.
53. Kogan JR, Hess BJ, Conforti LN, Holmboe ES. What drives faculty ratings of residents' clinical skills? The impact of faculty's own clinical skills. Acad Med 2010;85(10 Suppl):S25-S28.
54. Kogan JR, Conforti LN, Bernabeo EC, et al. Opening the black box of clinical skills assessment via observation: A conceptual model. Med Educ 2011;45(10): 1048-1060.
55. Yeates P, O'Neill P, Mann K, Eva KW. You're certainly relatively competent: Assessor bias due to recent experiences. Med Educ 2013;47(9):910-922.
56. Yeates P, O'Neill P, Mann K, Eva KW. Effect of exposure to good versus poor medical trainee performance on attending physician ratings of subsequent performances. JAMA 2012;308(21):2226-2232.
57. Yeates P, O'Neill P, Mann K, Eva KW. Seeing the same thing differently: Mechanisms that contribute to assessor differences in directly-observed performance assessments. Adv Health Sci Educ Theory Pract 2013;18(3): 325-341.
58. Govaerts MJ, van der Vleuten CPM. Validity in work-based assessment: Expanding our horizons. Med Educ 2013;47(12):1164-1174.
59. Govaerts MJ, van de Wiel MW, Schuwirth LW, et al. Work-based assessment: Raters' performance theories and constructs. Adv Health Sci Educ Theory Pract 2013;18(3):375-396.
60. Gingerich A, Regehr G, Eva KW. Rater-based assessments as social judgments: Rethinking the etiology of rater errors. Acad Med 2011;86(10 Suppl):S1-S7.
61. Landy FJ; Farr JL. Performance rating. Psych Bulletin 1980;87(1):72-107.
62. Holmboe ES, Fiebach NF, Galaty LA, Huot S. The effectiveness of a focused educational intervention on resident evaluations from faculty: A randomized controlled trial. J Gen Intern Med 2001;16(7):427-434.
63. Woehr DJ, Huffcutt AI. Rater training for performance appraisal: A quantitative review. J Occupational Org Psych 1994;67(3):189-205.
64. Hauenstein NMA. Training raters to increase the accuracy of appraisals and the usefulness of feedback. In Smither JW, ed. Performance Appraisal: State of the Art in Practice. San Francisco: Jossey-Bass, 1998: 404-442.
65. Stamoulis DT, Hauenstein NMA. Rater training and rating accuracy: Training for dimensional accuracy versus training for rater differentiation. J Appl Psych 1993; 78(6):994-1003.
66. AAMC. Core Entrustable Professional Activities for Entering Residency. <www.mededportal.org/icollaborative/resource/887>. Accessed February 7, 2015.
67. Holmboe ES, Hawkins RE, Huot SJ. Effects of training in direct observation of medical residents' clinical competence: A randomized trial. Ann Intern Med. 2004;140(11):874-881.
68. Cook DA, Dupras DM, Beckman TJ, et al. Effect of rater training on reliability and accuracy of mini-CEX scores: A randomized, controlled trial. J Gen Intern Med 2009;24(1):74-79.

69. Kogan JR, Bellini LM, Shea JA. Implementation of the mini-CEX to evaluate medical students' clinical skills. Acad Med 2002;77(11):1156-1157.
70. Norcini JJ, Blank LL, Arnold GK, Kimball HR. The mini-CEX (clinical evaluation exercise): A preliminary investigation. Ann Intern Med 1995;123(10):795-799.
71. Holmboe ES, Huot S, Chung J. Construct validity of the miniclinical evaluation exercise (miniCEX). Acad Med 2003;78(8):826-830.
72. Kogan JR, Holmboe ES, Hauer KE. Tools for direct observation and assessment of clinical skills of medical trainees: A systematic review. JAMA 2009;302(12):1316-1326.
73. Holmboe ES, Williams F, Yepes M, Huot S. Feedback and the mini-CEX. J Gen Intern Med. 2004;19(2):558-561.
74. Kogan JR, Conforti LN, Bernabeo EC, et al. Faculty perceptions of feedback to residents after direct observation of clinical performance. Med Educ 2012;46(2): 201-215.
75. Makoul G. The SEGUE framework for teaching and assessing communication skills. Patient Educ Couns 2001;45(1):23-34.
76. Cegala DJ, Lenzmeier Broz S. Physician communication skills training: A review of the theoretical backgrounds, objectives, and skills. Med Educ 2002;36(11): 1004-1016.
77. Lane JL, Gottlieb RP. Structured clinical observations: A method to teach clinical skills with limited time and financial resources. Pediatrics 2000;105(4 Pt 2):973-977.
78. Pangaro LN, Gibson K, Russell W, et al. A prospective, randomized trial of a six-week ambulatory internal medicine rotation. Acad Med 1995;70(6):537-541.
79. Hemmer PA, Grau T, Pangaro LN. Assessing the effectiveness of combining evaluation methods for the early identification of students with inadequate knowledge during a clerkship. Med Teach 2001;23(6):580-584.
80. Nasca TJ, Philibert I, Brigham T, Flynn TC. The next GME accreditation system: Rationale and benefits. N Engl J Med 2012;366(11):1051-1056.
81. Green ML, Aagaard EM, Caverzagie KJ, et al. Charting the road to competence: Developmental milestones for internal medicine residency training. J Grad Med Educ 2009;1(1):5-20.
82. Nabors C, Peterson SJ, Forman L, et al. Operationalizing the internal medicine milestones: An early status report. J Grad Med Educ 2013;5(1):130-137.

Chapter 10
Evaluating Medical Procedures: Evaluation and Transfer to the Bedside

Jeffrey H. Barsuk, M.D., M.S.
Eytan Szmuilowicz, M.D.

Our health care system, including the way we train physicians, is imperfect. This is especially the case for medical procedure training. We define medical procedures as any action done with the intent to achieve a particular patient care outcome. Procedures include actions that are minimally invasive (e.g., arterial puncture for blood gas analysis, central line insertion, thoracentesis, lumbar puncture, paracentesis) and non-invasive (e.g., difficult communication with patients). Medical procedures can have significant complications and are unsafe when performed by unskilled physicians. Medical errors account for more than one million injuries and up to 98,000 hospital deaths each year.[1]

Medical procedures are the second most common cause of iatrogenic patient complications.[2,3] This high rate of complications is unacceptable. Changes are needed in health care education and delivery. In response to these conditions, the Institute of Medicine (IOM) published *Crossing the Quality Chasm*.[4] The authors state six key principles of improved patient care: (a) safety, (b) effectiveness, (c) patient-centeredness, (d) timeliness, (e) efficiency, and (f) equity.[5] They emphasize that education of future health care practitioners needs to change in order to improve the health care system. Thus, safe and effective medical procedure education and evaluation are essential. Difficult communication training must also be accomplished, because communication skills are complex, require practice, and help clinicians to provide patient-centered care.

This chapter has five sections that address evidence-based methods for educating and evaluating medical student clinical skill acquisition:

1. Describes the current state of procedure and communication skills training.
2. Discusses mastery learning and how it contributes to learner evaluation.
3. Reveals the policies of the LCME and the AAMC on medical student skill acquisition.
4. Recommends specific procedural and communication skills that medical students should master.
5. Gives two examples of curricula designed to evaluate medical student procedural skill acquisition.
    A. Thoracentesis.
    B. Delivering bad news.

10.1. Current Procedure and Communication Skills Training

Medical learners are not usually trained to perform clinical procedures until they begin postgraduate education. Trainees traditionally learn clinical procedures, including difficult communication skills,[6] by relying on the apprenticeship "see one, do one, teach one" model involving real patients.[3,7] The apprenticeship model only ensures one thing - mistakes will be handed down across medical generations at the expense of patients and the health care system.[7] This model often subjects patients to invasive procedures before trainees are competent.[8,9] PGY-1 physicians may be expected to perform a procedure on the first internship day and are likely unprepared to provide safe patient care. In addition, many medical procedures done in teaching hospitals are performed by unsupervised medical trainees.[10,11] Rigorous procedural skill training in medical school would reduce the need for resident physicians to rely on "on-the-job" training.[12] There is no doubt that the current approach to procedural skill training in medicine must be changed and improved using new technology that can assure physician competence before working with patients.

Medical schools do not consistently educate their students about difficult communication skills.[13,14] In particular, end-of-life (EOL) communication has traditionally been taught poorly, either occurring early during the pre-clinical years or not using skills practice, reliable measurement, and feedback.[13-15] Some U.S. medical schools have introduced EOL care training into the pre-clinical curriculum but few have incorporated EOL training into clinical rotations. Not surprisingly, 29% of students completing the AAMC's Medical School Graduation Questionnaire report that instruction about "death and dying" is inadequate.[16] A majority of medical school administrative leaders now support adding more EOL care teaching into the undergraduate curriculum[17] but curriculum change is slow. More education, evaluation, and outcomes research is needed about which components of EOL communication are appropriate for undergraduate medical education and the best methods to train doctors in these difficult conversations.

We recommend rigorous, competency-based teaching and evaluation to ensure students are prepared to perform invasive and non-invasive clinical procedures with actual patients.

10.2. Mastery Learning

"Mastery learning"[18] is a rigorous form of competency-based[19] education and evaluation where knowledge and skills are acquired and measured against a high and uniform achievement standard. All learners must reach a preset standard so that educational results are equivalent. This is accomplished by allowing practice time to vary among individual learners as needed to achieve uniform results. This is especially relevant in medical education, because it assures that all learners reach a high-quality care standard before treating actual patients. Although medical trainees are typically high achievers, research indicates that learners may vary up to five times in the amount of time it takes to learn a task.[20] The mastery model may mitigate this temporal variability in skill learning.

The use of evidence-based achievement (competency) evaluation tools is a key feature of mastery learning. Checklists can be used to isolate important skill steps to evaluate competence on a procedure simulator or during communication with an SP. Checklists must be designed in an evidence-based[21] and stepwise manner.[22] Experts must review the checklist contents. Pilot testing is needed so that revisions can be made, because checklist design is an iterative process. Checklists are recommended instead of global rating scales, due to the dichotomous format of individual items and their advantage in assessing interobserver agreement.[8,23-25] Such a correct vs. incorrect dichotomy allows for easier standardized evaluation. By contrast, checklists may not be ideal for assessing unexpected learner actions, which are better captured by global ratings. Anchored global rating scales,[26] which contain a description of expectations for each score, and unanchored scales[27] may approach the reliability of checklists if there is rigorous instrument design, rater training, and testing.

Other medical educators have used students' self-assessments as evaluation tools. We do not recommend this form of evaluation because self-report of confidence or experience does not correlate with actual performance on simulated procedures.[8,23-25,28,29] Additionally, it is meaningless for a learner to report the degree of knowledge obtained during an educational intervention without evaluating learning objectively.

All training and testing sessions must be standardized. During checklist pilot testing, instructors need to be trained and calibrated so that data collection methods are rigorous and reliable.[30] For communication skills, evaluators can be instructors or SPs as long as checklist scoring is consistent between graders. This can be achieved by using the *kappa* coefficient to assess interrater reliability for scoring checklists. The *kappa* coefficient should be greater than 0.8, otherwise further calibration or revision is required on the most inconsistent checklist items. Standards can then be set for a minimal passing score (MPS) that a trainee must meet or exceed on a simulator-based skills assessment. (A discussion of standard setting can be found in Chapter 19.)

Once an MPS is determined, the trainees can be brought to the simulator or SP and given a pretest using the checklist. The pretest is a key feature of the educational intervention. If the trainees meet or exceed the MPS, they are considered competent and no further training is necessary. However, given the common failure of traditional methods for procedural training (or complete absence of training to this point), most trainees do not meet the MPS at pretesting.[8,23,24,28,31] If trainees fail to meet the MPS at pretesting, they undergo mastery learning with standardized lectures, videos, and deliberate skills practice. Pretesting is important because it gives the trainees opportunities to receive directed feedback before educational sessions. Pretesting heightens learner awareness of their deficiencies and allows focussed attention on improvement during subsequent training. A key component to mastery learning is feedback during practice sessions, so that trainees can immediately incorporate new knowledge into improved performance.[32] After training is complete, trainees are given a post-test using the checklist on the simulator or SP. All are expected to score at or above the MPS before performing procedures on actual patients. If the MPS is not reached, more deliberate practice occurs until each trainee reaches this score, the key feature of mastery learning.[8,23-25,28]

Educators must assess competency (mastery learning) to ensure that trainees are ready to perform procedures on actual patients. If not, patient care is compromised by increased medical errors and preventable in-hospital complications or miscommunications. A summary of mastery learning-based simulation education can be found in Table 10.1.

Table 10.1. Recommended Features of a Simulation-based Mastery Procedure Curriculum

1. Curriculum design should be evidence-based and standardized.
2. Curriculum framework should be used for both teaching and evaluation.
3. Teaching should be multi-modal, and include ample time for deliberate practice with directed feedback using simulation.
4. Minimum passing standards should be set.
5. Assessment should rely on observation with a dichotomous checklist for feedback at a pre- and post-training evaluation.
6. Evaluators should be calibrated so that they agree on scoring of checklist items.
7. Trainees must meet or exceed a minimal passing score before working with real patients.

10.2.1. Simulation-Based Mastery Learning, and Educational and Clinical Outcomes

Dougherty and Conway described translational science in terms of the 3T's roadmap.[33] T1 research moves basic laboratory science to the clinic.[33] T2 research shows clinical effectiveness for patient care, and T3 research translates to improvements in patients' health.[33] In several recent publications, McGaghie expanded the 3T's roadmap to medical education research.[34,35] As seen in Table 10.2, T1 educational research shows improved trainee skill and knowledge. T2 research shows improved patient care practices and T3 research demonstrates improved patient outcomes (Table 10.2).[34]

Table 10.2. Increasing Levels of "Translation" for which Research in Medical Education Documents Improvement (adapted from McGaghie[34]). T4 research extends the endpoint to skill retention, dissemination, and health policy, in which populations or targets other than research subjects benefit from improved health. Successful translational research incorporates all of these levels.

Level of Translation	T1	T2	T3	T4
Domain for desired improvement	Knowledge, skill, attitude, professionalism	Patent care practices	Patient outcomes	Unplanned populations or targets
Target Groups	Individuals and teams	Individuals and teams	Individuals and public health systems	Individuals, teams, public health systems
Setting	Simulation Lab	Clinic and bedside	Clinical and community	Clinic, bedside and community

All medical education assessment would ideally aim to incorporate patient-level outcomes, but this has been accomplished only in a few areas. Studies show that simulation-based education improves clinical outcomes in laparoscopic gallbladder surgery,[36,37] colonoscopy,[38,39] airway management during respiratory arrest,[40] bronchoscopy,[41] lumbar puncture,[42] advanced cardiac life support (ACLS),[43] paracentesis,[31,44] and central line insertion.[24,28,45] However, only a few of these studies used rigorous evidence-based assessment tools and few research groups have studied all translational science outcomes.[24,28,31,42-45]

10.2.2. Skill Retention

Procedural skills decay over time, which may dilute clinical outcomes. An advantage of using realistic high fidelity simulators and the mastery learning model is reduction of performance decay over time.[30,46-48] Our research group demonstrated that ACLS skills acquired on a simulator were robust up to fourteen months after the original educational intervention.[48] In the UK, use of a high fidelity obstetrics simulator to improve skills related to shoulder dystocia management showed skill retention at six months and one year follow up.[47] Furthermore, simulation-based education results in increased self-confidence regarding procedures.[8,24,29] Enhanced self-confidence may promote additional performance of clinical skills, which provides opportunities for additional deliberate practice in the patient care setting that enhances skill acquisition and retention.[49] Skill retention is also strengthened when the simulated environment closely resembles the actual training environment.[50] Despite the presence of factors that promote skill retention, we are unable to predict if an individual trainee will retain and demonstrate competence at follow-up testing. Clinical experience, self-confidence, and other demographic information do not correlate with follow-up performance.[46,48] Therefore, all learners should return to the simulation setting at fixed intervals for testing and refresher training.

10.3. Research Using Simulation-Based Mastery Learning

We have used simulation-based mastery learning (SBML) to promote medical knowledge, communication, and procedural skills in areas such as lumbar puncture,[42] thoracentesis,[8] code status discussions,[51] management of critically ill patients,[51] cardiac auscultation,[52] advanced cardiac life support,[43,53] paracentesis,[31,44] and central line insertion.[23,24,28,45] SBML improves quality of care, downstream patient outcomes, and has benefits for society.[54] To date, translational science results (T1 through T4) are available after SBML for ACLS, paracentesis, and central line insertion. Specifically, we found that SBML increases trainee skills (T1)[8,23-25,28] and improves patient care (T2), while reducing iatrogenic complications (T3).[24,28,43-45] Documented benefits of SBML also include skill retention (T4),[46,48] reduced hospital costs (T4),[44,55] and an improved patient safety culture (T4).[53,56]

10.4. Defining Required Procedures

Medical learners are often expected to perform procedures immediately after graduation, on the first day of internship.[12] Therefore, we believe that medical schools should be required to certify student competence on the procedures that students are expected to perform. Despite the 1999 AAMC recommendations for medical student procedural "competency," a publication by Fitch et al. surveyed 235 physicians who disagreed.[57] One hundred and eighty-four new physicians (just having completed internship) and 51 medical school teaching faculty had 32% agreement on the procedures identified as essential for medical student competence. Specifically, 90% believed that venipuncture and inserting an intravenous catheter were "must know" procedures before medical school graduation.[57] However, 77% reported arterial puncture as "must know," 21% thoracentesis, 44% lumbar puncture, 64% inserting a nasogastric tube, 46% inserting a Foley catheter (male patient), and 56% suturing lacerations.[57]

Based on the 1999 AAMC recommendations (Table 10.3), all graduating medical students should be competent in venipuncture, starting intravenous catheters, inserting nasogastric tubes, arterial puncture, urethral catheter insertion, suturing, and difficult conversations. Additionally, students would benefit from competency in central venous catheter insertion, intubation and mechanical ventilation, advanced cardiac life support, thoracentesis, chest tube insertion, arthrocentesis, paracentesis, and lumbar puncture (depending on their intended specialties). The fourth year of medical school is an ideal time to offer clerkships in these skills directed toward the specialty each student plans to enter. For communication skills, as recommended by the AAMC Medical School Objectives Project (MSOP), training should be integrated throughout all four years of medical school, with the first two years devoted to developing a basic foundation of general communication (including obtaining a patient history), and the final two years devoted to developing more difficult, context-specific skills, e.g., communicating with colleagues, obtaining informed consent for basic procedures, delivering bad news, clarifying goals of care, and EOL conversations.[58] Competency-based assessments should be performed and results presented to the intended residency programs. This assures these programs that interns are fit to perform procedures on the first day of residency. It also allows programs to target specific training for interns who have not mastered basic clinical procedures in medical school.

Table 10.3. Recommended Procedures for Medical Student Mastery
(italics indicate dependence on intended medical specialty)

Minimally-Invasive Procedures	Communication Skills
Venipuncture	Medical and surgical history
Intravenous catheter insertion	Social history (including occupational, spiritual, sexual, and substance use histories)
Nasogastric tube insertion	Informed consent for procedures
Arterial puncture	Communicating with colleagues (including patient hand-offs and requesting consultations)
Male and female urethral catheter insertion	Clarifying goals of care
Suturing	Delivering bad news
Central venous catheter insertion	Responding to emotion
Intubation and mechanical ventilation	
Advanced cardiac life support	
Thoracentesis	
Chest tube insertion	
Arthrocentesis (knee/shoulder)	
Paracentesis	
Lumbar puncture	

10.5. Examples of Simulation-Based Procedure Curricula

10.5.1. Example 1: Thoracentesis[59]

A curriculum was designed to ensure participants acquire the knowledge and skills necessary to perform a competent thoracentesis.[59] This curriculum was designed before ultrasound guided thoracentesis became common and has subsequently been revised to teach coincident ultrasound use. In the original curriculum, forty graduating third year internal medicine residents underwent baseline performance testing (pretest) on a thoracentesis simulator at the end of their residency training. A 23-item dichotomous checklist (Table 10.4) was designed to assess this clinical skill. Individual skill items were either marked correct or incorrect by one of two trained faculty graders and were rescored from video by a third evaluator to ensure interobserver agreement. In addition, two 20-question written exams, equally weighted for content and difficulty, were designed for administration pre- and post-training. An expert panel set an MPS for the skills exam and all residents were expected to meet or exceed this MPS (80%) before completing training. Angoff and Hofstee standard setting methods were used to establish the MPS (see Chapter 19).

Table 10.4. Thoracentesis Skills Checklist
(Key: A = Done Correctly; B = Done Incorrectly/Not Done)

Step	A	B
Recognize whether or not the procedure can be done at the bedside based on chest x-ray lateral decubitus	A	B
Informed consent obtained Benefits Risks Permission given	A	B
Identify the landmarks based on percussion	A	B
Mark the site	A	B
Clean area with sterilizing solution	A	B
Put on sterile gloves	A	B
Drape the area with the pregiven drape	A	B
Set up the kit using the catheter/tubing/stopcock system (making sure the flow is from needle to syringe, this is the default position)	A	B
Use 1 percent lidocaine to anesthetize the skin area above the rib (wheal)	A	B
Using lidocaine anesthetize to the bone and pleura with a longer needle	A	B
Aspirate pleural fluid with this needle	A	B
Using the thoracentesis needle (catheter/needle complex) enter the skin above the rib while aspirating	A	B
Once the catheter is about to enter the skin, nick the skin with a scalpel at the entry site and continue to advance the catheter/needle unit	A	B
Identify that the catheter and needle have entered the pleural space ... green change to red to green again and aspirate fluid	A	B
Advance the catheter over the needle until it is in the pleural space and withdraw the needle syringe unit	A	B
Turn the stopcock to direct flow from the catheter in the pleural space to the tubing	A	B
Connect the tubing to a vacuutainer, and control flow with the stop roller on the tubing	A	B
Aspirate no more than 1.5 liters of fluid (1 liter is acceptable) ASK: How much are you removing?	A	B
Withdraw catheter/syringe while pt exhales (resident must communicate)	A	B
Place dressing	A	B
Demonstrate knowledge as to whether to order a chest x-ray	A	B
Blood cx inoculated at the bedside (can verbalize)	A	B
Transfer fluid into appropriate vials and send for appropriate studies: LDH, protein, cell count, gram stain and culture, cytology and pH	A	B

After taking the baseline skills and written examinations, residents underwent two two-hour education sessions that included video recorded lectures on the indications, contraindications, interpretation, and complications of thoracentesis. A video recorded demonstration of a proper thoracentesis was also shown. Additionally, residents underwent deliberate practice on the thoracentesis simulator with directed feedback. After training, the residents completed a post-training skills exam using the checklist and the written post-test. Residents who did not meet the MPS underwent more deliberate practice until this score was achieved by further skills testing. An MPS was not set for the written examination.

Baseline performance among graduating residents was poor with mean checklist scores of 13/25 items correct (52%). After simulation training this increased by 71% to 22/25 (88%). Written exam scores improved 56% from pre- to post-test.

This study added significant evidence to the growing body of knowledge that traditional apprenticeship training involving "see one, do one, teach one" does not work. Traditional internal medicine training did not adequately prepare graduating residents to perform thoracentesis because they scored poorly on the pretest. More importantly, this study was conducted at a time when the ABIM required internal medicine residents to be competent in thoracentesis before graduating.

10.5.2. Example 2: Delivering Bad News (The SPIKES Framework for Delivering "Bad News")

Most of the EOL communication training programs for medical students have focussed on breaking bad news. Delivering bad news is a convenient and valuable communication task to teach medical students because it is a common type of procedure that provokes anxiety. However, the process can be broken down into smaller, individual tasks. Once these tasks are mastered, they can be used to carry out other types of difficult conversations.

There is no "one best way" to teach or evaluate a training program focussed on breaking bad news. To our knowledge there are no studies evaluating patient-related outcomes or mastery learning for communication skills. The most commonly used framework for delivering bad news is the SPIKES protocol developed by Baile and colleagues.[60] The SPIKES framework is used by many communication training programs focussing on learners of different experience and backgrounds. This type of "patient-centered" approach to communication has also been shown to lead to improved patient satisfaction and is the least likely to increase negative emotions after an encounter.[61]

The SPIKES protocol has six steps: (1) **S**etting up the Interview, (2) Assessing the **P**atient's Perception, (3) Obtaining the Patient's **I**nvitation (for Information), (4) Giving **K**nowledge and Information to the Patient, (5) Addressing the Patient's **E**motions with Empathic Responses, and (6) **S**trategy and Summary. For the purposes of observing and providing feedback on a simulated encounter, previous educators have focussed on the last five major steps. Within each of these five steps, there are a number of smaller steps that can be taught and evaluated.[60]

Students should be given opportunities to reflect and share previous experiences about witnessing the delivery of bad news or personal experiences with difficult conversations. Such discussions not only help to foster a safe learning environment but also can help to limit overconfidence[60] and to set an expectation that active participation is essential. Medical educators need to model effective use of the steps in addition to transmitting knowledge about the framework. Learning difficult conversation skills must include the opportunity to engage in deliberate practice and receive constructive feedback. Role-play involving peers or with an SP is a good way to have each learner practice skills in a controlled, structured, and supervised setting.[62] Use of SPs to teach and evaluate complex communication skills is also well received by students.[63]

Beyond using multiple modalities (small group discussion, didactics, modeling, skills practice, and feedback) to teach and reinforce key skills, educators should consider including training sessions in various clinical rotations and experiences. Yedidia and colleagues, for example, created a communication skills training program focussed on a number of different communication tasks (including breaking bad news) that was embedded into a number of different rotations during the third and fourth years.[64] Integrating communication skills curricula across different rotations in the clinical years not only allows for reinforcement but also strengthens the message that these are important, valued, and universal skills.

The best way to assess competence is by developing an evidence-based rating form or checklist with a definition of MPS as described earlier. This checklist should be based on the framework of the teaching materials, rely on observation of easily observable behaviors, and be simple to use. While educators may use a checklist that is specifically developed for breaking bad news, it is also possible to use a breaking bad news scenario to assess more general communication skills with other well-known communication frameworks, e.g., the Kalamazoo Consensus Statement,[65] the Macy Model,[66] and SEGUE.[67] An example checklist is provided below, adapted from work by Szmuilowicz et al. (Table 10.5).[68] Development of this checklist was based on expert opinion[69] and the SPIKES framework. An MPS has yet to be determined for this tool, but can be defined using conventional procedures.

10.6. Conclusion

Complications and miscommunications occur unnecessarily from procedures performed by medical trainees. Training policies need to change to ensure that medical students are competent to perform clinical procedures expected of new residents. Further research is needed to determine which procedural skills these students must acquire. Competency-based simulation assessment grounded in the mastery learning model has potential to decrease complications and miscommunications significantly, because medical schools will be able to certify trainees as competent before they perform procedures on real patients.

Table 10.5. Delivering Bad News Communication Skills Checklist

Communication Skills Training: Delivering Bad News	Behavior/Task Performed (check if Yes)
A. General Patient-Centered Interviewing Skills	
1. Creates initial rapport (within first 30 seconds)	
2. Explicitly elicits additional questions and/or concerns	
3. Makes an explicit expression of non-abandonment	
4. Uses summary statements to ensure understanding of patient's statements (e.g., "It sounds like...")	
	Subtotal
B. Delivering Bad News	
1. Assess patient's understanding of the illness	
2. Assesses patient's preferences for receiving information	
3. Gives a clear and concise "warning shot" with a pause prior to delivery of bad news	
4. Delivers bad news early in the conversation (within first 3 minutes)	
5. Delivers information clearly, concisely, and in plain language	
6. Allows at least 3 seconds of silence after delivery to allow patient to process information	
7. Suggests a plan for the next step	
8. Assesses patient's immediate safety and/or social support	
	Subtotal
C. Responding to Emotion	
1. Names, validates, or expresses understanding of the patient's emotional reaction	
2. Explores the emotional reaction in greater detail	
3. Appropriately uses silence to allow for patient to process and discuss difficult emotions	
	Subtotal
TOTAL SCORE	

References

1. Kohn LT, Corrigan JM, Donaldson MS, eds. Institute of Medicine. Committee on Quality of Health Care in America. To Err is Human: Building a Safer Health System. Washington, DC: National Academies Press, 2000.
2. Brennan TA, Leape LL, Laird NM, et al. Incidence of adverse events and negligence in hospitalized patients: Results of the Harvard Medical Practice Study I. N Engl J Med 1991;324(6):370-376.
3. Duffy FD, Holmboe ES. What procedures should internists do? Ann Intern Med 2007;146(5):392-393.

4. Institute of Medicine. Committee on Quality of Health Care in America. Crossing the Quality Chasm: A New Health System for the 21st Century. Washington, DC: National Academies Press, 2001.
5. Berwick DM. A user's manual for the IOM's "quality chasm" report. Health Aff (Millwood) 2002;21(3):80-90.
6. Tulsky JA, Chesney MA, Lo B. See one, do one, teach one? House staff experience discussing do-not-resuscitate orders. Arch Intern Med 1996;156(12):1285-1289.
7. Landro L. To reduce risks, hospitals enlist "proceduralists." Wall Street Journal, July 11, 2007. <www.wsj.com/articles/SB118410727844462566>. Accessed May 11, 2015.
8. Wayne DB, Barsuk JH, O'Leary KJ, et al. Mastery learning of thoracentesis skills by internal medicine residents using simulation technology and deliberate practice. J Hosp Med 2008;3(1):48-54.
9. Huang GC, Smith CC, Gordon CE, et al. Beyond the comfort zone: Residents assess their comfort performing inpatient medical procedures. Am J Med 2006; 119(1):71.e17-24.
10. Berns JS, O'Neill WC. Performance of procedures by nephrologists and nephrology fellows at U.S. nephrology training programs. Clin J Am Soc Nephrol 2008;3(4): 941-947.
11. Lucas BP, Asbury JK, Wang Y, et al. Impact of a bedside procedure service on general medicine inpatients: A firm-based trial. J Hosp Med 2007;2(3):143-149.
12. Wayne DB, Cohen ER, Singer BD, et al. Progress toward improving medical school graduates' skills via a "boot camp" curriculum. Simul Healthc 2014;9(1):33-39.
13. Billings JA, Block S. Palliative care in undergraduate medical education. Status report and future directions. JAMA 1997;278(9):733-738.
14. Ury WA, Berkman CS, Weber CM, et al. Assessing medical students' training in end-of-life communication: A survey of interns at one urban teaching hospital. Acad Med 2003;78(5):530-537.
15. Sullivan AM, Lakoma MD, Block SD. The status of medical education in end-of-life care: A national report. J Gen Intern Med 2003;18(9):685-695.
16. Barzansky B, Veloski JJ, Miller R, Jonas HS. Education in end-of-life care during medical school and residency training. Acad Med 1999;74(10 Suppl):S102-S104.
17. Sullivan AM, Warren AG, Lakoma MD, et al. End-of-life care in the curriculum: A national study of medical education deans. Acad Med 2004;79(8):760-768.
18. Block JH, ed. Mastery Learning: Theory and Practice. New York: Holt, Rinehart, and Winston, 1971.
19. McGaghie WC, Miller GE, Sajid AW, Telder TV. Competency-Based Curriculum Development in Medical Education: An Introduction. Public Health Paper No. 68. Geneva, Switzerland: World Health Organization, 1978. <apps.who.int/iris/bitstream/10665/39703/1/WHO_PHP_68.pdf?ua=1>. Accessed May 11, 2015.
20. Bloom BS. Time and learning. Am Psychol 1974;29(9):682-688.
21. McKinley RK, Strand J, Ward L, et al. Checklists for assessment and certification of clinical procedural skills omit essential competencies: A systematic review. Med Educ 2008;42(4):338-349.
22. Stufflebeam DL. Guidelines for Developing Evaluation Checklists: The Checklist Development Checklist (CDC). Western Michigan University Evaluation Center, July 2000. <www.wmich.edu/evalctr/archive_checklists/guidelines_cdc.pdf>. Accessed April 2, 2015.
23. Barsuk JH, Ahya SN, Cohen ER, et al. Mastery learning of temporary hemodialysis catheter insertion by nephrology fellows using simulation technology and deliberate practice. Am J Kidney Dis 2009;54(1):70-76.
24. Barsuk JH, McGaghie WC, Cohen ER, et al. Use of simulation-based mastery learning to improve the quality of central venous catheter placement in a medical intensive care unit. J Hosp Med 2009;4(7):397-403.
25. Wayne DB, Butter J, Siddall VJ, et al. Graduating internal medicine residents' self-assessment and performance of advanced cardiac life support skills. Med Teach 2006;28(4):365-369.

26. Adler MD, Vozenilek JA, Trainor JL, et al. Comparison of checklist and anchored global rating instruments for performance rating of simulated pediatric emergencies. Simul Healthc 2011;6(1):18-24.
27. Morgan PJ, Cleave-Hogg D, Guest CB. A comparison of global ratings and checklist scores from an undergraduate assessment using an anesthesia simulator. Acad Med 2001;76(10):1053-1055.
28. Barsuk JH, McGaghie WC, Cohen ER, et al. Simulation-based mastery learning reduces complications during central venous catheter insertion in a medical intensive care unit. Crit Care Med 2009;37(10):2697-2701.
29. Wayne DB, Butter J, Siddall VJ, et al. Mastery learning of advanced cardiac life support skills by internal medicine residents using simulation technology and deliberate practice. J Gen Intern Med 2006;21(3):251-256.
30. McGaghie WC, Issenberg SB, Petrusa ER, Scalese RJ. A critical review of simulation-based medical education research: 2003-2009. Med Educ 2010;44(1):50-63.
31. Barsuk JH, Cohen ER, Vozenilek JA, et al. Simulation-based education with mastery learning improves paracentesis skills. J Grad Med Educ 2012;4(1):23-27.
32. McGaghie WC, Siddall VJ, Mazmanian PE, Myers J. Lessons for continuing medical education from simulation research in undergraduate and graduate medical education: Effectiveness of continuing medical education. Chest 2009;135(3 Suppl):62S-68S.
33. Dougherty D, Conway PH. The "3T's" road map to transform US health care: The "how" of high-quality care. JAMA 2008;299(19):2319-2321.
34. McGaghie WC. Medical education research as translational science. Sci Transl Med 2010;2(19):19cm8.
35. McGaghie WC, Issenberg SB, Cohen ER, et al. Translational educational research: A necessity for effective health-care improvement. Chest 2012;142(5):1097-1103.
36. Andreatta PB, Woodrum DT, Birkmeyer JD, et al. Laparoscopic skills are improved with LapMentor training: Results of a randomized, double-blinded study. Ann Surg 2006;243(6):854-860; discussion: 860-863.
37. Seymour NE, Gallagher AG, Roman SA, et al. Virtual reality training improves operating room performance: Results of a randomized, double-blinded study. Ann Surg 2002;236(4):458-463; discussion: 463-464.
38. Cohen J, Cohen SA, Vora KC, et al. Multicenter, randomized, controlled trial of virtual-reality simulator training in acquisition of competency in colonoscopy. Gastrointest Endosc 2006;64(3):361-368.
39. Sedlack RE, Kolars JC. Computer simulator training enhances the competency of gastroenterology fellows at colonoscopy: Results of a pilot study. Am J Gastroenterol 2004;99(1):33-37.
40. Mayo PH, Hackney JE, Mueck JT, et al. Achieving house staff competence in emergency airway management: Results of a teaching program using a computerized patient simulator. Crit Care Med 2004;32(12):2422-2427.
41. Blum MG, Powers TW, Sundaresan S. Bronchoscopy simulator effectively prepares junior residents to competently perform basic clinical bronchoscopy. Ann Thorac Surg 2004;78(1):287-291; discussion: 291.
42. Barsuk JH, Cohen ER, Caprio T, et al. Simulation-based education with mastery learning improves residents' lumbar puncture skills. Neurology 2012;79(2):132-137.
43. Wayne DB, Didwania A, Feinglass J, et al. Simulation-based education improves quality of care during cardiac arrest team responses at an academic teaching hospital: A case-control study. Chest 2008;133(1):56-61.
44. Barsuk JH, Cohen ER, Feinglass J, et al. Clinical outcomes after bedside and interventional radiology paracentesis procedures. Am J Med 2013;126(4):349-356.
45. Barsuk JH, Cohen ER, Feinglass J, et al. Use of simulation-based education to reduce catheter-related bloodstream infections. Arch Intern Med 2009;169(15):1420-1423.
46. Barsuk JH, Cohen ER, McGaghie WC, Wayne DB. Long-term retention of central venous catheter insertion skills after simulation-based mastery learning. Acad Med 2010;85(10 Suppl):S9-S12.

47. Crofts JF, Bartlett C, Ellis D, et al. Management of shoulder dystocia: Skill retention 6 and 12 months after training. Obstet Gynecol 2007;110(5):1069-1074.
48. Wayne DB, Siddall VJ, Butter J, et al. A longitudinal study of internal medicine residents' retention of advanced cardiac life support skills. Acad Med 2006;81(10 Suppl):S9-S12.
49. Ericsson KA. Deliberate practice and the acquisition and maintenance of expert performance in medicine and related domains. Acad Med 2004;79(10 Suppl): S70-S81.
50. Arthur W, Bennett W, Stanush PL, McNelly TL. Factors that influence skill decay and retention: A quantitative review and analysis. Hum Perform 1998;11(1):57-101.
51. Cohen ER, Barsuk JH, Moazed F, et al. Making July safer: Simulation-based mastery learning during intern boot camp. Acad Med 2013;88(2):233-239.
52. Butter J, McGaghie WC, Cohen ER, et al. Simulation-based mastery learning improves cardiac auscultation skills in medical students. J Gen Intern Med 2010;25(8):780-785.
53. Didwania A, McGaghie WC, Cohen ER, et al. Progress toward improving the quality of cardiac arrest medical team responses at an academic teaching hospital. J Grad Med Educ 2011;3(2):211-216.
54. McGaghie WC, Issenberg SB, Barsuk JH, Wayne DB. A critical review of simulation-based mastery learning with translational outcomes. Med Educ 2014;48(4):375-385.
55. Cohen ER, Feinglass J, Barsuk JH, et al. Cost savings from reduced catheter-related bloodstream infection after simulation-based education for residents in a medical intensive care unit. Simul Healthc 2010;5(2):98-102.
56. Barsuk JH, Cohen ER, Feinglass J, et al. Unexpected collateral effects of simulation-based medical education. Acad Med 2011;86(12):1513-1517.
57. Fitch MT, Kearns S, Manthey DE. Faculty physicians and new physicians disagree about which procedures are essential to learn in medical school. Med Teach 2009;31(4):342-347.
58. AAMC. Medical School Objectives Project. Report III: Contemporary Issues in Medicine: Communication in Medicine. Washington, DC: AAMC, 1999.
59. Wayne DB, Barsuk JH, O'Leary KJ, et al. Mastery learning of thoracentesis skills by internal medicine residents using simulation technology and deliberate practice. J Hosp Med 2008;3(1):48-54.
60. Baile WF, Buckman R, Lenzi R, et al. SPIKES: A six-step protocol for delivering bad news: Application to the patient with cancer. Oncologist 2000;5(4):302-311.
61. Schmid Mast M, Kindlimann A, Langewitz W. Recipients' perspective on breaking bad news: How you put it really makes a difference. Patient Educ Couns 2005; 58(3):244-251.
62. Layat-Burn C, Hurst SA, Ummel M, et al. Telling the truth: Medical students' progress with an ethical skill. Med Teach 2014;36(3):251-259.
63. Fortin AH, Haeseler FD, Angoff N, et al. Teaching pre-clinical medical students an integrated approach to medical interviewing: Half-day workshops using actors. J Gen Intern Med 2002;17(9):704-708.
64. Yedidia MJ, Gillespie CC, Kachur E, et al. Effect of communications training on medical student performance. JAMA 2003;290(9):1157-1165.
65. Makoul G. Essential elements of communication in medical encounters: The Kalamazoo consensus statement. Acad Med 2001;76(4):390-393.
66. Kalet A, Pugnaire MP, Cole-Kelly K, et al. Teaching communication in clinical clerkships: Models from the Macy initiative in health communications. Acad Med 2004;79(6):511-520.
67. Makoul G. The SEGUE framework for teaching and assessing communication skills. Patient Educ Couns 2001;45(1):23-34.
68. Szmuilowicz E, el-Jawahri A, Chiappetta L, et al. Improving residents' end-of-life communication skills with a short retreat: A randomized controlled trial. J Palliat Med 2010;13(4):439-452.
69. Roter DL, Larson S, Fischer GS, et al. Experts practice what they preach: A descriptive study of best and normative practices in end-of-life discussions. Arch Intern Med 2000;160(22):3477-3485.

Chapter 11
Assessing Clinical Reasoning

Steven Durning, M.D.
Joseph Rencic, M.D.
Lambert Schuwirth, M.D.

11.1. Clinical Reasoning and Clinical Decision Making

Clinical reasoning is central to a physician's performance, and this chapter deals with attempts to define and measure it. Despite present limitations in our ability to do this, there are still important points for educators to understand, and in any case, there is the practical but very necessary problem of assessing it. This chapter reviews approaches to this problem, in order for educators to make their own decisions about how to incorporate available methods into their curriculum.

Though definitions and descriptions of clinical reasoning differ, enough similarity exists for educators to approach the problem. They all converge on the idea that clinical reasoning entails cognitive operations allowing clinicians to observe, collect, and analyze information, resulting in actions that take into account a patient's specific circumstances and preferences.[1,2] Thus, clinical reasoning involves steps up to and including establishing the diagnosis (understanding the nature of the patient's problem, which entails recognition and classification as well as knowing the solution or diagnosis, all referred to as "diagnostic reasoning"), as well as deciding on a treatment plan specific to the patient's circumstances and preferences ("therapeutic reasoning"). "Decision making" in this sense means that the decision is a proposed action, such as to order a test or to initiate a therapy.

Indeed, clinical reasoning encompasses nearly all aspects of what physicians do in practice.[2,3] Clinical reasoning enables physicians to take "wise" action, or the best-judged action in a specific situation or *context*.[4,5] The complex nature of clinical reasoning has been previously described.[4] It involves, among other things, the need to develop tolerance for ambiguity and reflection on the practice.[6]

Assessing the phenomenon of clinical reasoning is not simple, mainly because cognitive operations cannot be observed directly and therefore always need to be inferred from observable behavior.[7] This has always been the "Achilles heel" of assessments of clinical reasoning, because in the sequence of cognitive processes to eventual observable behaviors (diagnoses and plans) various factors may interfere. This is where clinical reasoning differs from clinical decision making.

Reasoning leads to statements or propositions that are results of the process of obtaining, filtering, and synthesizing clinical findings. Clinical decision making is the aspect of the clinical reasoning process that arrives at conclusions, which are proposed or intended actions, and these entail observable behavior. Each of these two phases of reasoning may be inferred and/or observed for the purpose of evaluation.

11.2. Limitations in the Assessment of Clinical Reasoning

Two assessment purposes may apply to clinical reasoning and the related process of clinical decision making: summative and formative. On the assumption that "correct" diagnoses and treatment plans can be identified for specific clinical problems, summative assessment of clinical decision making is used routinely on standardized tests in the form of vignette-based MCQs. Developmentally, however, assessing learners - especially students - solely on the correctness of their diagnosis or treatment plan may fail to provide meaningful feedback that can lead to improvement (it entails just the last step of the clinical reasoning process). Therefore, educators have spent considerable effort in developing additional assessment tools. Unfortunately, as alluded to above, the idiosyncratic, context-specific nature of processes of clinical reasoning means that there often is no single correct or generalizable approach for "solving" a clinical case.[8-10] How does one score these clinical reasoning processes in a standardized, reliable manner when, other than a final step (does the participant arrive at the correct diagnosis and/or treatment?), no gold standard exists?

There are other challenges that merit consideration. For example, an additional difficulty for assessment of clinical reasoning, which is noted above, is that judgments about clinical reasoning are usually not directly observed, and are typically inferential. Indeed, one area for the future of clinical reasoning assessment is developing tools that may better capture these non-observable, or difficult to observe, processes, so that we can enhance our understanding of what clinical reasoning entails, and so improve upon our teaching, assessment, and research practices. Second, because many cognitive processes are subconscious, retrospective attempts to acquire and understand the reasoning processes from participants may not accurately reveal the processes that had been used to solve the clinical case. This is particularly believed to be true when participants use non-analytic reasoning (entailing automatic or pattern-recognition techniques) as opposed to collecting actively and analyzing patient data (referred to as analytic reasoning).[11] The former, we believe, may lead to rationalizations that do not accurately explain actual cognitive processes. Third, within all that is encompassed by "clinical reasoning," the assessment of *therapeutic* reasoning (clinical decision making) is particularly challenging because there are usually several - and at times many - "answers" derived from this reasoning, which can be viewed as "reasonable" management strategies for a given problem (as opposed to a single correct diagnosis).

11.3. Case Context Specificity

Correlation of a given individual's diagnostic performance across different case presentations with the same underlying diagnosis is low, suggesting that other factors (i.e., environmental factors) may be important for clinical reasoning. This lack of correlation, known as "context specificity," emphasizes that more than the clinical content of the patient's findings is influencing reasoning.[2,12] Indeed, several contemporary educational theories argue that clinical reasoning is not merely personal (inside the decision maker's head), but rather is social (wherein physician, patient, and environment may contribute to the reasoning process) with leading theories such as situated cognition, ecological psychology, and distributed cognition.[2]

In this section, we begin with a brief review of the history of clinical reasoning theories and assessments. We then discuss contemporary means of assessing clinical reasoning with emphasis on practical examples, highlighting the reliability of these methods. Finally we present future avenues of research and assessment. We also provide a number of readings on each subject area to assist the reader, to include weaving concepts and understanding from educational fields relevant to the topic of assessing clinical reasoning.

11.4. A Brief History of Clinical Reasoning Theories and Assessments

Over the past several decades, a number of approaches to the assessment of clinical reasoning have been explored in parallel with prevailing hypotheses. Here we briefly outline highlights of these themes and the underlying theoretical perspectives that shaped assessment in each period. Unfortunately, as in many areas of research, previous assumptions about understanding both the process of clinical reasoning and its assessment have often been shown to be wrong.[5] Nevertheless, research has resulted in tremendous gains in our understanding of clinical reasoning, and some presumably outdated assessment methods for clinical reasoning are making a comeback. Therefore, we believe that outlining this history provides a perspective for readers and encourages them to review the provided references in more detail.

11.4.1. Expertise as a General Problem Solving Process: The Age of Patient Management Problems

In the 1960s, medical education scholars were convinced that experts in clinical reasoning were also experts in general problem solving, which could be measured and demonstrated superior in experts as opposed to novices. Problem solving was conceived as a general teachable skill that would result in superior performance, regardless of a patient's disease presentation.

11.4.1.a. Patient Management Problems (PMPs)

To assess patient management, educators developed "long" clinical problems (or cases) as opposed to single MCQs, which were meant to mimic on paper actual clinical problems (usually an evolving patient presentation). Assessment experts believed that these cases were more valid than short cases, and would reveal an expert's thinking, as well as demonstrate general problem solving differences between experts and novices. One such assessment method was the patient management problem (PMP).[13] Thirty years ago the ABIM used PMPs on certifying exams for internal medicine. They consisted of three to six clinical problems with thirty to sixty diagnostic and/or management options per problem. In a typical PMP, the relevant history and physical exam information of a realistic patient problem are presented, and then the examinee sequentially chooses essential tests and management options, with the goal to be as thorough but as efficient as possible. Examinees would use yellow felt-tipped pens to highlight latent answers to the information sought, then, based on these answers, would choose their next step. A test development committee ("experts") would rank the thirty to sixty options into one of six categories with differing numeric weights from "indicated and essential" (+10 points) to "not indicated and dangerous (-12 points)." A composite score would then be determined for all test answers.[14] Examinees' responses were compared, in both their answers and their sequence or "path" to the "solution" of the case, with the expert panel's approach.

11.4.1.b. Lessons Learned from the Problem Management Approach

It turned out that PMPs and other long case studies demonstrated that a score derived from one problem did not predict performance on another, establishing the concept of "case *content* specificity." In other words, the fact that someone could diagnose a cardiac case did not allow the inference that this person could diagnose a neurologic problem.[15] The broader term now preferred is "*context* specificity," meaning that something more than the facts of a patient's presentation, or case, impacts clinical reasoning performance.[16-18]

Intercase correlations of performance among these cases ranged on the order of 0.1 to 0.3 (as a reference, the goal for a reliable test is at least 0.6-0.8).[19,20] Expertise was found to be highly domain-specific or, stated another way, the correlation among cases even for a single expert was poor.[21] The long time needed to complete a single PMP in an open-ended format also limits reliability of a set of PMPs, which is in part an issue of sampling.[22] Furthermore, expert panels did not always agree with each other on the correct pathway to the answer. In other words, the correlation among experts on the same case was low. Finally, experienced clinicians performed not better or sometimes even poorer than less experienced clinicians, because PMP mainly rewarded proficiency or selecting all the intermediate steps.[23,24] This finding conflicts with the literature about expertise, which shows that experts are more efficient in their collection of information but not more proficient, and that they want to work according to their own scripts, not predefined pathways.[5] Therefore, intermediates outperformed experts because the long simulation is flawed in its construct validity.[16] All of these findings cast doubt on the use of this type of assessment tool for measuring clinical reasoning.

A particular body of work during this time was that of Elstein and colleagues, who studied clinical reasoning as a problem solving process.[19,25] This work led to the important conclusion that we could not establish an expert *process* of clinical reasoning. It showed that experts were not necessarily better at a "process" of problem solving; i.e., experts and novices generated a similar number of hypotheses; it was just that experts were more likely to choose the correct hypothesis (or diagnosis) for a given presentation. This finding, that experts were not better than novices in certain observable steps in problem solving, and the doubt created as to whether a generic "problem solving skill" exists, was one factor in abandoning long cases in favor of multiple shorter cases to improve the reliability and potentially also the validity of findings.[26] This was consistent with the expertise literature from multiple fields demonstrating that expertise is more about efficiency than completeness and that experts make better "first moves," or better leading diagnostic or therapeutic impressions, than novices.

Since the 1990s, long cases, such as PMPs, have been rarely used to assess clinical reasoning, because of concerns about sampling (to approach defensible reliability with this method it is estimated that the learner needs to be examined for eight hours or more, completing eight or more cases).[27]

11.4.2. Expertise as Knowledge Organization: The Era of Key Features

Following the exploration (and shortcomings) of PMPs, investigation of assessment of clinical reasoning focussed in a new direction. About the same time as the emergence of the computer and artificial intelligence, an information processing model based on programming logic was applied to medical education with the goal of enhancing our understanding of clinical reasoning.[28] Information processing theory led to further work on knowledge organization (how knowledge is organized in memory), on the development of illness scripts (automated or aggregated mental models of a certain diagnosis), and on cognitive load (the limitations of human capacity to process information at once). Thus, "good" knowledge representation in memory, and processes that could lead to enhanced knowledge in memory (knowledge acquisition or clinical reasoning expertise as acquisition) became the prevailing question for clinical reasoning research.

11.4.2.a. Knowledge Organization

The clinical reasoning concept of knowledge organization argues that experts not only have more knowledge than novices on a given topic, but also that this knowledge is more interconnected or "more readily accessible and usable" in memory. This led to work by Bordage and others on knowledge organization, and to the formulation that knowledge could be: reduced or absent; dispersed ("can't connect the dots"); elaborated; or compiled, concise, or condensed.[29] Also resulting from this approach was the concept that accurate clinical reasoning was, in part, "semantic competence," the ability to apply descriptive pairs of terms, ("semantic qualifiers") such as "acute" vs. "chronic," "monoarticular" vs. "polyarticular," and "symmetric" vs. "asymmetric." The contrasting characterizations of symptoms constitute "axes," which are believed to reflect how well the learner can efficiently and accurately represent the problem. Success in problem representation (and knowledge organization) was determined by the use of such key descriptive terms, and a clinician's or learner's semantic competence was illustrated in their spoken and written (free text) case presentations and reports.

11.4.2.b. Scripts

With the emphasis on knowledge organization, script theory also emerged.[20,30] Illness scripts refer to the mental representation of the "story" of a disease, such as its typical epidemiology, signs, symptoms, laboratory data, and natural history. Illness scripts are believed to contain all the relevant information about a diagnosis as well as the needed interconnections among other relevant clinical information, so that the diagnosis can be rapidly identified as the script becomes more robust.[23] The semantic qualifiers mentioned above are believed to be part of such illness scripts. Thus, the script for a diagnostic entity contains key features (the symptoms and findings that are needed to establish the diagnosis), the range of these findings for each feature that can be seen and still be consistent with the diagnosis, as well as the most likely presentation for each symptom and finding (feature) as the "default" value. Importantly, scripts are believed to be evolving mental representations, and can be modified each time that a physician sees a patient with a given diagnosis.

11.4.2.c. Cognitive Load

A related line of research pertains to cognitive load. Cognitive load theory (CLT) is based upon the known limits of human cognitive architecture - we can only hold so many pieces of information in our short-term or working memory, much like a computer processor.[31] CLT proposes that expertise in clinical reasoning develops through "chunking" information into related units (e.g., scripts) within long-term memory, which are essentially limitless in content. Each of these chunks occupies a single "slot" of working memory. Using the computer metaphor, these "slots" can be thought of as word documents. Each word document, or slot, or script, can be limitless; but for the sake of argument, the processor (i.e., short-term memory) can only open a limited number (e.g., 4-7) of documents at one time. Thus, clinical reasoning expertise from a CLT perspective entails building larger scripts (or documents) so that the processor (short-term memory) can be freed up and more information units can be taken in (or processed).

11.4.2.d. Key Features

In light of the cognitive psychology literature described above, regarding information processing theory (we have only described a sample of these concepts) and the shortcomings of PMPs, assessment of clinical reasoning shifted to key features.[32] The prevailing belief and focus became describing the "hard drive" memory; improving memory acquisition, efficiency, and "processor speed" through knowledge organization and building illness scripts; and providing knowledge acquisition of the important facts to store in memory toward establishing the diagnosis (key features).

Key features emerged several decades ago out of an international conference of experts on clinical reasoning. Investigators argued that any clinical problem has one or more features crucial to its diagnosis and management: the so-called "key features."[33] In essence, the key features approach argues that any clinical problem can be simplified to a series of key components or features, which lead to arriving at the correct diagnosis and treatment. In other words, each clinical presentation has a lot of unneeded information, and the task for the clinician (and teacher) is to help to identify these essential key components. This assessment methodology derived directly from script theory. Educators hoped that assessment would promote more detailed and robust script development in learners.

11.4.2.e. Lessons Learned from the Key Features Approach

Information processing is still a major prevailing theoretical perspective in assessment of clinical reasoning today, and the metaphor is that our brain is like a computer. Thus, these theories propose that knowledge organization differs between more and less experienced clinicians; and that such organization enables more experienced ones to accomplish tasks such as diagnosis and management more efficiently. In other words, successful diagnosis and treatment involves the organization of knowledge in memory in such a way that it can be recalled efficiently and effectively in practice.

Work exploring knowledge organization[34-36] suggests that physicians actually use multiple cognitive models in practice.[5] These cognitive models are often grouped into analytic (actively collecting and analyzing data to make decisions) and non-analytic (automatic, based on prior experiences). Research shows that experts use both cognitive models in different situations or contexts.[1,19]

Unfortunately, studies attempting to demonstrate that the participant category based on semantic competence (qualifiers) is associated with clinical reasoning success have been largely unfruitful.[37] Assessments of cognitive load[38-40] are beginning to emerge as a component of clinical reasoning assessment. These assessments entail questioning the participant, typically on a 1-10 scale regarding their current cognitive effort.[38]

There has been resurgence of interest in the key feature approach, and we discuss this in further detail later in this chapter. However, results with this approach indicated that performance for clinicians at the end of their training was superior to that of experienced clinicians, which again raised concern about the validity of this approach.[41]

11.4.3. Clinical Reasoning Expertise as a State: Context Specificity and Situativity Theory

With the difficulties in demonstrating case or content specificity, work has recently explored the issue of expertise as a trait (a general skill within a field) as opposed to a state (a given set of patient circumstances).[22] Investigators have found that a physician or trainee can see two patients with the same diagnosis, presenting with the same or similar chief complaint, yet arrive at different diagnoses and therapeutic plans. In other words, the content of the cases is nearly identical, yet different conclusions (or solutions) are reached. Thus "case or content specificity" has been renamed as "context specificity" to capture the notion that something besides the content of a case (symptoms, physical examination findings) influences diagnoses and therapy.[42]

This work has developed largely in parallel with contemporary educational psychology theory, which argues that clinical diagnostic performance is "situated" in a specific set of circumstances, and that the importance of the environment (patient or case, setting, and interactions among the physician, setting, and patient) is critical in decisions and actions. This "situativity" theory suggests that authentic assessments, multifaceted measures (taking into account these different factors), and qualitative assessments are needed.

Context specificity in clinical reasoning argues that one should sample broadly to assess clinical reasoning expertise (sample many situations) and that reliability and validity are more difficult to establish due to the number of potential factors impacting a given clinical situation.[2]

11.5. Assessment Methods

There are a variety of assessment methods for clinical reasoning, and we focus on methods used with trainees, especially medical students. Because clinical reasoning entails multiple steps, several of which can occur subconsciously, it is probably not surprising that there is no single "best method" for assessing clinical reasoning. We believe that educators should use authentic measurements (clinical cases in the form of paper, video, SPs, or actual patients) and that learners should be assessed with multiple cases (≥ 8) in different subject areas, in order to provide broad sampling.[43] This approach is necessary to overcome the phenomenon of context specificity and because physicians use multiple strategies when reasoning, as discussed above.

It is important to keep in mind that any of these assessments can be given on paper, by video or audio presentation of the same material, or by using an SP. Recent studies suggest that, as the authenticity of the vignette format increases (paper to SP), more cognitive load is induced in the learner.[43] The assessment methods discussed below can be applied to a variety of emerging platforms, including virtual patients.[44] This chapter does *not* compare and contrast these different platforms for presenting the vignette.

11.5.1. Multiple Choice Examination

MCQs depicting patient scenarios are a validated, reliable method to assess clinical reasoning,[45,46] Asking students higher order questions, which require synthesis, better enable MCQs to assess clinical reasoning (see Chapter 18). For example, rather than asking, "Select the item that best matches Charcot's triad," the examination question would present a case of a patient presenting with RUQ pain, fever, and jaundice, and thus assess the student's ability to synthesize these findings into the diagnosis of cholangitis.

Brevity of individual cases within an examination allows broader sampling. In an exam with multiple, brief clinical vignettes, the learner can complete many "cases," and defensible reliability can be achieved.[46] The reasonable psychometric properties of MCQs have led most licensing bodies to use them to assess clinical reasoning. It is important to recognize that MCQs can assess high level cognitive activities (e.g., synthesis, analysis), provided the appropriate stem/stimulus.[47,48] MCQs' disadvantage is that they do not mimic the reality of seeing a patient. They provide students with a limited differential diagnosis, including one right answer: an effect called "cueing."[49]

To counteract the cueing effect, a variation on the theme of MCQs has been developed, i.e., extended matching questions (EMQs). An EMQ lists more than the typical five options used in an MCQ and some work has shown that EMQs can be superior for assessing clinical reasoning by reducing the likelihood of being correct by guessing.[50,51] The set of EMQs is usually preceded by a list of plausible clinical diagnoses. Examples of MCQs and EMQs may be found in Chapter 18.

11.5.2. Script Concordance Testing

Script concordance testing (SCT) represents a modification of MCQs.[52] Charlin *et al.* developed SCT to assess decision making under uncertainty, a common situation in clinical reasoning. They challenged the premise used in MCQs that a given clinical problem must have a single solution.[53] SCT is founded in script theory.

An SCT item provides the examinee with a very brief clinical vignette, a diagnosis, and subsequently adds an additional fact to consider (e.g., the presence of an abnormal finding).[11] The examinee then determines how much more or less likely the additional fact or finding makes the diagnosis that the question provides. In essence, SCT asks the examinee whether the additional fact is concordant (consistent) with the script provided. Such an examination allows for testing multiple cases in rapid fashion. The same lead-in vignette can be used to test an examinee's understanding of numerous diagnoses and additional facts. Research has found that defensible reliability can be found in a shorter period of time than MCQs.[53]

A difficult issue, from a psychometric perspective, is that an SCT question typically has multiple possible answers. SCT items typically have five choices: much more likely (+2), more likely (+1), unchanged (0), less likely (-1), or much less likely (-2). However, unlike MCQs, where there is a single correct answer, a test taker receives some credit for any choice that an expert panel of judges (e.g., clinicians deemed to have outstanding knowledge in the content area) has selected. The amount of points allotted for a given response is based on the number of judges who chose it. To determine a number value for each choice, credit is calculated by dividing the total number of judges selecting that choice by the mode for each question. Consider a question where six of ten judges rate "much more likely" as the answer, while the four others rate "more likely" as the answer. The mode is six. Therefore, a test taker would receive full credit (1 point) for a "much more likely" response (6/6). Partial credit (0.66 (4/6) would be given for a "more likely" response. The other options would result in a score of zero. This approach guarantees that each item is worth 1 point only (Figure 11.1).

Figure 11.1. Example of Script Concordance Test

| A 27-year-old man presents with pleuritic chest pain and shortness of breath. ||||||||
If you were thinking of the following diagnosis ...	... and the following new information was to become available ...	... then this hypothesis would become ...				
Pneumonia	Cough with purulent sputum production	-2	-1	0	+1	+2
Interstitial lung disease	Hemoptysis	-2	-1	0	+1	+2
Pneumothorax	Decreased breath sounds on left side	-2	-1	0	+1	+2

In part to dampen the potential subjectivity of expert judging and improve the ability to assess earlier learners, a modified version of the SCT (Figure 11.2) has emerged that uses three options and can have one best answer (i.e., 100% credit for one answer and 0% credit for the other two answers).[54]

The values in the example in Figure 11.2 can vary. The key distinction is that the learner only has three choices: more likely, less likely, or unchanged.

Figure 11.2. Modified Script Concordance Problem

A 27-year-old man presents with pleuritic chest pain and shortness of breath.					
If you were thinking of the following diagnosis ...	... and the following new information was to become available ...	... then this hypothesis would become ...			
Pneumonia	Cough with purulent sputum production	-2		0		+2
Interstitial lung disease	Hemoptysis	-2		0		+2
Pneumothorax	Decreased breath sounds on left side	-2		0		+2

11.5.3. Key Features Examination

This examination format focusses on the ability of the learner to identify clinical findings in a patient presentation of sufficient sensitivity or specificity to be important or essential in making a correct diagnosis; these are the "key features."[55] A series of subsequent questions can be generated for each key feature. This assessment method has been incorporated into the Canadian Qualifying Examination in Medicine based on favorable reliability and validity data.[32,56] Practical advice on writing key features questions has been published[57,58] and an example is provided in Figure 11.3.[59]

11.5.4. Clinical Integrative Puzzle

The clinical (comprehensive) integrative puzzle (CIP) is like a clinical crossword puzzle. It asks examinees to compare and contrast a group of related diagnoses (typically four to seven) on a variety of domains such as history, physical examination, laboratories, etc. For each domain, descriptions are provided which fit a given diagnosis (Figure 11.4). The learner matches the appropriate domain description to the diagnosis (e.g., episodic, chest pressure with exertion relieved by rest would be matched with stable angina). It assesses the learner's ability to determine the key elements, or features, that discriminate one diagnosis from another. Experts believe that CIPs may be particularly beneficial for early learners (to assess in individual domains) and their strength is the ability to integrate a variety of different domains or disciplines into a single exam format. Additional research is needed to confirm the reliability and validity of this assessment method. Early work suggests that this tool has favorable psychometric characteristics.[62]

11.5.5. Qualitative Assessment Methods

11.5.5.a. Free Text Questions

Learners can be given a brief vignette and then asked to complete a variety of free text questions. These questions can entail many clinical reasoning domains, such as: generating a problem list, differential diagnosis, leading diagnosis, justification for leading diagnosis, and work-up or therapeutic plan. The form may be given without subsequent information or can be based on an examinee's answers; more data can be provided (clinical reasoning problem or multi-step examination). The practical challenge of grading large numbers of written exams as well as low interrater and intrarater reliability prevent free text questions from becoming the sole method used on standardized testing of clinical reasoning. However, free text responses can provide valuable qualitative insights into a learner's thinking. Question 1 of the key features example in Figure 11.3 could also be classified as a free text question. The number of options to list is generally specified, but no further direction is given (e.g., no list, however long, from which to choose).

Figure 11.3. Key Features Examination

A 35-year-old mother of three presents to your office at 1700h with complaints of severe, watery diarrhea. On questioning, she indicates that she has been ill for about 24 hrs. She has had 15 watery bowel movements in the past 24 hours, has been nauseated, but has not vomited. She works during the day as a cook in a long-term care facility, and she left work to come to your office. On her chart, your office nurse notes a pulse of 110/minute), a blood pressure of 105/50 mm Hg supine, 90/40 standing, and an oral temperature of 36.8°C. On physical examination, you find she has dry mucous membranes and active bowel sounds. A urinalysis (urine microscopy) was normal, with a specific gravity of 1.030.

1. What clinical problems are most important to focus on in the immediate management of this patient? List up to three.

_____
_____
_____

2. What is the most appropriate treatment for this patient at this time? Select up to three.
   - Antidiarrheal medication
   - Antiemetic medication
   - Intravenous 0.9% NaCl
   - Intravenous 2/3 to 1/3
   - Intravenous gentamicin
   - Intravenous metronidazole
   - Intravenous Ringer lactate
   - Nasogastric tube and suction
   - Nothing by mouth
   - Oral ampicillin
   - Oral chloramphenicol
   - Oral fluids
   - Rectal tube
   - Send home with close follow-up
   - Surgical consultation
   - Transfer to hospital

3. After management of the patient's acute condition, what additional measures, if any, are indicated? Select up to four or select #11, None, if none is indicated.
   - Avoid dairy products
   - Colonoscopy
   - Enteric precautions
   - Gastroenterology consultation
   - Give immune serum globulin to patients at long-term care facility
   - Infectious disease consultation
   - Notify Public Health Authority
   - Stool cultures
   - Strict isolation of patient
   - Temporary absence from work
   - None

Figure 11.4. Clinical Integrative Puzzle (CIP) Example (from Ber[79])

Diagnosis	I: Medical history	II: Physical exam	III: Chest x-ray and ECG	IV: Laboratory and other tests	V: Treatment and follow-up	VI: Pathology
Unstable angina						
Myocardial infarction						
Rheumatic mitral stenosis						
Acute pericarditis						
Infective endocarditis						
Hypertrophic cardiomyopathy						

Selected matching items for inserting into table:

Medical History:
a. A 28-year-old woman, in her third month of pregnancy, arrived at the emergency room because of severe shortness of breath (dyspnea). She complains of exertional fatigue from the beginning of her pregnancy, and increasing shortness of breath during the last week.
b. A 25-year-old man complains of shortness of breath and dizziness on exertion. Both his grandfather and elder brother died suddenly at the age of 32 years.

Physical Exam:
a. Pale, sweating, apprehensive. BP 80/60 mmHg, pulse 95/minute, with slight irregularity - premature beats? Lungs - alveolar breathing, no additional sounds. On palpation - hyperdynamic cardiac point of maximum impact (PMI), and on auscultation - accentuated first heart sound.
b. Excellent general condition. BP 130/80 mmHg, pulse 78/minute, regular, abrupt pulse wave. Jugular venous pulse shows marked 'a' wave. Lungs - alveolar breathing, no additional sounds. On palpation - presystolic lift of the PMI, on auscultation - heart sounds normal, harsh systolic murmur increases on sitting and decreases upon squatting.

11.5.5.b. Free Text Paragraph

Learners can also be given a brief vignette and asked to complete a paragraph on diagnosis and therapeutic decisions (Figure 11.5). This can also take the form of an oral examination, which is still used for some specialty boards in many countries. When used as part of an oral examination, the trainee is given a vignette that typically changes over time, based on the answers, and involves verbal reply. Another platform for the verbal or written free text paragraph is a chart stimulated recall (CSR) examination.[63] In this examination, the trainee is asked to review a patient's record (typically one already seen) and then to answer diagnostic and therapeutic decisions retrospectively.

Figure 11.5. Free Response Question

A 62 year old patient with recently diagnosed colon cancer presents with acute onset shortness of breath and right-sided pleuritic chest pain. Her exam is unremarkable (normal lung exam) other than her vital signs which are significant for a heart rate of 126, blood pressure of 80/40, respiratory rate of 20, and a oxygen saturation of 89% on room air. Your pre-test probability is high for pulmonary embolism (80%).
a. Would you perform a CT pulmonary angiogram prior to initiating heparin therapy? Explain why or why not based on the concepts of thresholds to test and treat.
b. Would you perform a CT pulmonary angiogram prior to giving thrombolytic therapy? Explain why or why not based on the concepts of thresholds to test and treat.

11.5.5.c. Oral Examinations

Oral examinations continue to be employed by health professions schools, licensing examiners, and boards. They can be administered in a valid and reliable way, but many challenges exist.[64] The high resource utilization of oral examinations makes undersampling a common problem.[65] Furthermore, stringency (e.g., strict vs. lenient construct) or irrelevant variance (e.g., appearance or manner of examinee) can impact validity.[66] To overcome these challenges, multiple carefully designed cases and well-trained examiners should be used to assess a broad array of content knowledge and skills.

11.5.5.d. Think-Aloud Protocol

In the think-aloud protocol, the examinee is asked to work aloud through a problem with a defined task (e.g., to establish the diagnosis for this patient). The goal is to hear the participant's unfiltered thoughts approaching the problem. If the participant stops speaking, the examiner reminds her/him to "think aloud." This protocol has been well described.[67,68] Its method has been extremely valuable in cognitive psychologists' quest to understand clinical reasoning; however, its labor-intensive nature makes it impractical for large scale assessment of students. For example, a participant could be given a scenario (on paper, DVD, etc.), then asked to state how to arrive at the diagnosis, saying whatever comes to mind for the task without analyzing thoughts. The person (e.g., a research assistant) conducting the protocol will ask the participant to "think-aloud" if he/she makes no utterances after a set period of time (e.g., ten seconds).

11.5.6. Other Methods to Assess Clinical Reasoning

Some methods use inferences to assess the reasoning process. These include faculty questions, oral case presentations, and written notes. Questions about a student's clinical reasoning are a traditional way by which faculty gain insight into a student's reasoning process, and this insight informs global summative evaluations. Although these assessments provide the backbone of student assessment in clinical rotations, standardizing faculty assessments is challenging, due to variation among individual faculty's clinical reasoning ability and limited sampling opportunities. Two published studies have evaluated the value of oral case presentation assessment. Lewin *et al.* developed a tool for clinical reasoning assessment using oral case presentations.[68] However, they showed limited interrater reliability for the items that most closely related to clinical reasoning. Another study used checklists,[70] but checklists have not been shown to be correlated with increasing levels of expertise.[71] To our knowledge, there are no well-studied tools for assessing clinical reasoning quality in written admission or progress notes.

11.5.7. Emerging Methods in Assessing Clinical Reasoning

Additional methods are emerging to assess the process of clinical reasoning. These methods include: assessing cognitive load, emotional engagement, facial feature analysis (disclosure of emotions on the face implying inner thoughts), and functional MRI and PET scanning. Furthermore, Web-based virtual case platforms (e.g., MedU) allow opportunities for clinical reasoning assessment as cases evolve, and for large data set analysis, which may provide further insights into the clinical reasoning process.[72] We believe that, with these new methods, which can largely and more directly "sample" the knowledge structure and cognitive processes involved in clinical reasoning, new understandings to advance the field of clinical reasoning assessment and research will be brought to light.

11.6. Implications for Practice, Research and Application to Assessment

There is no single way to assess clinical reasoning. Since it is clear that clinical reasoning is a key component of competence, choices must be made. The educator has leeway in choosing which (or multiple) measures to use. It is also important to point out that while assessment drives learning, even with imperfect measures, formative assessment can potentially help learners. We have compiled Table 11, which highlights advantages and disadvantages of various clinical reasoning assessment instruments. These instruments should be selected based on local expertise and resource availability.

1. Multiple assessments for each learner are needed;[41,22] that is, there should be broad sampling of a learner's clinical reasoning in terms of case types and contexts. Given the phenomenon of context specificity and the notion that expertise in clinical reasoning appears to be a state, as opposed to a trait, multiple cases should be given in order to improve reliability.
2. Low tech can be good tech. High fidelity presentations are not better than low fidelity[73] Studies have not demonstrated superiority in the assessment of clinical reasoning with using highly authentic (i.e., virtual patients or SPs) as opposed to low fidelity methods (i.e., paper cases).[74]
3. Physicians use multiple processes when engaging in clinical reasoning. Some of these processes, such as nonanalytic reasoning, are very difficult, if not impossible with current methods, to assess reliably. Sample multiple domains and contexts.
4. More theory-driven research and more direct methods for assessing cognitive processes are needed. Fortunately, gains are being made in these areas. This makes clinical reasoning a ripe area for research.
5. As assessment drives curriculum, it is important to point out that experts do not agree on how to teach clinical reasoning, if it can be taught at all.

Table 11. Selected Clinical Reasoning Assessment Approaches

Assessment Approach	Pros and Cons	Reliability for Different Testing Times: 1 hr -- 2 hr -- 4 hr -- 8 hr
MCQs (Case and Swanson 1993[51])	Pros: Broad sampling, strong validity and reliability, readily available standardized tests, low resource utilization. Cons: Cueing effects, difficult to construct items that assess higher order thinking, difficult to come up with "creative" items.	0.62 -- 0.76 -- 0.93 0.93 (Norcini 1985[75])
Extended Matching Questions (EMQs)	Pros: Reduced cueing, broad sampling, good face validity. Cons: All vignettes in a set have to be written such that they relate to the same question. Less variability across the different types of decisions per test (as opposed to key feature approaches).	0.80 (Beullens et al. 2002[76])
Free text short answer / essay questions (Downing 2009[64])	Pros: No cueing effects, qualitative insights into critical thinking. Cons: Low interrater reliability, resource-intensive, often used inappropriately merely to test factual recall ("regurgitation" rather than analysis/synthesis).	Variable based on methodology
Key Features Examination (Farmer and Page 2005[58])	Pros: Good face validity, no cueing effects. Cons: Time and expertise to design tests.	0.32 -- 0.49 -- 0.66 0.79 (Hatala and Norman 2002[77])
SCT (Lubarsky et al. 2013[78])	Pros: Assessment of judgment under uncertainty, good validity and reliability. Cons: No "right answer," answer dependent on judges' quality, assesses only data interpretation.	0.80 (Charlin and van der Vleuten 2004[53])
Comprehensive Integrative Puzzles (CIP) (Ber 2003[79])	Pros: Assess multiple domains of knowledge and disease presentations, low resource utilization. Cons: Lack of reliability data.	Unavailable / Unknown
Oral examinations	Pros: Good validity and reliability if structured - i.e., each interviewer asks same questions. Cons: Resource-intensive, stressful to learner.	0.50 -- 0.69 -- 0.82 0.90 (Swanson 1987[24])
OSCEs (general assessments of performance which can include clinical reasoning)	Pros: Greater authenticity than other methods, assesses data collection. Cons: Resource-intensive, checklist scores correlate poorly with experience.	0.54 -- 0.69 -- 0.82 0.90 (van der Vleuten et al., 1998[80])
mini-CEX	Pros: Authentic clinical experience, assesses data collection. Cons: Resource-intensive.	0.73 -- 0.84 -- 0.92 0.96 (Norcini et al., 2003[81])

References

1. Eva KW. What every teacher needs to know about clinical reasoning. Med Educ 2005;39(1):98-106.
2. Durning SJ, Artino AR, Pangaro LN, et al. Redefining context in the clinical encounter: Implications for research and training in medical education. Acad Med 2010; 85(5):894-901.
3. Higgs J, Jones MA, Loftus S, Christensen N, eds. Clinical Reasoning in the Health Professions - third edition - Boston: Elsevier, 2008.
4. Cervero RM. Effective Continuing Education for Professionals. San Francisco: Jossey-Bass, 1988.
5. Norman G. Research in clinical reasoning: Past history and current trends. Med Educ 2005;39(4):418-427.
6. Bleakley A, Farrow R, Gould D, Marshall R. Making sense of clinical reasoning: Judgement and the evidence of the senses. Med Educ 2003;37(6):544-552.
7. Schuwirth LW. Is assessment of clinical reasoning still the Holy Grail? Med Educ 2009;43(4):298-300.
8. Elstein AS. Thinking about diagnostic thinking: A 30-year perspective. Adv Health Sci Educ Theory Pract 2009;14(Suppl 1):S7-S18.
9. Eva KW. On the generality of specificity. Med Educ 2003;37(7):587-588.
10. Swanson DB, Norcini JJ, Grosso LJ. Assessment of clinical competence: Written and computer-based simulations. Assess Eval High Educ 1987;12(3):220-246.
11. Humbert AJ, Miech EJ. Measuring gains in the clinical reasoning of medical students: Longitudinal results from a school-wide script concordance test. Acad Med 2014;89(7):1046-1050.
12. van der Vleuten CPM. When I say ... context specificity. Med Educ 2014;48(3): 234-235.
13. McCarthy WH, Gonnella JS. The simulated patient management problem: A technique for evaluating and teaching clinical competence. Brit J Med Educ 1967;1(5):348-352.
14. Norcini JJ, Swanson DB, Grosso LJ, Webster GD. Reliability, validity, and efficiency of multiple choice question and patient management problem item formats in assessment of clinical competence. Med Educ 1985;19(3):238-247.
15. Schmidt HG, Boshuizen HPA, Hobus PPM. Transitory stages in the development of medical expertise: The "intermediate effect" in clinical case representation studies. In: Proceedings of the Tenth Annual Conference of the Cognitive Science Society. Hillsdale, NJ: Erlbaum, 1988: 139-145.
16. Schmidt HG, Norman GR, Boshuizen HP. A cognitive perspective on medical expertise: Theory and implication. Acad Med 1990;65(10):611-621.
17. van der Vleuten CPM, van Luijk SJ, van Beckers HJM. A written test as an alternative to performance testing. Med Educ 1989;23(1):97-107.
18. van der Vleuten CPM, Newble D, Case S, et al. Methods of assessment in certification. In: Newble D, Jolly B, Wakeford R, eds. The Certification and Recertification of Doctors: Issues in the Assessment of Clinical Competence. Cambridge: Cambridge University Press, 1994: 105-125.
19. Elstein AS, Shulman LS, Sprafka SA. Medical Problem Solving: An Analysis of Clinical Reasoning. Cambridge, MA: Harvard University Press, 1978.
20. Bland JM, Altman DG. Statistics notes: Cronbach's alpha. BMJ 1997;314(7080): 572.
21. Eva KW, Neville AJ, Norman GR. Exploring the etiology of content specificity: Factors influencing analogic transfer and problem solving. Acad Med 1998;73(10 Suppl):S1-S6.

22. van der Vleuten CPM, Schuwirth LW. Assessing professional competence: From methods to programmes. Med Educ 2005;39(3):309-317.
23. Schmidt HG, Boshuizen HP. On the origin of intermediate effects in clinical case recall. Mem Cognit 1993;21(3):338-351.
24. Swanson DB. A measurement framework for performance-based tests. In: Hart IR, Harden RM, eds. Further Developments in Assessing Clinical Competence. Montreal: Can-Heal, 1987: 13-45.
25. McGaghie WC. Medical problem solving: A reanalysis. J Med Educ 1980;55(11): 912-921.
26. Norman GR. Objective measurement of clinical performance. Med Educ 1985; 19(1):43-47.
27. Holmboe ES, Hawkins RE. Methods for evaluating the clinical competence of residents in internal medicine: A review. Ann Intern Med 1998;129(1):42-48.
28. Pauker SG, Gorry GA, Kassirer JP, Schwartz WB. Towards the simulation of clinical cognition: Taking the present illness by computer. Am J Med 1976;60(7): 981-996.
29. Bordage G. Elaborated knowledge: A key to successful diagnostic thinking. Acad Med 1994;69(11):883-885.
30. Schmidt HG, Rikers RM. How expertise develops in medicine: Knowledge encapsulation and illness script formation. Med Educ 2007;41(12):1133-1139.
31. Sweller J, van Merriënboer JJG, Paas FGWC. Cognitive architecture and instructional design. Educ Psych Rev 1998;10(3):251-296.
32. Page G, Bordage G. The Medical Council of Canada's key features project: A more valid written examination of clinical decision-making skills. Acad Med 1995; 70(2):104-110.
33. Bordage G, Page G. An alternative approach to PMPs: The "key features" concept. In: Hart IR, Harden RM, eds. Further Developments in Assessing Clinical Competence. Montreal: Can-Heal, 1987: 59-75.
34. Schallert DL. The significance of knowledge: A synthesis of research related to schema theory. In: Otto W, White S, eds. Reading Expository Prose. New York: Academic, 1982: 13-48.
35. Barrows HS, Feltovich PJ. The clinical reasoning process. Med Educ 1987;21(2): 86-91.
36. Custers EJ, Regehr G, Norman GR. Mental representations of medical diagnostic knowledge: A review. Acad Med. 1996;71(10 Suppl):S55-S61.
37. Nendaz MR, Bordage G. Promoting diagnostic problem representation. Med Educ 2002;36(8):760-766.
38. Sweller J, Chandler P. Why some material is difficult to learn. Cogn Instr 1994; 12(3):185-233.
39. van Merriënboer JJG, Sweller J. Cognitive load theory and complex learning: Recent developments and future directions. Educ Psych Rev 2005;17(2):147-177.
40. van Merriënboer JJG, Sweller J. Cognitive load theory in health professional education: Design principles and strategies. Med Educ 2010;44(1):85-93.
41. Bordage G, Brailovsky CA, Cohen T, Page G. Maintaining and enhancing key decision-making skills from graduation into practice: An exploratory study. In: Scherpbier AJJA, van der Vleuten CPM, Rethans JJ, van der Steeg AFW, eds. Advances in Medical Education. Dordrecht: Kluwer Academic;1997: 128-130.
42. Hobus PP, Schmidt HG, Boshuizen HPA, Patel VL. Contextual factors in the activation of first diagnostic hypotheses: Expert-novice differences. Med Educ 1987;21(6):471-476.
43. Williams RG, Klamen DA, McGaghie WC. Cognitive, social, and environmental

sources of bias in clinical performance ratings. Teach Learn Med 2003;15(4): 270-292.
44. Cook DA, Triola MM. Virtual patients: A critical literature review and proposed next steps. Med Educ 2009;43(4):303-311.
45. Schuwirth LWT, Verheggen MM, van der Vleuten CPM, et al. Do short cases elicit different thinking processes than factual knowledge questions do? Med Educ 2001;35(4):348-356.
46. Schuwirth LWT. An approach to the assessment of medical problem solving: Computerised case-based testing. Universiteit Maastricht (thesis), 1998.
47. Schuwirth LWT, van der Vleuten CPM, Donkes HHLM. Open-ended questions versus multiple choice questions. In: Harden RM, Hart IR, Mulholland H, eds. Approaches to the Assessment of Clinical Competence. Norwich, UK: Page Brothers, 1992: 486-491.
48. Ward WC. A comparison of free-response and multiple choice forms of verbal aptitude tests. Appl Psychol Meas 1982;6(1):1-11.
49. Hurlburt D. The relative value of recall and recognition techniques for measuring precise knowledge of word meaning, nouns, verbs, adjectives. J Educ Res 1954; 47(8):561-576.
50. Beullens J, Struyf E, van Damme B. Diagnostic ability in relation to clinical seminars and extended matching questions examinations. Med Educ 2006;40(12):1173-1179.
51. Case SM, Swanson DB. Extended matching items: A practical alternative to free-response questions. Teach Learn Med 1993;5(2):107-115.
52. Charlin B, Roy L, Brailovsky C, et al. The script concordance test: A tool to assess the reflective clinician. Teach Learn Med 2000;12(4):189-195.
53. Charlin B, van der Vleuten CPM. Standardized assessment of reasoning in contexts of uncertainty: The script concordance approach. Eval Health Prof 2004;27(3):304-319.
54. Bland AC, Kreiter CD, Gordon JA. The psychometric properties of five scoring methods applied to the script concordance test. Acad Med 2005;80(4):395-399.
55. Bordage G, Page G. An alternative approach to PMPs: The "key features" concept. In: Hart IR, Harden RM, eds. Further Developments in Assessing Clinical Competence. Montreal: Can-Heal, 1987: 59-70.
56. MacRury KA. Testing key features of the clinical case: A written format for a pre-clerkship examination. In: Rothman AI, Cohen R, eds. Proceeedings of the Sixth Ottawa Conference on Medical Education. Toronto: University Bookstore, 1994: 201-202.
57. Schuwirth LWT. How to write short cases for assessing problem-solving skills. Med Teach 1999;21(2):144-150.
58. Farmer EA, Page G. A practical guide to assessing clinical decision-making skills using the key features approach. Med Educ 2005;39(12):1188-1194.
59. Page G. Writing Key Features Problems for the Clinical Reasoning Skills Examination. 1999. <www.idealmed.org/workshop/SectionD-KeyFeatures.pdf>. Accessed May 14, 2015.
60. Groothoff JW, Frenkel J, Tytgat GA, et al. Growth of analytical thinking skills over time as measured with the MATCH test. Med Educ 2008;42(10):1037-1043.
61. Solomon DJ, Reinhart MA, Bridgham RG, et al. An assessment of an oral examination format for evaluating clinical competence in emergency medicine. Acad Med 1990;65(9 Suppl):S43-S44.
62. Davis MH, Karunathilake I. The place of the oral examination in today's assessment systems. Med Teach 2005;27(4):294-297.
63. Turnbull J, Danoff D, Norman G. Content specificity and oral examination

certification. Med Educ 1996;30(1):56-59.
64. Downing SM, Yudkowsky R, eds. Assessment in Health Professions Education. New York: Routledge, 2009.
65. Fonteyn ME, Kuipers B, Grobe SJ. A description of think aloud method and protocol analysis. Qual Health Res 1993;3(4):430-441.
67. Ericsson KA, Simon HA. How to study thinking in everyday life: Contrasting think-aloud protocols with descriptions and explanations of thinking. Mind, Culture, and Activity 1998;5(3):178-186.
68. Lewin LO, Beraho L, Dolan S, et al. Interrater reliability of an oral case presentation rating tool in a pediatric clerkship. Teach Learn Med 2013;25(1):31-38.
69. Kakar SP, Catalanotti JS, Flory AL, et al. Evaluating oral case presentations using a checklist: How do senior student-evaluators compare with faculty? Acad Med 2013;(9):1363-1367.
70. Hodges B, Regehr G, McNaughton N, et al. OSCE checklists do not capture increasing levels of expertise. Acad Med. 1999;74(10):1120-1134.
71. Fall LH, Berman NB, Smith S, et al. Multi-institutional development and utilization of a computer-assisted learning program for the pediatrics clerkship: The CLIPP project. Acad Med 2005;80(9):847-855.
72. Norman G, Dore K, Grierson L. The minimal relationship between simulation fidelity and transfer of learning. Med Educ 2012;46(7):636-647.
73. LaRochelle, JS, Durning SJ, Pangaro LN, et al. Authenticity of instruction and student performance: A prospective randomised trial. Med Educ 2011;45(8): 807-817.
74. Case SM, Swanson DB. Constructing Written Test Questions for the Basic and Clinical Sciences - third edition - Philadelphia: National Board of Medical Examiners, 2000.
75. Norcini JJ, Swanson DB, Grosso LJ, Webster GD. Reliability, validity, and efficiency of multiple choice question and patient management problem item formats in assessment of clinical competence. Med Educ 1985;19(3):238-247.
76. Beullens J, van Damme B, Jaspaert H, Janssen PJ. Are extended-matching multiple choice items appropriate for a final test in medical education? Med Teach 2002;24(4):390-395.
77. Hatala RM, Norman GR. Adapting the key features examination for a clinical clerkship. Med Educ 2002;36(2):160-165.
78. Lubarsky S, Dory V, Duggan P, et al. Script concordance testing: From theory to practice: AMEE guide no. 75. Med Teach 2013;35(3):184-193.
79. Ber R. The CIP (comprehensive integrative puzzle) assessment method. Med Teach 2003;25(2):171-176.
80. van der Vleuten CPM, van Luijk SJ, Swanson DB. Reliability (Generalisability) of the Maastricht Skills Test. Proc Annu Conf Res Med Educ 1988;27:228-233.
81. Norcini JJ, Blank LL, Duffy FD, Fortna GS. The mini-CEX: A method for assessing clinical skills. Ann Intern Med 2003;138(6):476-481.

Chapter 12
The Search for a Meaningful Evaluation of Professionalism

Emily E. Anderson, Ph.D., M.P.H.
Mark Kuczewski, Ph.D.

Professionalism has consumed a fair amount of attention in the medical and medical education literature over the past decades. There is widespread agreement that fostering professionalism is an important aspect of medical training. As a result, professionalism is among the enumerated competencies that must be demonstrated by all medical students.[1]

12.1. Definitions of Professionalism

Professionalism has many meanings. It is viewed as a competence that enables physicians to deliver patient-centered care and be sensitive to patients' psychosocial, cultural, and spiritual needs.[2] This overlaps with competence in basic clinical ethics and the delivery of compassionate end-of-life care. Professionalism is valued as a way to preserve the "doctoring" aspect of medicine that can easily be usurped by an increasing focus on technical and procedural excellence. Professionalism is also invoked as an antidote to systemic and financial pressures that can compromise patient care.[3] Others see professionalism as rooted in the social contract between society and the medical profession.[4,5]

Given this diversity of definitions, it is not surprising that there are no clear standard best practices for assessing professionalism in physicians-in-training or practicing physicians. Of course, some aspects of professionalism are more relevant to, or more easily assessed at, a particular developmental stage. Depending on which aspect of professionalism is deemed most important, a medical school might track only negative behaviors, promote certain actions or interactions, assess knowledge of clinical ethics or the workings of the health care system, or foster, support, and measure particular attitudes toward patients and interprofessional colleagues.

12.2. Why Evaluate Professionalism?

The LCME Standards for Accreditation of Medical Education Programs[1] require assessment of medical student performance as it relates to professional behavior. Professionalism as defined by the LCME includes communication; ability to work on interprofessional health care teams; cultural competence; and medical ethics and human values.[1] As is the case with many accreditation standards, implementation can take a wide variety of forms. Individual medical schools have discretion to define professionalism for their own purposes and to develop and implement appropriate student assessments. ABIM's *Project Professionalism*,[6] the AAMC's *Learning Objectives for Medical Student Education: Guidelines for Medical Schools*,[7] and the ACGME's *Common Program Requirements*[8] and others[9] provide additional guidance regarding definitions of professionalism and professional attitudes, attributes, and behavior (see Table 12).

Table 12. Overview of Definitions of Professionalism

Swick (2000), Toward a Normative Definition of Medical Professionalism	ABIM Project Professionalism	AAMC Learning Objectives for Medical School Education[7]	ACGME Common Program Elements
Physicians subordinate their own interests to the interests of others.	Altruism	Altruism	Altruism
Physicians adhere to high ethical and moral standards.	Integrity Honor		Integrity Sound ethics
Physicians respond to societal needs, and their behaviors reflect a social contract with the communities served.	Duty	Duty	Responsiveness to others' needs
Physicians evince core humanistic values, including honesty and integrity, caring and compassion, altruism and empathy, respect for others, and trustworthiness.	Respect for Others Integrity Honor		Respect Compassion Sensitivity (to culture, age, gender, disability, etc.) Integrity
Physicians exercise accountability for themselves and for their colleagues.	Accountability		Accountability
Physicians demonstrate a continuing commitment to excellence and a commitment to scholarship and to advancing their field.	Excellence	Knowledge Skill	Commitment to excellence
Physicians deal with high levels of complexity and uncertainty.	Excellence	Knowledge Skill	Commitment to excellence
Physicians reflect upon their actions and decisions.	Accountability		Accountability

In part, LCME requires medical schools to assess professionalism because assessment communicates the importance of professionalism. Assessment motivates students to learn what is important by signifying that performance in certain areas "counts" for something. Teaching - yet failing to measure -

professionalism can send mixed messages regarding its importance. If a particular competency (or aspect of professionalism) is not graded, students infer that it is not important.[10]

The 2002 AAMC guidelines suggest that information about professionalism be included in the "Academic Progress" section of the Medical Student Performance Evaluation (MSPE, formerly called "dean's letters") and that an appendix include assessment details. Summative assessment of professionalism may be useful for the early detection of potential long-term behavioral and character issues. Preliminary research has shown incidents of unprofessional behavior in medical school to be correlated with disciplinary action for unprofessional behavior in practice.[11,12] A growing body of research also suggests that the clerkship years are characterized by moral erosion, increases in stress, moral distress, and burnout.[13-15] These realities make evaluating and fostering professionalism in clerkships all the more important.

However, assessment should do more than simply identify weaknesses. Much of the current interest in professionalism revolves around a desire to strengthen the character of the physician so that he or she may be an effective caregiver in the face of competing and potentially corrupting influences. This can involve fostering positive habits and traits, identifying and remediating students whose character can be seen to fall short of the professional ideal, and offsetting potentially negative influences. A key tenet of medical professionalism is commitment to lifelong, self-directed learning. Formative assessment of professionalism during clerkship can provide an introduction to this practice, which requires learning to incorporate constructive feedback and apply it for self-improvement.[16]

12.3. Defining Professionalism in Clerkship

Professionalism is a complex, multifaceted construct. A universally accepted definition is lacking and likely always will be. However, it is clear that a set of considerations have emerged to focus the definition of professionalism (see Table 12). Professionalism consists of several "clusters" that might be assessed: (1) adherence to ethical principles; (2) effective interactions with patients and with people who are important to patients; (3) effective interactions with people working within the health system; (4) reliability; (5) commitment to autonomous maintenance of improvement of competence in oneself, others, and systems;[3] and (6) commitment to advocacy and social responsibility.[4,5]

We need not only a working definition, but also to determine what should specifically be assessed during the clerkship years. How professionalism is defined affects not only *what* things are measured but *how* these things are measured.[10] As with all competencies, these considerations have knowledge, skill, and attitudinal elements. But professionalism is distinctive in that virtues *and* behaviors are also included. Schools should not settle for ensuring that students simply demonstrate knowledge of what professional behavior entails or produce that behavior in a single trial. Professionalism must be judged upon typical behavior patterns. A propensity of character to act appropriately, i.e., virtue, is the outcome of professional formation.

It is clear that these considerations - for instance, one's interactions with other health care team members - will necessarily be lived differently at different points in one's career. As a result, assessment must also differ. We therefore endorse a stage-specific or developmental approach to defining and assessing professionalism.[17] Characteristics of the clerkship stage include: (1) being oriented toward learning what is required (as opposed to the more external orientation of the experienced medical professional); (2) exhibiting increasingly principled moral decision making; and (3) exercising reflective judgment, particularly in cases of complex and ambiguous problems that require consideration of multiple viewpoints and evaluation of multiple solutions. As medical students enter clerkships, they become increasingly responsible for their own learning. Professional development during medical school, particularly the clerkship years, should then focus on "meta-skills" such as reflection and self-directed learning, including students' own observations of their learning experience.[18]

During the clerkship years, medical students' relationship to authority becomes increasingly complicated. Openness to constructive feedback must coexist with the self-confidence to speak up when one see that things are not right. The clerkship is a particularly vulnerable time for students, often characterized by the mantra: "Go along to get along."[19] During this period, students are aware that there is sometimes a disconnect between what they are seeing and what they have learned about appropriate norms, but they often feel powerless to do anything about it. Thus, professionalism in clerkships is postulated as a set of habits that enable students to direct their learning in a fruitful way and to discard the negative influences that can easily produce moral erosion.

The good of the patient is given primacy in our definition of professionalism in clerkships.[20] Interactions and multiple relationships are at the core of professionalism, and those relationships change significantly as students ascend the training ladder. At the clerkship stage, this is marked by openness to feedback but speaking up when something is wrong in patient care.

12.4. Approaches to the Assessment of Professionalism

Approaches that evaluate observable behavior, behaviors in relation to multiple relationships, and appropriate attitudes are most promising for assessing medical students at the clerkship level. Clerkships are characterized by learning to work in a team to benefit patients. They are also an intense socialization process in which the informal and hidden curricula play important roles in student development. As a result, assessment of exhibited behavior as well as attitude development will ensure that students are developing appropriate attitudes that will guide them in lifelong professional development in the service of the good of patients.

The summative and formative purposes of assessment must be carefully considered and balanced given finite resources. The desired aim of each assessment must be clearly articulated to students and evaluators. The goal of any professionalism assessment should be not only to measure but ultimately to improve, and this is especially the case in clerkships.[21] Of course, it is important to ensure that students display minimally acceptable behaviors and therefore it may be desirable to implement summative evaluation. But if there are multiple goals, then there should be multiple, separate, and *independent* tools, data, and systems of evaluation.[22]

Observation is a necessary component of any evaluation of professionalism. Observers must be able to assess accurately the meaning of their observations. This requires significant faculty preparation, time, and effort. Describing what is being seen is especially challenging, given that the "demonstration" of professionalism can be subtle and complex and requires the development of observational skills as well as skills in writing up evaluations.[10] Faculty members and others involved in assessing students' professionalism must be appropriately trained.[23-25]

Context matters. Evaluation of professionalism should involve situations that include conflict and are representative of the kinds of dilemmas that occur in everyday practice.[10] To ensure validity, any hypothetical scenario used in the evaluation of professionalism needs to be realistic concerning social desirability, personal values, and organizational hierarchy. Meaningful evaluation also requires rater understanding of the effects of situations on behavior and on the rating itself.

High-quality evaluation requires multiple assessments, but opportunities to observe behaviors related to professionalism in real-world settings are rare. Unprofessional behaviors do not happen frequently. This makes quantification difficult and requires reliance on hypothetical scenarios. Many professional behaviors (e.g., respectful interaction with a colleague) cannot be meaningfully assessed by observing a single interaction. The number of settings in which we observe professionalism-related behaviors - and the number of observers - must be large in order to achieve an adequate and representative sample of observed behaviors. Additionally, multiple observers are required in a single setting, given that professionalism assessments are subjective (and often qualitative) in nature and triangulation is fundamental to validity of the data.[10]

Observed student behavior alone may not be representative of professionalism.[26] Attitudes are not representative of potential behavior and vice versa; the two are often independent and therefore each should be measured.[27] Students may express positive behaviors in clerkships to succeed but may simultaneously be suffering the effects of moral erosion from the stress and contradictory messages of the environment.

It is clear that few, if any, medical schools have the resources necessary for robust evaluation involving observing behaviors and assessing attitudes across multiple relationships and dimensions. Given limited resources, subjective and labor-intensive educational efforts may be rejected in favor of things that are standardized, reproducible, easily measured, and documented. However, quantitative tools that are good at documenting unacceptable behavior (e.g., checklists) are not as good at encouraging positive action. On the other hand, programs that aim to develop character (e.g., formation programs) do not easily generate data that assure minimal competency on some standard measure of professionalism.[20] It is tempting to oversimplify the concept of professionalism to satisfy the need for *assessment* of professionalism to be simple, expedient, and consistent. This may lead to a very narrow - and dangerous - definition of professionalism as essentially the avoidance or absence of bad behavior. However, if the evaluation of professionalism becomes simply "counting" unprofessional behavior and documenting small transgressions, professionalism becomes trivialized.

12.5. Assessment Methods and Tools

The research on assessing professionalism has not kept pace with that on measurement of clinical skills.[22] Few validated measurement tools exist. Several reviews of existing tools and instruments for evaluating professionalism have been published, although none of these are specific to assessment in clerkship. Each review categorizes tools in somewhat different terms, highlighting the variety of instruments. An older yet still often cited review by Arnold[28] categorizes instruments developed during a thirty-year period according to whether they assess professionalism as part of clinical performance, assess it as a comprehensive entity, or assess separate elements of professionalism (e.g., ethical decision making). Arnold found that while many tools exist, they are weak in terms of validity and reliability and are primarily quantitative in nature.

Veloski *et al.*[29] reviewed studies published between 1982 and 2002 related specifically to the assessment of professionalism in medical students and residents. A national panel of experts reviewed 134 studies and, like Arnold, they identified few instruments with sufficient content validity, reliability and practicality to recommend their use for summative or formative evaluation (rather, most instruments were better used for program evaluation). Approximately half of the empirical studies relied solely upon self-administered instruments. However, they noted an increase in published papers near the final years of their search, signifying a growing interest in the topic and potentially useful works-in-progress.

Ginsburg et al.[17] reviewed twenty years of research on the assessment or evaluation of professionalism in medical school and residency, including instruments to measure professional behavior, professionalism, humanism, values, and attitudes. They found that most tools focussed on observable behaviors and therefore categorized existing assessment tools in terms of raters (e.g., peers, supervisors, nurses, patients). Interestingly, they noted that papers calling for new and better methods of evaluating professionalism outnumbered research reporting specific efforts to do so.

Lynch et al.[30] built on the work of Arnold and Ginsburg, reviewing techniques used to assess professionalism across the career continuum (medical students, residents, and practicing physicians). Searching 1992-2002, they identified 88 tools, which were categorized by content area (ethics, personal characteristics, comprehensive professionalism, diversity) and type of outcome examined (affective, cognitive, behavioral, environmental). Like Arnold, they recommended improving existing tools, particularly in terms of predictive validity, and more research on the use of existing tools for formative purposes.

Noting that other reviews focussed on professional behaviors and skills, Jha et al.[31] reviewed studies specifically assessing medical students' *attitudes* toward professionalism. They found that most of these 97 studies used instruments that measured attitudes toward specific attributes of professionalism (e.g., doctor-patient relationship, ethical or cultural issues), rather than professionalism broadly or as a whole. Those that took a holistic approach lacked validity and reliability. They recommended operationalization of a "generic" definition of professionalism as integral to future research. Defining it as a developmental process, they also urged the importance of measuring attitudes toward professionalism throughout the curriculum rather than at a single time.

Based on our synthesis of these reviews, we focus on those we believe to be most innovative and promising: structured reflection; assessments by supervising physicians; multisource (sometimes called "360 degree") assessments; OSCEs; and professional development portfolios.

12.5.1. Structured Reflection

Development of reflective capacity, the "expertise-enhancing, metacognitive, tacit process whereby personal experience informs practice" (p. 41),[32] can enhance professionalism.[22] Reflective capacity is integral to lifelong, self-directed learning. Research has also shown an association between analytic reflective reasoning and improved diagnostic accuracy in difficult cases.[33]

Reflection has *prima facie* appeal in formative assessment. Clerkships have a strong resocialization aspect, because the immersion experience helps students to absorb the formal, informal, and hidden curricula and to form ways of thinking and behaving. These influences are varied and the experience can significantly impact students' formation. Concerns about negative attitude formation have been expressed specifically about moral erosion and jadedness.[34,35] As a result, written and oral reflections have been used to give the learners self-control over their attitude development. For instance, in a recent study conducted by the authors and colleagues, students reflected on their care for a dying patient.[36] Without prompting, many students noted changes they saw in themselves, such as becoming more desensitized to tragedy and suffering. The reflective writing exercise enabled them to articulate an ideal of balancing the desensitization necessary to encounter tragedy and suffering routinely with a sensitivity to the needs of each particular patient. Students typically articulated a commitment to this ideal and to advancing their skills and attitudes. In the last decade, there has been a proliferation of reflective writing in medical school curricula across the country[37] and an "increased interest in formal assessment of level of reflection as an indicator of professional development of medical students."[32] However, tools to aide in the summative and formative assessment of reflective writing have been slower to come. One promising rubric for evaluating reflective writing, the REFLECT tool (Reflection Evaluation for Learners' Enhanced Competencies Tool) has been developed and tested at Brown.[32,38]

Braun et al.[39] aimed to evaluate the use of student reflective writing about a palliative care clinical assessment to teach and assess professionalism. Conversely, they found that the reflective essays had limited usefulness for summative evaluation of professionalism competencies. Student essays revealed useful information about student's progress toward a few professional competencies, specifically demonstrating awareness of one's own perspectives and biases; and caring, compassion, empathy, and respect. However, reflective essays did not shed much light on students' progress toward displaying self-awareness of performance or recognizing and taking action to correct deficiencies in behavior, knowledge, and skills.

Reflective exercises are proliferating because of their potential to offset negative influences on attitude development and to enable learners to take control of their developmental agenda. More research is needed on ways to structure and assess such exercises in order to achieve the desired outcomes.[40] We do not know if written reflection alone might produce the desired results or if reflection is more effective when embedded within small group discussion or accompanied by one-on-one oral feedback.[41] Feedback from mentors is important, but more research is needed on effective methods of assessing reflective competency[42,43] and providing feedback.[44,45]

12.5.2. Multisource ("360 Degree") Assessments

Teams deliver contemporary health care. Medical students must learn to navigate among the multiple relationships necessary to provide effective care. A student may be more adept at working with some kinds of professionals (e.g., residents) than others (e.g., nursing staff). As a result, assessing the student's professionalism during the clerkship years involves several key relationships. A holistic, multisource, sometimes called a "360 degree" approach to assessment has gained favor over the past decade in corporate environments, including health care.[46] The literature on the use of 360 degree assessments of professionalism in physicians-in-training is limited,[47,48] but we believe that this approach holds promise because it aligns with the developmental phase of clerkships and a relationship-based definition of professionalism. Use of multisource feedback is growing in other areas, such as patient communication and clinical competence.

A multisource assessment of professionalism in a clerkship is resource-intensive. It requires many evaluators from different groups, including supervisors, medical student peers, other health professionals (e.g., nursing), and patients as well as self-evaluation.[30] Such an approach also requires collecting many evaluations in a timely manner and interpreting the data in a meaningful way. Evaluators will require training to ensure reliability and must be incentivized to perform meaningful assessments. Many, possibly most, of those performing assessments of medical students in a 360 degree model are not medical school faculty members and it is not likely a part of their job description to assess medical students. Meaningful observation rather than volume of observation should be the key consideration.[28]

If students perceive that they are constantly being watched, this can diminish their enjoyment of learning and encourage false behavior ("Hawthorne effect").[49] Further, 360 degree assessments generally use quantitative scales, which are limited in terms of their ability to capture nuance or account for particular circumstances. However, multisource feedback allows students to compare their own self-ratings with those of peers and patients, prompting reflection and, ideally, commitment to improvement. Each of the parties potentially involved in 360 degree assessment will be discussed in more detail below.

12.5.3. Assessments by Supervising Physicians

Physicians supervising clerkships may provide global ratings, but structured observations using checklists are preferred. In a recent study using the mini-CEX format, twenty-four professionalism behaviors were culled from a set of 142 observable behaviors, converted into an evaluation instrument (the P-MEX) designed for use in multiple clerkship settings, and tested in medicine, surgery, obstetrics/gynecology, psychiatry, and pediatrics.[50] Preliminary testing revealed adequate content and construct validity, but ideally ten to twelve independent raters are needed to achieve dependability. This early research suggests that the P-MEX is a feasible format for professionalism evaluation in clerkship settings if sufficient faculty effort is given. Four items frequently marked "below expectations" may be particularly useful to identify problem students: (a) "demonstrated awareness of limitations," (b) "solicited feedback," (c) "was on time," and (d) "addressed gaps in own knowledge and skills." Interestingly, three of these four items are closely related to reflective skills.[50]

Written global ratings of professionalism may be limited by the wiliness of teacher to be honest *on the record*. Face-to-face conversation has in some settings been shown to enhance detection of students' deficiencies.[51]

12.5.4. Peer Assessment

Peer assessment is used independently or as part of multisource feedback. Peer assessment can potentially measure students' interpersonal skills, which are hard to reach by other methods. Students value peer feedback, which is important for professional formation.[52] Peer assessment has the added benefit of training students over time to evaluate peers, offer constructive feedback, and judge important professional competency.[53] Peer assessments correlate weakly with faculty assessments of professionalism.[54] The extent to which peer assessment can effectively identify students who may not be demonstrating appropriate professional behavior is unclear, but this is a problem inherent in many methods of assessing professionalism. More research is needed.

In a study of students across all four years of medical school, Arnold and colleagues[55] found peer assessment to be a useful approach that provides unique information. Students expressed concerns about participating and were afraid of the negative impact that positive and negative assessments might have on relationships with other students. The authors suggest that negative assessments should have a formative intent while positive assessments should have a summative purpose. An impartial counselor should receive information about unprofessional behavior and work with students toward corrective action without penalty in a safe environment. Information about professional behavior should be reported to students directly. Arnold *et al.* suggested that such information could be used as the basis of selection into a professionalism honor society. This approach has been used by chapters of the Gold Humanism Honor Society (GHHS).[55]

12.5.5. Patients' Assessments of a Learner's Professionalism

The role of patients in multisource feedback assessment of medical students is less explored than other potential parties. Britain leads the way in involving patients in medical student assessment.[56] A study conducted by Lyons et al.[57] found that students were as likely to take patient feedback into account as feedback from supervising physicians. While they did not attempt to correlate patient ratings with performance on the OSCE, they did find that students who participated in the study of patient feedback were more likely to pass all portions of an OSCE. More work is needed to assess and improve the reliability and validity of patient feedback instruments. A real concern is that patients may be overly positive in their ratings and induce false confidence or reinforce unprofessional behaviors.

12.5.6. Assessment by Nurses and Other Health Care Professionals

A robust 360 degree assessment of medical students' professionalism should include participation by nurses and other health care professionals. No studies involving nurse assessment of medical students were found. One study of nurses' assessments of first-year internal medicine residents' "humanistic qualities" suggests that patients, attending physicians, program supervisors, and nurses all contribute different viewpoints, and that nurses' ratings are more reproducible, thereby requiring fewer raters, compared with patients and attending physicians. However, the same study also found that nurses' perceptions correlate more closely with those of patients than physician raters, which raises questions about the added utility of including an additional group of raters for whom this exercise would be beyond the limits of their usual responsibilities.[58]

12.5.7. Self-Assessment

The popularity of self-assessments is probably due, in part, to the fact that observational assessments are so resource-intensive. Self-assessment allows formative assessment to be accomplished more efficiently. Furthermore, self-assessment skills are potentially important as a means to lifelong professional development. While observational feedback over the course of a career will be intermittent at best, self-assessment can and should be ongoing. Self-assessments are also useful for comparison with the assessments of others. However, studies have shown that the accuracy of self-assessments is poor and that self-assessment methods suffer from a variety of methodological weaknesses.[59]

12.5.8. Objective Structured Clinical Examinations (OSCEs)

While multisource assessments provide feedback on students' generalized, "real-world" behavior, OSCEs assess student behavior in a controlled setting. The few studies that have used OSCEs to assess professionalism have produced varied results. Mazor et al.[60] compared the observations of physician preceptors, SPs, and lay individuals (as proxies for "average" patients). They found variance both among and within rater categories during assessment of students' professionalism. Their findings highlight the fact that different raters (even within groups) pay attention to different verbal and nonverbal behaviors, even when given the same instructions and rating forms.

12.5.9. Professional Development Portfolios

Professional development portfolios, which can be developed and managed using an online Web-based platform, use a narrative-based approach to emphasize critical self-reflection with review and feedback by faculty mentors.[61] Portfolios enable the learner to self-direct the construction of their professional development narrative. Program leaders identify areas of professionalism that are valuable to the learner, defining the required elements of the portfolio. Thus, a professional development portfolio is similar to a list of required clinical procedures that a student must complete. A professionalism portfolio does not necessarily demonstrate mastery of required elements, but does show familiarity with those elements and some degree of progress. Portfolio assessment requires significant time and effort from faculty mentors who provide feedback about diverse sets of portfolios. Portfolio development has waned in popularity recently, likely due to growing awareness that the approach requires significant mentor effort and faculty development.

12.6. Key Recommendations

Despite assessment challenges, inherent ambiguities, and equivocations in meanings, professionalism is a competency around which the ideals of medicine coalesce. Given resource constraints, the future of assessing professionalism will likely continue to emphasize self-assessments and reflective exercises. Such approaches are more congruent with formative aims. Given the intense resocialization experience of the clinical clerkships, emphasizing the formation of professionalism is paramount.

Professionalism is a matter of lifelong learning. Students on clerkships must receive feedback on their behaviors from a variety of team members, and possibly patients. Students must learn to conform behavior to the interpersonal and ethical norms of the health care delivery team. Students must also develop appropriate attitudes to match these clinical behaviors which will guide future development.

Specific recommendations include:
1. Formative processes should take precedence over summative ones. This is simply because the professionalism of medical students, especially during their clerkships, is in formation. Student understanding of the norms of the clinical environment and their adaptation to the interpersonal skills needed and the attitudes to sustain those skills are likely to be in flux. Thus, we must provide formative assessment that helps students grow as health care professionals.

2. The resource-intensive nature of observational assessments tempts educators to use quantitative tools like checklists that provide a "quick and dirty" assessment of a students' professionalism. However, approaches that emphasize qualitative methods[60,62] or focus on improving the clinical context and environment to ameliorate the effects of the informal and hidden curricula should be prioritized.
3. As we seek to foster an environment more conducive to reinforcing professionalism, we should emphasize patient-centeredness as the heart of professionalism. Our recent study of medical students addressing the spiritual needs of dying patients found students reporting that making personal connections with these patients by discussing shared general interests was more important to some patients than trying to discuss death meaningfully or directly.[36] Such insights bring the picture of what professionalism looks like into focus.

12.7. Future Research on Assessing Professionalism

The potential of reflection as a means to teach and assess professionalism should be explored. Reflection is pragmatic and does not necessarily require the resource intensity of observational exercises. We have also noted that interest in reflection has been motivated by a concern for the negative effects of the informal and hidden curricula on students. We need to understand the informal and hidden curricula better and to acknowledge their existence as legitimate sources of learning and socialization, even though they may teach both positive and negative lessons about the ideals of professionalism. Such an understanding is necessary to improve the environment and to develop better methods of teaching and assessing professionalism.

More research is also needed to determine specific attitudes, characteristics, and behaviors exhibited in clerkship that predict unprofessional behavior in clinical practice. Research aimed at connecting what happens in the training years with later clinical practice has the potential to contribute significantly to improving patient outcomes and preventing harm.

Standardization of teaching and assessing professionalism is a key question for the future. There is not sufficient agreement about the key behaviors and attitudes that every medical student should exhibit before entering residency, nor is there an established means of measurement. Therefore, we cannot at this time recommend a standardized approach among medical schools. This lack of consensus has enabled many schools to pilot a variety of different measures. It is reasonable to expect that more standardization will take place in the future, because behavioral expectations are not completely open-ended, even at this early stage in a physician's development. But we believe that it is ideal if the teaching and assessment of professionalism always retains some area for the creativity of individual schools. Keeping space available for experimentation will produce important innovations to help to develop professionalism as social responsibility or as addressing dying patients' spiritual needs. Achieving the appropriate balance is an ongoing task for medical educators.

References

1. LCME. Functions and Structure of a Medical School: Standards for Accreditation of Medical Education Programs Leading to the M.D. Degree, 2015. <www.lcme.org/publications/2016-17-functions-and-structure-april-2015.doc>. Accessed May 16, 2015.
2. Coulehan J. Viewpoint: Today's professionalism: Engaging the mind but not the heart. Acad Med 2005;80(10):892-898.
3. Wilkinson TJ, Wade WB, Knock LD. A blueprint to assess professionalism: Results of a systematic review. Acad Med 2009;84(5):551-558.
4. Rothman DJ. Medical professionalism: Focusing on the real issues. N Engl J Med 2000;342(17):1284-1286.
5. Cruess SR, Cruess RL. Professionalism: A contract between medicine and society. Can Med Assoc J 2000;162(5):668-669.
6. ABIM. Project Professionalism. 2001. <www.abimfoundation.org/~/media/Foundation/Professionalism/Project%20professionalism.ashx?la=en>. Accessed May 16, 2015.
7. AAMC. Medical School Objectives Project. Report I. Learning Objectives for Medical Student Education: Guidelines for Medical Schools. 1998. <members.aamc.org/eweb/upload/Learning%20Objectives%20for%20Medical%20Student%20Educ%20Report%20I.pdf>. Accessed May 16, 2015
8. ACGME. Common Program Requirements, 2013. <www.acgme.org/acgmeweb/tabid/429/ProgramandInstitutionalAccreditation/CommonProgramRequirements.aspx>. Accessed May 11, 2015.
9. Swick HM. Toward a normative definition of medical professionalism. Acad Med 2000;75(6):612-616.
10. Stern DT. A framework for measuring professionalism. In: Stern DT, ed. Measuring Medical Professionalism. New York: Oxford University Press, 2006: 3-14.
11. Papadakis MA, Hodgson CS, Teherani A, Kohatsu ND. Unprofessional behavior in medical school is associated with subsequent disciplinary action by a state medical board. Acad Med 2004;79(3):244-249.
12. Papadakis MA, Teherani A, Banach MA, et al. Disciplinary action by medical boards and prior behavior in medical school. N Engl J Med 2005;353(25):2673-2682.
13. Dyrbye LN, Massie FS, Eacker A, et al. Relationship between burnout and professional conduct and attitudes among US medical students. JAMA 2010; 304(11):1173-1180.
14. Ginsburg S, Regehr G, Lingard L. Basing the evaluation of professionalism on observable behaviors: A cautionary tale. Acad Med 2004;79(10 Suppl):S1-S4.
15. Reddy ST, Farnan JM, Yoon JD, et al. Third-year medical students' participation in and perceptions of unprofessional behaviors. Acad Med 2007;82(10 Suppl):S35-S39.
16. Epstein RM. Assessment in medical education. N Engl J Med 2007;356(4):387-396.
17. Ginsburg S, Regehr G, Hatala R, et al. Context, conflict, and resolution: A new conceptual framework for evaluating professionalism. Acad Med 2000;75(10 Suppl):S6-S11.
18. Hilton SR, Slotnick HB. Proto-professionalism: How professionalisation occurs across the continuum of medical education. Med Educ 2005;39(1):58-65.
19. Myers MF, Herb A. Ethical dilemmas in clerkship rotations. Acad Med 2013; 88(11):1609-1611.
20. Kuczewski MG. The problem with evaluating professionalism: The case against current dogma. In: Wear D, Aultman JM, eds. Professionalism in Medicine: Critical Perspectives. New York: Springer, 2006: 185-198.

21. Inui TS. A Flag in the Wind: Educating for Professionalism in Medicine. 2003. <members.aamc.org/eweb/upload/A%20Flag%20in%20the%20Wind%20Report.pdf>. Accessed May 16, 2015.
22. Stern D, Papadakis M. The developing physician: Becoming a professional. N Engl J Med 2006;355(17):1794-1799.
23. Frohna A, Stern D. The nature of qualitative comments in evaluating professionalism. Med Educ 2005;39(8):763-768.
24. Steinert Y, Cruess S, Cruess R, Snell L. Faculty development for teaching and evaluating professionalism: From programme design to curriculum change. Med Educ 2005;39(2):127-136.
25. Wang KE, Fitzpatrick C, George D, Lane L. Attitudes of affiliate faculty members toward medical student summative evaluation for clinical clerkships: A qualitative analysis. Teach Learn Med 2012;24(1):8-17.
26. Hafferty F. Measuring professionalism: A commentary. In: Stern DT, ed. Measuring Medical Professionalism. New York: Oxford University Press, 2006: 281-306.
27. Rees CE, Knight LV. Viewpoint: The trouble with assessing students' professionalism: Theoretical insights from sociocognitive psychology. Acad Med 2007;82(1):46-50.
28. Arnold L. Assessing professional behavior: Yesterday, today, and tomorrow. Acad Med 2002;77(6):502-515.
29. Veloski JJ, Fields SK, Boex JR, Blank LL. Measuring professionalism: A review of studies with instruments reported in the literature between 1982 and 2002. Acad Med 2005;80(4):366-370.
30. Lynch DC, Surdyk PM, Elser AR. Assessing professionalism: A review of the literature. Med Teach 2004;26(4):366-373.
31. Jha V, Bekker HL, Duffy SR, Roberts TE. A systematic review of studies assessing and facilitating attitudes towards professionalism in medicine. Med Educ 2007;41(8):822-829.
32. Wald H, Reis S. Beyond the margins: Reflective writing and development of reflective capacity in medical education. J Gen Intern Med 2010;25(7):746-749.
33. Mamede S, Schmidt HG, Penaforte JC. Effects of reflective practice on the accuracy of medical diagnoses. Med Educ 2008;42(5):468-475.
34. Feudtner C, Christakis DA, Christakis NA. Do clinical clerks suffer ethical erosion? Students' perceptions of their ethical environment and personal development. Acad Med 1994;69(8):670-679.
35. Rentmeester CA, Brack AB, Kavan MG. Third and fourth year medical students' attitudes about and experiences with callousness: The good, the bad and the ambiguous. Med Teach 2007;29(4):358-364.
36. Kuczewski MG, McCarthy MP, Michelfelder A, et al. "I will never let that be ok again": Student reflections on competent spiritual care for dying patients. Acad Med 2014;89(1):54-59.
37. Chaffey LJ, de Leeuw EJ, Finnigan GA. Facilitating students' reflective practice in a medical course: literature review. Educ Health (Abingdon) 2012;25(3):198-203.
38. Wald HS, Borkan JM, Taylor JS, et al. Fostering and evaluating reflective capacity in medical education: Developing the REFLECT rubric for assessing reflective writing. Acad Med 2012;87(1):41-50.
39. Braun UK, Gill AC, Teal CR, Morrison LJ. The utility of reflective writing after a palliative care experience: Can we assess medical students' professionalism? J Palliat Med 2013;16(11):1342-1349.
40. Stark P, Roberts C, Newble D, Bax N. Discovering professionalism through guided reflection. Med Teach 2006;28(1):e25-e31.
41. Baernstein A, Fryer-Edwards K. Promoting reflection on professionalism: A comparison trial of educational interventions for medical students. Acad Med 2003;78(7):742-747.

42. Howe A, Barrett A, Leinster S. How medical students demonstrate their professionalism when reflecting on experience. Med Educ 2009;43(10):942-951.
43. Aukes LC, Geertsma J, Cohen-Schotanus J, et al. The development of a scale to measure personal reflection in medical practice and education. Med Teach 2007;29(2/3):177-182.
44. Aronson L, Niehaus B, Hill-Sakurai L, et al. A comparison of two methods of teaching reflective ability in year 3 medical students. Med Educ 2012;46(8):807-814.
45. Reis SP, Wald HS, Monroe AD, Borkan JM. Begin the BEGAN (The Brown Educational Guide to the Analysis of Narrative): A framework for enhancing educational impact of faculty feedback to students' reflective writing. Patient Educ Counsel 2010;80(2):253-259.
46. Lockyer J. Multisource feedback in the assessment of physician competencies. J Contin Educ Health Prof 2003;23(1):4-12.
47. Wood J, Collins J, Burnside ES, et al. Patient, faculty, and self-assessment of radiology resident performance: A 360-degree method of measuring professionalism and interpersonal/communication skills. Acad Rad 2004;11(8):931-939.
48. Brinkman WB, Geraghty SR, Lanphear BP, et al. Effect of multisource feedback on resident communication skills and professionalism: A randomized controlled trial. Arch Pediatr Adolesc Med 2007;161(1):44-49.
49. Rees C, Shepherd M. The acceptability of 360-degree judgements as a method of assessing undergraduate medical students' personal and professional behaviours. Med Educ 2005;39(1):49-57.
50. Cruess R, McIlroy JH, Cruess S, Ginsburg S, Steinert Y. The professionalism mini-evaluation exercise: A preliminary investigation. Acad Med 2006;81(10 Suppl):S74-S78.
51. Hemmer PA, Hawkins R, Jackson JL, Pangaro LN. Assessing how well three evaluation methods detect deficiencies in medical students' professionalism in two settings of an internal medicine clerkship. Acad Med. 2000;75(2):167-173.
52. Dannefer EF, Henson LC, Bierer SB, et al. Peer assessment of professional competence. Med Educ 2005;39(7):713-722.
53. Cottrell S, Diaz S, Cather A, Shumway J. Assessing medical student professionalism: An analysis of a peer assessment. Med Educ Online 2009;11:8. <med-ed-online.net/index.php/meo/article/view/4587>. Accessed May 8, 2015.
54. Kovach R, Resch D, Verhulst S. Peer assessment of professionalism: A five-year experience in medical clerkship. J Gen Intern Med 2009;24(6):742-746.
55. Arnold L, Shue CK, Kalishman S, et al. Can there be a single system for peer assessment of professionalism among medical students? A multi-institutional study. Acad Med 2007;82(6):578-586.
56. Berlin A, Seymour C, Johnson I, Cupit S. Patient and Public Involvement in the Education of Tomorrow's Doctors. London: University College London, 2011.
57. Lyons O, Willcock H, Rees J, Archer J. Patient feedback for medical students. Clin Teach 2009;6(4):254-258.
58. Woolliscroft JO, Howell JD, Patel BP, Swanson DB. Resident-patient interactions: The humanistic qualities of internal medicine residents assessed by patients, attending physicians, program supervisors, and nurses. Acad Med 1994;69(3):216-224.
59. Eva KW, Regehr G. Self-assessment in the health professions: A reformulation and research agenda. Acad Med 2005;80(10 Suppl):S46-S54.
60. Mazor KM, Zanetti ML, Alper EJ, et al. Assessing professionalism in the context of an objective structured clinical examination: An in-depth study of the rating process. Med Educ 2007;41(4):331-340.
61. Kalet AL, Sanger J, Chase J, et al. Promoting professionalism through an online professional development portfolio: Successes, joys, and frustrations. Acad Med 2007;82(11):1065-1072.
62. Ginsburg S, Regehr G, Mylopoulos M. From behaviours to attributions: Further concerns regarding the evaluation of professionalism. Med Educ 2009;43(5):414-425.

Chapter 13
Feedback

Lisa E. Leggio, M.D.
T. Andrew Albritton, M.D.

According to Standard 9 (formerly Educational Program Standard ED-30) of the LCME, "The directors of all courses and clerkship rotations in a medical education program must design and implement a system of fair and timely formative and summative assessment of medical student achievement in each course and clerkship." Even without this mandate, there is no question that providing feedback to students is one of the most important responsibilities of an educator. "Feedback has been described as the cornerstone of effective clinical teaching"[1] and is essential to the improvement of skills through deliberate practice.[2]

This chapter discusses how providing effective feedback about a learner's performance supports educational processes. There are many discussions of this topic in educational textbooks[3,4] and medical journals.[5] The main focus of this chapter is practical advice in giving feedback to learners, but we also discuss how a culture of feedback allows a flow of information "upward" to supervisors.

13.1. The Importance of Feedback

Without feedback students can, at best, only gauge performance by trial and error. Frequently, the student learns about problems at the end of an educational experience when it is too late to make corrections. Feedback should follow directly from formative evaluation in which a student's performance is judged against expectations; then it reinforces appropriate behaviors and corrects mistakes and misconceptions. There are several useful definitions and discussions of feedback available.[6] All convey that feedback is information provided to improve or optimize performance. Van de Ridder et al. have proposed a definition derived from a literature review: "feedback is specific information about the comparison between a trainee's observed performance and a standard, given with the intent to improve the trainee's performance."[7] This definition makes explicit that there is a standard of comparison against which current performance is judged.

Most definitions of feedback refer to "improving performance," and imply that there is something to improve. Therefore, they address "corrective" feedback, sometimes called "negative" feedback, from an analogy with engineering models that imply correction of the system's desired output. However, medical education also emphasizes "reinforcing" or "positive" feedback, so that learners will know what they did correctly. Therefore, the van de Ridder definition should be expanded to state that feedback intends "to improve or sustain" the trainee's performance.

13.2. Elements and Characteristics of Effective Feedback

13.2.1. Timeliness and Setting

The classic article by Ende[8] in 1983 outlined the characteristics of effective feedback that have been frequently cited by others. Feedback should be *timely* and take place as close as possible to when the learning event occurred. This timeliness allows both learners and teachers to recall events and specifics clearly. However, teachers must also consider each student's *emotional state,* and postpone giving feedback if the student is under a lot of stress, such as just before an exam or when ill. Teachers should also consider their own emotional state and not give immediate feedback if angry or when they lack adequate time to provide thoughtful feedback. Always use an *appropriate location* for feedback. A private area should be used, and do not provide feedback when others are present unless giving general feedback to a group. The general maxim has been, "Praise in public, but critique in private." Of course, there are exceptions, such as when an error to be corrected is typical of all learners, and all can profit from hearing the general feedback. Sometimes a gross breach of professional demeanor has been universally observed, and a faculty member has to remind the group of general standards.

Effective feedback must be *timely and occur on a regular basis*. After a specific incident, provide feedback as soon as possible after the event, rather than waiting until the end of the clerkship. In addition, explicitly *labeling feedback* sessions as that (e.g., "I'd like to give you some feedback about this progress note") will help students to realize that in fact they are receiving feedback. Be supportive when giving feedback.

13.2.2. Specificity and Behaviorally Oriented

Feedback should be *specific*, not just general statements about performance, such as "Good job." The learner, especially a beginner, may not know what it was that he or she did correctly; therefore, being specific about what the learner did applies as much to what went right, as to corrective feedback (what went wrong). General statements are less helpful in improving performance than specific statements based on observation, such as, "The way you described the plan to the patient was clear and used lay terms, giving the patient a good understanding of what to expect."

Feedback should be *descriptive, non-judgmental,* and *based on observations*. Talk about "what" the students did, rather than "who" they are, and focus on the specific behavior that you, the teacher, observed, and not the person. The purpose of feedback, much like coaching or parenting, is to *reinforce the good* behaviors or actions and to *correct errors*.

13.2.3. Based on Observations Rather Than Inferences

Feedback is most clear when it is about *observed* actions or about explicit *decisions and actions*, not assumed intentions or interpretations. Rather than inferring intentions, it is often useful to use the device of interactive feedback to allow learners themselves to express what they intended in saying or doing something. For instance, the teacher says, "I noticed that you raised your voice and crossed your arms when asking the patient about smoking. What did you intend by that?"

Remembering that learners may be novices and that confidence may be slow to develop, feedback should be *supportive,* with focus on areas that the student can control or change. This will help the student to improve while maintaining self-respect. Feedback should be given in such a way that the student understands it and knows how to take the next step.

13.2.4. Focus and Prioritize

The amount of feedback given at one time should be *limited*, to avoid "feedback overload," which may be caused by providing too many suggestions during a single session. Make two or three important points and schedule additional feedback sessions, if needed, to address other areas for improvement. Generally, prioritization in order to avoid feedback overload can be based on the goals most appropriate for a learner's level of training. The focus, for instance, for an early clerkship student might be on improving basic interviewing skills, rather than on a detailed discussion of management options in an area of medical controversy.

13.2.5. Trust and Learning Climate

From the beginning the teacher must create a climate of *mutual trust and respect*. Eva et al. emphasize[9] that feedback should be given within an established relationship "from a position of beneficence and non-maleficence." Relationships matter when giving feedback.[10] Faculty can foster trust and respect by creating a positive learning climate. Behaviors that foster relationships include simple actions like using the student's preferred name, including students in patient discussions, and demonstrating interest in their learning. Effective feedback should take place in a private location.

13.2.6. Feedback Is Based on Explicit Goals

The teacher and student should be sure that they have *common goals*. Make sure that students clearly understand the expectations for the clerkship. Review the goals and objectives, and the criteria for evaluation during the clerkship orientation. If confusion or resistance is anticipated, have the clerkship goals, objectives, and criteria available in writing during the feedback session. They should also be posted on the clerkship Web site or learning management system. During the educational experience, students usually want to know about their performance in terms of a projected grade. What steps are necessary to reach a desired grade? If a student perceives that a teacher's assessment is based on personal preferences, then feedback may seem arbitrary or even unfair. Making a direct connection between feedback and the explicit learning objectives and goals of the clerkship can provide clarity for students, whenever there is any question about whether students see the feedback as relevant.

13.2.7. Formative Information vs. Summative Judgment

Feedback is best presented as information provided for the learner's benefit. Any explicit evaluation is formative and provisional, because it allows for future improvement. Feedback is clearer when teachers use verbs and nouns. In contrast, summative evaluation (grading) is presented as a judgment and uses adverbs and adjectives to relate observations to performance standards. An example of formative evaluation with feedback is, "Your differential diagnosis did not include leukemia, which should be considered in a patient with easy bruising." An example of summative evaluation is, "Your differential diagnoses on the last few patients were inadequate."

Evaluation and feedback are often paired. While useful as an evaluation, "Your differential diagnoses were inadequate" is not helpful for learner improvement. Coupling evaluation with feedback that the student can use to improve will be perceived by the student as beneficial.

13.3. Guidelines for Giving Feedback

The following steps will foster the efficacy of feedback:

13.3.1. Encourage Self-Assessment

When there is time, ask students to self-assess their performance. Feedback can be solicited from a student by asking questions like, "How did things go?" or "What went well?" Self-assessment is often inaccurate when asking students to rate their overall performance. However, asking about the students' impressions of their success in a specific task with a specific patient can start the feedback session and foster the relationship. Eva *et al.*[9] and Chou *et al.*[10] assert that this plays an important role in how well feedback is received.

13.3.2. Share Your Direct Observations

Explicitly describe the skills, attitudes, or behaviors that the student is performing well. Direct observation is critical. Eva and colleagues[9] found that students discount feedback from those who had not actually observed their performance.

13.3.3. Have an Action Plan

Help the student to identify specific areas for improvement and suggest next steps to improve performance. For example, "If you had an opportunity to do it again, what would you do differently?" Per Eva,[9] it may be helpful to tailor the feedback to make it more palatable, based on student perceptions. Planning a way to observe again for improvement supports a trusting learning climate.

13.3.4. Clarify Understanding

Ask students if they understand or have any questions. Interactive feedback has two helpful benefits: (a) It allows students to verbalize the problem, and (b) creates opportunities to see if students have any insight into their performance. Students may not be willing to admit that they did not grasp what you were trying to say. Have a clear vision about ways that students' understanding of your feedback will be evident.

13.3.5. Structuring a Session to Include Feedback

Among many strategies which may be helpful to share with teaching faculty and residents are the classic "feedback sandwich" and the STOP technique published by Gigante and colleagues.[11] The "feedback sandwich" has the preceptor begin by telling students what they did well, followed by what they need to improve, and ends with another activity that they are doing well. Some feel that this technique has been overused, causing students to brace themselves for bad news when they hear what they are doing well. The STOP mnemonic is a helpful way to remember that feedback should be **S**pecific, **T**imely, **O**bjective, and include a **P**lan for improvement. The One-Minute Preceptor[12] includes giving feedback as one of five key micro-skills to be used in a clinical teaching session. The structured clinical observation (SCO),[13] developed for pediatrics, also expects the teaching encounter will be concluded with feedback for the learner.

13.4. Types of Feedback Sessions

Three types of feedback sessions described by Branch and Paranjape[14] may be used at various times.

13.4.1. Brief Focussed Session *During* a Patient Encounter

Opportunities for giving *brief feedback* (brief, but still labeled "feedback," and delivered within the context of learning) occur frequently. For example, after observing a student's physical exam on a child with congenital heart disease, first ask the student how she or he felt that the encounter went (self-evaluation and interactive feedback). If the student expresses concern about not having heard the heart murmur, say, "Talking to the child about her new puppy seemed to make her more comfortable in the beginning" - (*something specific that was done well*). "After you examined her ears, she was crying and you were not able to hear her heart murmur" - (*something specific that could have been done better*). "Try listening now to the heart first, while the child is calm and quiet, before looking in the ears" - (*action plan*).

13.4.2. Formal Review Session after an Encounter

"Recap" and review after a teaching session can provide an effective time for feedback. The session is fresh in the learner's mind. Consider this a situation for giving *formal feedback*, a brief time set aside specifically for explicit feedback. A student presents a patient during rounds or in clinic. The presentation includes the pertinent information, but was lengthy and disorganized. In an appropriate setting, at the end of rounds or at the end of the clinic session, ask the student how she or he felt about the presentation (*encourage self-assessment*). The student self-assessment helps frame the session. Tell the student that you are giving feedback about the presentation on that particular patient (*labeling feedback*). "Your presentation earlier this morning included all the pertinent information" - (*positive feedback*). "To streamline the organization of the presentation, there was extraneous information you could have omitted. For example, while it is important that you had more information available, it was not critical for me to hear it at that time" - (*based on observation*, and *suggestions for improvement*). Ask the student if the feedback was helpful and if he or she has any questions. Help the student, if appropriate, to develop an action plan to improve (*making sure that the learner understands the feedback*).

13.4.3. Major Summative Feedback, Planned Session

The third feedback category described by Branch and Paranjape is *major feedback*. This is a scheduled session, often at the midpoint of a learning experience, and adequate time is reserved. According to LCME Standard ED-31, "Each medical student in a medical education program should be assessed and provided with formal feedback early enough during each required course or clerkship (or, in Canada, clerkship rotation) to allow sufficient time for remediation." *Major feedback* should occur during a mid-clerkship feedback session. Depending on the length and structure of the clerkship, the mid-rotation feedback may need to occur more than once during different parts of the clinical experience. Consider creating a standardized form for mid-rotation feedback that correlates with the final evaluation form and maps to the course competencies and objectives. This gives students insight about their progress toward common clerkship goals.

13.5. Challenges in Giving Feedback

13.5.1. The Student Who Does Not Improve with Feedback

First, determine why the student failed to incorporate prior feedback. Was the barrier was cognitive or emotional? Did the student not recognize that he or she was receiving feedback? Does "not responding to feedback" mean that the student is resistant to receiving or incorporating feedback? Was the barrier on the teacher's side; i.e., was the feedback not provided effectively? By always labeling feedback explicitly as "feedback," we expect the student to recognize it, and that it is something to be incorporated into future performance. Asking the student if she or he "understands" the feedback may only prompt a deferential "yes" to the teacher. It is wise to have a follow-up question to confirm the desired understanding.

Resistant students can be challenging. One strategy is giving "feedback about the feedback." The process is the same as giving feedback alone, but with an emphasis on the importance of incorporating feedback. Students who consistently fail to respond to feedback from faculty or residents should be reported to the clerkship director. Students who are actively disrespectful about feedback should be counseled about their lack of professionalism and referred to the appropriate dean's office.

13.5.2. "Second-Hand" Feedback

Faculty and residents who see a behavior needing improvement may not have provided first-hand feedback to the student, but rather have contacted the clerkship director. As clerkship director, you may then have to provide what is called "second-hand feedback," i.e., feedback about something which you did not observe directly. When providing second-hand feedback it is important to have a clear understanding of the issues before meeting with the student. Request that the individual(s) who raised the concern document the issue(s) in writing. When meeting with the student, ask him or her to describe what happened from his or her perspective. Try giving feedback about behaviors and how they were perceived by the teachers who reported them to you. Do not make judgments about the learner's personality or assumed intent. Discussing behaviors in this way provides opportunities to help students gain insight into how they are perceived.

On the other hand, the term "second-hand feedback" is not always pejorative. Sometimes "direct" or first-hand feedback from a teacher working with the student might reflect the teacher's preferences, rather than be based on students' priority goals. In this case, feedback provided to the student by the clerkship director may be "second-hand" but synthesized and prioritized and therefore more important. Further, the second-hand feedback provided to students through the clerkship director may be more valid because it is based on priority goals for students. Second-hand feedback may reflect patterns distilled from the observations of several teachers that are integrated into multisource feedback provided by the clerkship director.

13.5.3. Issues Regarding Professionalism

Giving feedback on professionalism issues can be especially challenging, even for experienced clerkship directors. When there is a serious lapse in professionalism, it is important for the clerkship director to follow a consistent process. The clerkship director should gather as much information as possible about the concerning behavior, then meet with the student to hear the student's perspective about the possible deficiency. An action plan should be discussed, and the student should be held accountable for improvement. Depending on the nature of the offense, further action may be warranted (see also Chapter 12).

A second aspect of this issue is working with your faculty and residents to recognize professionalism issues and to help them learn how to provide corrective feedback. Professionalism issues are best handled promptly by the person who observed the behaviors in question. Always document in writing what took place during meetings regarding professional concerns and consider forwarding them to the dean's office. With serious or recurrent problem behaviors, strongly consider having a representative from the office of student affairs attend the meeting.

Finally, remember that teachers may have important observations about a student's professional behavior that have not been discussed with the student, or have not been written down on an evaluation form.[15] Therefore, a key aspect when preparing to give a student feedback is that current observations may be provisional. The key issue is student improvement following the feedback.

13.5.4. The Angry Learner

Before attempting to give feedback to an angry student, clarify with the student what you, as the clerkship director, perceive. The cause of anger should be addressed. Open approaches such as, "You seem angry; would you like to talk about it?" may be effective. Sometimes the student's behavior escalates to the point of being inappropriate. When this happens, it is critical to take control of the situation. There are several possible strategies. Talking with the student in a private setting is paramount. Have the student calm down and get control of emotions before the situation can be discussed. It is important to provide immediate feedback about how the anger or emotion impacts upon others' perceptions of the student's professionalism. Be prepared to answer the question, "What do you mean?" This is the opportunity to give the learner feedback about how to handle this type of situation in a more professional manner. It may be helpful to have a second person (e.g., clerkship administrator or chief resident) available to witness or take notes during emotional situations. In the rare situation when there is risk for escalation to a dangerous level, it may be wise to have someone ready to notify security. Eva and colleagues[9] found that some students go through a process similar to Kübler-Ross' stages of grief when hearing feedback which they perceive as unflattering: anger, denial, bargaining, depression, and finally acceptance. Within a supportive relationship, faculty can help the student to work through these stages, emphasizing their desire to help the student improve.

13.6. System Aspects of Feedback

13.6.1. Planning and Receiving Feedback about the Clerkship

In addition to having a feedback session to provide feedback to students at the end of the clerkship, periodically obtaining feedback from the students during the clerkship experience is also important. By soliciting feedback, students' concerns can be identified before major problems develop. Be open and receptive to their problems and even criticisms. Consider scheduling a time to meet with the students, or spend a few minutes before a conference, asking for feedback about how things are going or if there are any concerns or problems. Students are more likely to be open and honest in a group than individually. Group feedback gives you an opportunity to determine whether the issues are related to one or a few students, or if they are of a more general concern. It is a powerful improvement tool for the clerkship.

13.6.2. Feedback for Faculty

One of the most challenging and difficult situations for a clerkship director is to give feedback to senior faculty members.[16] The principles for providing the feedback are the same as for students. However, providing feedback in this setting will depend on your relationship with the colleague. If the person is receptive to feedback, focus the feedback on how the person can improve and not on interpersonal issues. If the person is not receptive, it may be best not to give feedback yourself, but to convey students' written evaluations of the teacher. One may simply forward students' written evaluations about their teachers to the faculty members with a comment containing reinforcing feedback ("very nice comments!") or a prompt to corrective action ("Are you surprised by this?").

A strategy to open the conversation might include: "As the clerkship director, I have a perspective of how students perceive your role as an attending physician. Would you like me to give you some feedback about their perceptions?" Focus the feedback on specific examples and observations. A key to providing effective feedback in this setting is your desire to help your colleagues improve. Try to concentrate on specific actions or behaviors that would help them improve, just as you would for a student. In 2013 van der Leeuw et al.[17] described how faculty responded to feedback from learners. In order to change in response to learner feedback, certain 'tipping points" must be reached which include recognition of need for change, developing a commitment to change, and emotional acceptance of the feedback. Faculty may also need help from clerkship directors and other educational leaders to facilitate setting goals and strategies for improvement. Clerkship directors can coach during faculty feedback sessions, much like the faculty coach the students.

13.6.3. Developing a Culture of Feedback

A common complaint from students is that they "never receive feedback." Changing the culture about feedback may be one of the most challenging endeavors for clerkship directors. Finding time for feedback is becoming more difficult. Consider encouraging faculty to have planned "feedback rounds" once a week ("Friday is for feedback") instead of teaching rounds. This provides the team with an opportunity to talk about what went well in the care of the patients for that week. In the case of an unexpected death or a transfer to the intensive care unit, the team can explore what, if anything, might have been done differently in patient care. Feedback rounds offer a chance to address issues or concerns that the team may be encountering. Attending physicians can also obtain feedback about their roles. With weekly feedback rounds, attendings can also meet individually with students and residents to give and receive feedback. Requiring the supervising faculty to complete and submit mid-rotation feedback forms is another way to ensure that all students receive feedback before the end of the clerkship.

13.6.4. Supporting Faculty

The same barriers that affect teachers' honest assessments of student performance affect their giving feedback to students. Clerkship directors and department chairs have to be alert to barriers in giving helpful feedback. These include cognitive barriers such as understanding student learning objectives and understanding educational terminology (e.g., competencies and milestones). Logistic barriers include having time for direct observation of students and time for feedback. Finally, acknowledge emotional barriers such as mentoring relationships with students and not wanting the learner to "feel bad."

Students are not always receptive to honest feedback. In a study by Boehler et al.,[18] one group of students was given specific suggestions to improve skills and another group received vague praise without specific improvement guidelines. Faculty who gave non-specific praise were rated more favorably by the students than those who gave specific suggestions in a neutral way without praise. Student satisfaction does not necessarily correlate with the quality of feedback, but feedback is correlated with learning.

The department chair is responsible to support teachers who provide honest assessment and feedback. The clerkship director is responsible to alert the chair about the time and training needed to support a culture of feedback.

References

1. Cantillon P, Sargeant J. Giving feedback in clinical settings. BMJ 2008;337:a1961.
2. Ericsson KA. Deliberate practice and the acquisition and maintenance of expert performance in medicine and related domains. Acad Med 2004;79(10 Suppl): S70-S81.
3. Westberg J, Jason H. Fostering Reflection and Providing Feedback: Helping Others Learn from Experience. New York: Springer, 2001.
4. Whitman NA, Schwenk TL. The Physician as Teacher - second edition - Salt Lake City: Whitman Associates, 1997.
5. Hewson MG, Little ML. Giving feedback in medical education: Verification of recommended techniques. J Gen Intern Med 1998;13(2):111-116.
6. Veloski J, Boex JR, Grasberger MJ, et al. Systematic review of the literature on assessment, feedback and physicians' clinical performance: BEME guide No. 7. Med Teach 2006;28(2):117-128.
7. van de Ridder JM, Stokking KM, McGaghie WC, ten Cate OT. What is feedback in clinical education? Med Educ. 2008;42(2):189-197.
8. Ende J. Feedback in clinical medical education. JAMA 1983;250(6):777-781.
9. Eva KW, Armson H, Holmboe ES, et al. Factors influencing responsiveness to feedback: On the interplay between fear, confidence, and reasoning processes. Adv Health Sci Educ Theory Pract 2012;17(1):15-26.
10. Chou CL, Masters DE, Chang A, et al. Effects of longitudinal small-group learning on delivery and receipt of communication skills feedback. Med Educ 2013;47(11): 1073-1079.
11. Gigante J, Dell M, Sharkey A. Getting beyond "Good job": How to give effective feedback. Pediatrics 2011;127(2):205-207.
12. Neher JO, Gordon KC, Meyer B, Stevens N. A five-step "microskills" model of clinical teaching. J Am Board Fam Pract 1992;5(4):419-424.
13. Lane JL, Gottlieb RP. Structured clinical observations: A method to teach clinical skills with limited time and financial resources. Pediatrics 2000;105(4 Pt 2):973-977.
14. Branch WT, Paranjape A. Feedback and reflection: Teaching methods for clinical settings. Acad Med 2002;77(12 Pt 1):1185-1188.
15. Hemmer PA, Hawkins R, Jackson JL, Pangaro LN. Assessing how well three evaluation methods detect deficiencies in medical students' professionalism in two settings of an internal medicine clerkship. Acad Med. 2000;75(2):167-173.
16. Litzelman DK, Stratos GA, Marriott DJ, et al. Beneficial and harmful effects of

augmented feedback on physicians' clinical-teaching performances. Acad Med 1998;73(3):324-332.
17. van der Leeuw RM, Slootweg IA, Heineman MJ, Lombarts KMJMH. Explaining how faculty members act upon residents' feedback to improve their teaching performance. Med Educ 2013;47(11):1089-1098.
18. Boehler ML, Rogers DA, Schwind CJ, et al. An investigation of medical student reactions to feedback: A randomised controlled trial. Med Educ 2006;40(8):746-749.

Section Three

Chapter 14
Introduction to Section Three: Structured Assessments for Clerkships

William C. McGaghie, Ph.D.

This section has four chapters that together address structured assessments for clerkships in medical education. The term, "structured," is used liberally, chiefly to mean that these assessments typically take place in controlled classroom or simulation center settings. This contrasts with medical student assessments covered in Section Two that usually occur in inpatient or outpatient clinical environments. The separation of student assessments in classrooms vs. clinics is deliberate because variation in control within assessment settings affects data reliability and the accuracy of the decisions that the data allow. As a general rule, greater environmental control leads to higher data reliability and the ability to make more granular decisions about medical student achievement.

Chapter 15, by Thomas Sisson and Cyril Grum, addresses clerkship examinations, which are typically composed of MCQs, measures of medical student knowledge acquisition. This chapter discusses the purposes of clerkship examinations and two principal sources of these tests: (a) NBME subject examinations, a.k.a., shelf tests; and (b) faculty generated examinations (FGEs). We are reminded that FGEs may be composed not only from MCQs but also from other test procedures, including essays and other open-ended formats, oral examinations, OSCEs, and script concordance tests. The chapter concludes with a set of six "lessons learned" from research on clerkship examinations.

Chapter 16, by Ruth-Marie Fincher and Robert Nesbit, is about writing MCQs. The ubiquity of MCQs demands that their preparation, editing, tryout, and use should be done with great care and attention to detail to ensure accurate medical student assessment. Fincher and Nesbit provide simple, useful rules for constructing MCQs in a variety of formats. They provide examples of both good and flawed MCQs to teach readers how to discriminate useful test items from questions having little or no value. The chapter concludes with a tabular presentation of MCQ writing guidelines and suggestions for clerkship educators who evaluate medical students using this technology.

Chapter 17, by Michael Ainsworth and Karen Szauter, covers SP-based assessment of clinical skills in clerkships. The word "standardized" is especially important here because it denotes uniformity of patient presentations in the context of medical student assessment which contributes to data reliability and valid decisions about students. Ainsworth and Szauter focus on the utility of SP-based assessments to evaluate students' clinical skills, reminding readers of the importance of matching evaluation goals and tools. The authors describe how to design an SP-based assessment, detail resource requirements for these tests, address benefits and limitations of SP test formats, discuss costs, and briefly cover SP-based assessment research and how to build SP-based assessments into a comprehensive medical student evaluation program.

Chapter 18, "Assessment Using Simulation Technologies," is by Keith Muccino and Viva Jo Siddall. Medical simulation is a recent addition to the family of medical student assessment technologies, so the chapter serves as a primer for most readers. Muccino and Siddall begin by locating medical simulation in its educational context and proceed to cover optional ways to use simulation for student assessment. They continue with a rationale for simulation-based assessment; the notion that evaluation form follows function; and discussions about feasibility, novel driving forces, and simulation to evaluate student readiness for residency. They complete the chapter by describing the utility of simulation to address the Milestones Project and the AAMC-endorsed EPAs movement, then offering concluding remarks.

The four chapters in Section Three on structured assessments for clerkships give practical advice to medical educators who evaluate students routinely. They remind readers that routine assessments should also be robust, whether they are used for formative (evaluation for learning) or summative (evaluation of learning) purposes.

Chapter 15
Clerkship Examinations

Thomas Sisson, M.D.
Cyril Grum, M.D.

End-of-clerkship examinations should be part of the evaluation process for all medical students in core clerkships. This chapter discusses the use of written examinations, whether MCQ format examinations or exams requiring constructed responses. The context is clinical clerkships, yet the general considerations here are applicable to the pre- and post-clerkship periods. These examinations should complement students' clinical evaluations by attending physicians, preceptors, and house officers. Clerkship directors agree that observed clinical performance should contribute the greatest weight to each student's overall grade, with the end-of-clerkship objective examinations constituting a smaller (e.g., 20%-35%) part of a comprehensive evaluation process.

15.1. Purposes of Clerkship Examinations

Clerkship examinations motivate students to study and practice essential clinical skills. Assessment methods and their content drive student learning more than any other stimulus; therefore, assessment methods and content should reflect clerkship learning objectives. Clerkship directors should test memory and recall if the goal for students is to memorize and recall clinical facts. The NBME subject tests motivate students to read and improve their knowledge base. These examinations also emphasize that having a core knowledge base and the ability to apply knowledge to clinical situations is a critical part of clinical competence. However, many skills, including history taking, physical examination, communication, and procedural proficiency, cannot be assessed using multiple choice tests. Thus different test formats are needed to assess and to motivate acquisition of these skills.

Beyond motivating students to study, end-of-clerkship examinations are needed to evaluate key features of students' competence. For example, examinations covering electrocardiogram (ECG) and chest x-ray (CXR) interpretation, and recognition of heart sounds can show that students are learning these core competencies. Many clerkship directors require students to pass these examinations. Clerkship examinations also separate students (i.e., identify the top and bottom performers) for grading and other purposes. Finally, in addition to evaluating students, end-of-clerkship examinations are useful to judge the effectiveness of the clerkship curriculum and the extent to which a local curriculum meets national standards.

This chapter does not discuss the requirements for support of examinations within a larger assessment system. Department chairs or the medical school dean's office should provide clerical support for examination administration, security, and recordkeeping in addition to securing faculty time and money needed to purchase or administer external examinations.

15.2. Assessment Options

Clerkship directors in the U.S. typically have two categories of assessment options for written examinations: (a) nationally developed examinations, such as the subject examinations from the NBME, and (b) faculty generated examinations (FGEs).

15.2.1. NBME Subject Examinations

The NBME subject tests are high-quality, psychometrically sound, clinical-vignette-based multiple choice examinations. They are nationally recognized tests that assess student knowledge in a clinical specialty. Tests are available for all core clinical disciplines. The exams focus on knowledge application and integration rather than recall of isolated facts. The NBME subject exams reflect each medical specialty's priorities for the USMLE Step 2 CK examination. For instance, the NBME subject exam in internal medicine identifies medical students who are at risk of poor performance on USMLE Step 2 CK.[1] A key feature of the subject tests is that they have excellent psychometric properties. The reliability (typically, 0.75 to 0.85), validity, and standardization of these examinations add to their desirability as an assessment method.[2] Since these exams are administered on computers, their results are available to clerkship directors very quickly. Furthermore, the use of a national examination allows clerkship directors to gauge the performance of their students against national norms.

The NBME subject examination program makes subject tests available to all 141 (as of May 8, 2015) U.S. medical schools. In 2013, 145,000 subject examinations were administered in the clinical sciences <www.nbme.org/PDF/Publications/2013Annual-Report.pdf> (accessed May 8, 2015). Based on the 2007 and 2009 surveys of internal medicine (IM) clerkship directors, about 90% of IM clerkships use the NBME medicine subject exam at the end of the clerkship.[3,4]

Subject examinations for core clinical clerkships (neurology, family medicine, medicine, obstetrics/gynecology, pediatrics, psychiatry, surgery) have been available for decades. The NBME also offers adult ambulatory medicine and adult and pediatric ambulatory medicine examinations. Recently added are advanced clinical examinations in internal medicine, surgery, pediatrics, and emergency medicine, designed to measure the effectiveness of subinternship or M4 experiences.

Questions often arise about how the NBME subject tests are developed and who writes the questions. Using internal medicine as an example, a committee of clerkship directors and residency program directors generate the questions. These medical educators have extensive experience with students and residents. The goal of the writing committee is to create questions that a new intern in internal medicine should answer correctly. This intern has graduated from medical school and is ready for specialty training supervised by more senior residents and attending physicians.

A description of the NBME subject examination program can be found at <www.nbme.org/PDF/SubjectExams/subexaminfoguide.pdf> (accessed May 8, 2015). The distribution of subject test questions is confidential to preserve test integrity. A general scheme about the distribution of subject exam questions and sample questions can be found at <www.nbme.org/PDF/SubjectExams/SE_ContentOutlineandSampleItems.pdf> (accessed May 8, 2015).

The NBME subject examination program provides extensive feedback to schools and students. The *Score Interpretation Guide* for examinees gives information about the exam, the precision of scores, and a performance profile of the major content areas of the exam. For schools, the *Score Interpretation Guide* includes national means and data about the rise in scores as the academic year progresses. For the first quarter of academic year 2012-2013, the national mean score for examinees taking the internal medicine exam was 78.1 ± 8.1, which rose to 79.4 ± 8.0 for students taking the test during the last academic quarter. Grading guidelines assist clerkship directors to set passing scores, although a passing standard is always at the discretion of individual schools. A 2009 standard-setting study of twenty-five internal medicine clerkship directors recommended a passing score of 65 using the modified Angoff procedure and a score of 66 using the Hofstee compromise procedure.[5] The content area item analysis report describes the content of each item, along with the percentage of examinees from each medical school answering the item correctly. This allows clerkship directors to identify specific areas where their students are strong or weak. Fees for the administration of the 2015-2016 Clinical Subject exam are $42.00 per test per examinee. The fee structure is posted at <www.nbme.org/Schools/Subject-Exams/Fees2.html> (accessed May 8, 2015).

NBME exams must be proctored. Extensive information is available at the NBME Web site for subject exams: <www.nbme.org/Schools/Subject-Exams/index.html> (accessed May 8, 2015).

The NBME has moved all of its subject exams to a Web-based format. Paper versions of the subject examinations will continue to be available through 2015. Multiple forms of each exam are available for use in successive courses or clerkships <www.nbme.org/Schools/Subject-Exams/index.html> (accessed May 8, 2015).

Clerkship directors need to recognize areas of competency that NBME subject tests do *not* address. Specifically, the NBME subject exams do not cover clinical skill acquisition and professional or personal attributes. Subject tests permit student comparison with a national standard, but do not evaluate whether the local curriculum is delivered effectively. Therefore, clerkship directors should consider supplementing the NBME subject test with locally generated examinations that are tailored to the goals and objectives of their individual clerkships.

The number of clerkship directors who use the NBME medicine subject test has increased over the past twenty years.[3,6-8] Reasons for using NBME subject tests include the hard work and time needed to create local examinations that yield reliable data to contribute to student evaluation. It is difficult to link the content of NBME subject exam questions to core clerkship objectives. However, agreement between NBME test committees and local medical educators is likely, because both groups feel that students should be tested on common problems that they are likely to see in an undifferentiated U.S. medical practice. The subject test template and the learning objectives identified in the *Core [Internal] Medicine Clerkship Curriculum Guide* are similar.[9] The Society for General Internal Medicine (SGIM)'s and the CDIM's *Core Medicine Clerkship Curriculum Guide* (2006) can be found at <www.im.org/p/cm/ld/fid=657>, <connect.im.org/p/cm/ld/fid=385>, or <connect.im.org/d/do/2285> (all accessed May 12, 2015).

The NBME has expressed interest in working with clerkship directors to develop examinations that satisfy clerkship needs.[10] Clerkship directors often serve on NBME item-writing committees. Involvement of clerkship directors in the development of subject exams ensures that questions are relevant and target the appropriate difficulty level.

The NBME subject exam contributes 20%-25% of each student's final grade in most internal medicine clerkships.[3,4] Eighty-nine percent of clerkships allow students to retake the exam if they fail it on the first attempt.[3] Most clerkships forbid additional retests after a second failure. Students who fail a subject exam taken again often receive a failing clerkship grade and undergo remediation.

15.2.2. Faculty-Generated Examinations (FGEs)

There are several options available within FGEs including (a) one-best answer multiple choice examinations, (b) essay and other open-ended formats, (c) oral examinations, (d) OSCEs, and (e) SCT. Here we discuss examination formats; standard setting for FGEs is discussed at length in Chapter 19.

15.2.2.a. One-Best-Answer Multiple Choice Examinations

Faculty-generated written examinations to test knowledge and its application can be based on multiple choice or extended matching item formats. Both formats use patient case vignettes. These locally generated examinations have the advantage of testing specific knowledge and clinical skills relevant to a single clerkship within a singular curriculum. Therefore, local examinations should have high local content validity (e.g., tick-borne RMSF in the southeast U.S.). On the other hand, assuring acceptable reliability and validity from in-house examinations is difficult. We emphasize that assessments should be included in an annual review process in which data for reliability, validity, and impact are reviewed as they relate to curricular planning and educational goals.[11] Are the exams sufficiently reliable and valid for their purpose? Would additional resources improve the exams or not? These considerations apply whether the exams are written, oral, or practical.

Another attractive feature of locally generated examinations is that they may be based on different premises and may test different characteristics than NBME subject tests. As one example, a locally generated diagnostic pattern recognition examination, administered at the end of the clerkship, featured brief patient vignettes that described classic presentations of common diseases seen in the local community.[12] Students identified the correct diagnosis from an extended matching list of between sixteen and twenty-six diagnoses. The overall correlation with the NBME medicine subject test was quite high, although about 10% of students performed about a standard deviation higher and 10% a standard deviation lower than on the subject test. This suggests that student ability to recognize common diagnostic problems may be independent of their ability to perform well on a knowledge-based examination, such as the NBME medical subject test.

There are several potential disadvantages of locally generated examinations, e.g., the psychometric characteristics (especially reliability) are often poor, questions may be included that have not been previously validated, and question quality may vary. Test construction and grading demand faculty time and effort, which may be difficult to fund. Furthermore, many faculty have not been trained in examination development or question writing and cannot be expected to write high-quality questions. Poor questions that do not reflect important content help only testwise students and do not assess overall student knowledge or knowledge application. Finally, local examinations cannot be used to determine student performance against national standards.

Despite these drawbacks, having an examination process that includes both the NBME subject exam and a locally generated examination has pedagogic appeal. Local examinations have content validity and may make students confident that they are being examined about material that their own faculty judges important. In addition, use of local examinations reinforces the educational mission of all medical centers and reminds faculty that student evaluation is a key part of the overall teaching mission. In a 2009 survey of internal medicine clerkship directors, 33% indicated they used locally developed exams, most using these faculty-written exams *in addition to* the NBME subject exam. Most (70%) reported using locally developed exams to cover content felt to be underrepresented by the NBME.[13]

Chapter 16 provides guidance about writing examination questions. Clerkship directors who want to build a local multiple choice examination can use a manual that informs writing quality questions: *Constructing Written Test Questions for the Basic and Clinical Sciences* - third edition, revised - (2002), available for free at the NBME Web site <www.nbme.org/publications/item-writing-manual.html> (accessed May 12, 2015). This manual covers issues about technical item flaws and problems with item content, helps staff to review statistical indices of item quality after test administration, and provides an overview of standard setting techniques.

The NBME also presents item-writing workshops to help faculty write high-quality MCQs. These workshops are available by special arrangement and usually take place at a host medical school.

15.2.2.b. Essay and Other Open-Ended Formats

Faculty-generated essay questions and other open-ended question formats have educational appeal. Since the students are not selecting from among preset choices, these may be referred to as constructed response formats.

However, unless there is only a small group of students per rotation, or faculty who are extremely motivated to grade examinations, the time-intensive nature of these examinations makes them less feasible. In addition, it is very difficult to ensure reliability in scoring open-ended responses.[14,15]

15.2.2.c. Oral Examinations

Faculty-administered oral examinations were once used exclusively as the end-of-clerkship assessment. They are now used rarely, due to the difficulty of achieving sufficient reliability and because of faculty time demands, whether for rater training or to administer the exam.

Oral examinations can assess a student's ability to reason and solve problems. This approach can also assess overall factual knowledge. However, factual knowledge assessment by oral examinations is less precise than by written examinations, whether they are from the NBME or generated locally. The logistics of giving an oral examination, estimating reliability, and judging score validity can be daunting. Low reliability has many sources. Oral examinations usually allow time for students to tackle only one or two clinical scenarios. Student ability to perform well in these scenarios may reflect only student experience with a similar patient during a clinical rotation.

Overall class performance on oral examinations may be an indicator of the class's experience and level of competence. In contrast, an individual student may score high or low on the examination, based on prior exposure to clinical material, which may have been random, and the results may be a poor reflection of overall ability. Oral examinations are often given by many faculty, leading to variability in student assessment by examiners.[16] Furthermore, few faculty examiners have been trained to administer oral examinations, and typically, limited effort has been made to ensure examiner standardization. These factors all contribute to low interrater reliability. The time-consuming nature of oral examinations for faculty and students adds to their unpopularity. On the other hand, oral examinations can be a powerful motivating force for students to study and review core material.

If an oral examination is used, it is wise to limit its scope and boost its standardization. For example, students may be asked to submit a list of patient problems encountered on a particular rotation. The faculty member limits the oral examination to questions about these specific clinical problems. Oral examinations are currently used much less frequently than NBME subject tests or local written examinations. When oral examinations are used, they are usually weighted less for determining grades than other examinations.

15.2.2.d. Objective Structured Clinical Examinations (OSCEs)

An OSCE is a practical examination that assesses student performance of specific clinical skills and often involves the use of SPs. This assessment method is now in widespread use. An OSCE is a viable method for assessing clinical and interpersonal skills that cannot be assessed using multiple choice examinations.[17] Further discussion of examinations using SPs and other methods is in Chapters 17 and 18. (Standardized observation of procedural skills is discussed in Chapter 10.)

OSCEs are becoming increasingly popular to assess clinical skills at the end of clerkships, because attending physicians and house officers perceive them as being more objective than subjective ratings.[18,19] The addition of an OSCE component to the USMLE Step 2 CS during 2004-2005 underscores the popularity and acceptance of this technique. The presence of the USMLE Step 2 CS exam has encouraged development of OSCEs at medical schools. Background research by the NBME before implementation of the clinical skills exam indicated that the public feels strongly that clinical skills are necessary for each physician and should be tested.

Students, faculty, and the public have the perception that OSCEs test essential clinical skills for physicians. As a result, OSCE face validity is high.[20] In addition, OSCE high face validity is because the cases simulate experiences that students have encountered during clinical rotations and address core competencies necessary for internship and beyond. OSCEs can be designed to test any facet of student clinical skills, including ability to take a directed history, perform various aspects of the physical exam, interpret laboratory and x-ray studies, and make decisions about specific clinical problems.[21] In their simplest form, OSCEs can present clinical case scenarios, including laboratory data, chest x-rays, EKGs, and photographs of clinical findings, without including SPs.

OSCEs are labor-intensive and costly, because SPs must be recruited, trained, and compensated. SPs are individuals taught to simulate a particular disease presentation or who have stable physical findings. Although many clerkships have added an OSCE as an end-of-clerkship examination, it may be less expensive and time-consuming to administer a cross-clerkship OSCE at the end of the third year. In addition, a centralized, multidisciplinary examination is likely to be of higher quality than a department-based end-of-clerkship examination.

15.2.2.e. Script Concordance Testing

In addition to assessing medical knowledge and clinical competence, clerkship directors may choose to evaluate the development of clinical reasoning skills among students. SCT is a mechanism to address this goal. These tests are standardized, objective, and evaluate reasoning about clinical data interpretation. In SCT, examinees are presented with a clinical scenario and are asked to make diagnostic, investigative, or therapeutic decisions as additional information is revealed. The clinical data are typically ambiguous, and there is no one best answer, even among experts presented with the same information. Possible answers, or decisions, that an examinee might select in response to the clinical information are determined by a panel of experts (typically ten to twenty experienced physicians). All answers individually chosen by experts are accepted as valid. The particular answer chosen by the most experts is given the highest score and the answer chosen by the second most experts is given the next highest score, and so on. How closely the decision making of the examinee matches a panel of experts who are presented with the same clinical information determines the score. Thus, SCT is an assessment that compares the degree of agreement among answers selected by examinees with answers selected by an expert panel. Ultimately, this test has appeal because the cognitive tasks used to evaluate the ambiguous clinical scenarios are the same tasks employed daily in practice.[22]

For clerkship directors wishing to administer SCT, we refer them to articles which detail the key elements of question development.[23,24] In general, the first step in writing questions is to determine the purpose of the exam. For example, is SCT evaluating professional development or is it designed to assess learning achievement at the end of a clerkship? It is also important to decide whether the test is meant to discriminate among the examinees. If student discrimination is the goal, SCT should include questions of medium difficulty, so that the variance of examinees' scores will be maximized. By contrast, if SCT is designed to identify areas of weakness among low-ability students, then the test should be composed mostly of relatively easy questions.

A second important step in designing SCT is to write questions that contain uncertainty. Research shows that questions which lead to variable answers within the expert panel are more effective to detect levels of clinical experience in a group of examinees. The desire for uncertainty in SCT is different from that in MCQs, where uncertainty results in poor quality.

A third issue in developing SCT is the size and composition of the expert panel to score the exam. Studies have shown that fifteen panel members are required to obtain acceptable reliability estimates for high-stakes exams. On the other hand, a smaller panel with less than ten members may be reasonable for a lower-stakes exam. The composition of the panel is also important. Student or resident performance should be compared with that of a group of physicians who best represent the target area of competency. For example, if one wishes to assess the decision making of a student on an internal medicine rotation with respect to a pulmonary scenario, it may be more reasonable to populate the panel of experts with general internists or perhaps internal medicine residents, but not pulmonologists.

The performance of SCT to assess clinical decision making has been evaluated in several studies. For example, SCT was used to evaluate medical decision making among twenty poorly performing family practitioners in Québec.[25] These physicians underwent a structured daylong interview to assess their competence and were also given SCT. Three investigators reviewed the structured interviews and rated the physicians as being above or below the median for the group. The examinees were also divided into two groups, based on their SCT performance. Investigators then assessed the correlation between the two methods of evaluation. Agreement between the two methods of evaluation occurred in thirteen of twenty cases, but disagreement in the other seven. Overall, the poorly performing physicians, with one exception, scored two standard deviations below the panel of experts on SCT, indicating significant deficiencies. The investigators concluded that adding SCT to other evaluations is helpful in discerning decision making weakness in physicians. Evidence for its use at the student level is still preliminary.

15.3. Lessons from Research on Clerkship Exams

15.3.1. Clerkship Characteristics and Student Examination Performance

Griffith and colleagues at seventeen medical schools studied which clerkship characteristics were associated with enhanced student exam performance on the NBME subject exam and USMLE Step 2 exam.[5] These authors also analyzed the characteristics relative to the change in a student's score from USMLE Step 1 to USMLE Step 2. In their study, the factors associated with a higher mean exam score included a larger number of small group hours per week and the use of community-based preceptors. Significant improvements in USMLE Step 1 to USMLE Step 2 scores were associated with a greater number of patients per day cared for by the third year medical students. In addition, higher NBME subject exam scores were associated with greater length of rounds with the attending and the use of computer-based instruction. Also, higher USMLE Step 2 scores were associated with longer attending rotations (four weeks vs. two weeks) and the use of hospitalists. The most consistent finding was the association of more patients cared for per day with higher exam performance.

15.3.2. Relevance of NBME Subject Tests

Although the clinical relevance of NBME subject tests has not been directly assessed, the similarities between USMLE Step 2 and the subject exam allow several inferences. The validity of USMLE Step 2 CK has been analyzed by addressing the degree to which experts view exam content as clinically relevant and appropriate to the level of examinee.[26] The underlying principle of USMLE Step 2 is to assess whether an individual can apply medical knowledge, skills, and an understanding of clinical science material to the provision of safe and effective patient care under supervision. The prototype person is a new intern on the first day of internship. Cuddy and colleagues[26] asked 27 experts to rate the clinical relevance and propriety of 150 questions individually. They demonstrated that 92% of these experts saw the item content as clinically relevant, 90% saw it as appropriate for Step 2, and 85% recognized its use in clinical practice. A regression analysis indicated that difficult items and frequently used items were considered more appropriate for Step 2. Overall, the results showed that the majority of content is clinically relevant and appropriate, providing important validation for the USMLE Step 2 exam.

The NBME subject examination performance from six clerkships was correlated with the USMLE Step 1 and Step 2 CK examination scores of 507 students. A moderate to large correlation between subject exam performance and USMLE scores provides reassurance that subject exam scores are associated with USMLE performance.[27]

15.3.3. NBME Subject Exam to Assess Knowledge Acquisition

NBME subject examinations and end-of-clerkship examinations reflect cumulative knowledge, including knowledge acquired from basic science courses and prior clinical experiences. Therefore, they are not simply assessments of knowledge acquired during particular clerkships. To determine what knowledge was acquired during a clerkship itself, assessment of prior knowledge or control for prior experience must be determined. In practice, this is usually done only for medical education research purposes. One approach to this issue is to evaluate student subject test performance based on the timing of the clerkship and use a "normative" method to compare one student with others taking the clerkship at the same time. Research on this subject has produced uneven results.

In one study, different versions of the NBME subject test were given on the first and last day of a medicine clerkship to all students over two consecutive years.[8] Students' mean scores were equally low at the start of the clerkship, regardless of when they took the clerkship or which other clerkships they had previously taken. However, students in the second half of the year had greater improvement in performance from the beginning to the end of the clerkship than their colleagues in the first half of the year. The experience of many clerkship directors nationally has shown that student performance on the NBME subject tests and other exams tends to be better as students progress through their clinical year.[2,28-30] Since this reflects higher student achievement later in the year, a "criterion-based" system of evaluation would accept a rise in clerkship grades later in the year as a reflection of more student experience.

15.3.4. NBME Subject Exam as an Evaluation Tool

The NBME subject examination might be one of the more discriminating indicators for calculating student grades.[31] In an ob/gyn clerkship, a student's final grade was calculated by weighing clinical performance 60%, formal presentation 10%, an oral exam 10%, and the NBME subject test score 20%. Of these four indicators, only the NBME subject exam score was normally distributed. The clinical performance score and the formal presentation scores were highly skewed, while the oral examination scores were slightly skewed. The NBME subject exam was the most highly correlated ($r = 0.86$) with the overall clerkship performance, much higher than the clinical performance, formal presentation score, or oral examination. The NBME subject exam explained 74% of the variance in the overall clerkship performance. The results are likely applicable to other clerkships.

Despite the practice in most internal medicine clerkships to weigh the NBME subject exam about 20% to 25% of each student's final grade, grading committees might give excessive weight to exam scores. One study proposed that clerkship grading committees should derive students' clinical scores while blinded to examination scores.[32]

15.3.5. Multimedia Formats

Since the advent of computer-based testing for USMLE in 1999, the NBME has worked toward increasing the authenticity with which patient situations are described by incorporating multimedia into test questions. Holtzman and colleagues examined the impact of presenting cardiac auscultation findings in a multimedia format vs. text format.[33] The multimedia items were significantly more difficult for students than matched text versions. Multimedia items were also less discriminating and required more testing time. Multimedia presentations were introduced into the USMLE licensing exam in 2007. As the NBME has changed subject exams to a Web-based format, we expect multimedia formats to become an increasing part of the subject exam series.

15.3.6. Timing

The NBME subject exams are designed for standardized administration. They must be proctored and have a set time limit. The time limit on NBME subject exams is comparable to that on USMLE Step 2. Adherence to the time prescription allows the test results to be compared on a national level. Clerkships that allow students more time than prescribed for the exam need to recognize that they cannot compare their results to national standards. Cuddy and colleagues have shown that examinees who receive more time per item generally outperform examinees who receive less time per item.[34]

15.3.7. In-Clerkship Examinations

In-clerkship exams have been assessed to see if they can identify students with insufficient knowledge during the medicine clerkship.[35-37] This concept is similar to the in-training evaluation that is a common feature in internal medicine residency programs. In-clerkship tests have identified students who are at risk of failing an end-of-clerkship examination. Unfortunately, counseling did not improve final examination pass rates.[36]

References

1. Ripkey DR, Case SM, Swanson DB. Identifying students at risk for poor performance on the USMLE Step 2. Acad Med. 1999;74(10 Suppl):S45-S48.
2. Ripkey DR, Case SM, Swanson DB. Predicting performance on the NBME surgery subject test and USMLE Step 2: The effects of surgery clerkship timing and length. Acad Med. 1997;72(10 Suppl):S31-S33.
3. Torre D, Papp KK, Elnicki M, Durning S. Clerkship directors' practices with respect to preparing students for and using the National Board of Medical Examiners Subject Exam in Medicine: Results of a United States and Canadian survey. Acad Med. 2009;84(7):867-871.

4. Fazio SB, Papp KK, Torre DM, DeFer TM. Grade inflation in the internal medicine clerkship: A national survey. Teach Learn Med 2013;25(1):71-76.
5. Griffith CH, Wilson JF, Haist SA, et al. Internal medicine clerkship characteristics associated with enhanced student examination performance. Acad Med 2009; 84(7):895-901.
6. Hemmer PA, Szauter K, Allbritton TA, Elnicki DM. Internal medicine clerkship directors' use of and opinions about clerkship examinations. Teach Learn Med 2002;14(4):229-235.
7. Magarian GJ, Mazur DJ. A national survey of grading systems used in medicine clerkships. Acad Med 1990;65(10):637-639.
8. Magarian GJ, Mazur DJ. Does performance on the NBME Part II medicine examination when used as a clerkship examination reflect knowledge acquired during the medicine clerkship? J Gen Intern Med. 1991;6(2):145-149.
9. Bass EB, Fortin AH, Morrison G, et al. National survey of clerkship directors in internal medicine on the competencies that should be addressed in the medicine core clerkship. Am J Med 1997;102(6):564-571.
10. Elnicki DM, Lescisin DA, Case S. Improving the National Board of Medical Examiners internal medicine subject exam for use in clerkship evaluation. J Gen Intern Med 2002;17(6):435-440.
11. van der Vleuten CPM, Schuwirth LW. Assessing professional competence: From methods to programmes. Med Educ 2005;39(3):309-317.
12. Grum CM, Case SM, Swanson DB, Woolliscroft JO. Identifying the trees in the forest: Characteristics of students who demonstrate disparity between knowledge and diagnostic pattern recognition skills. Acad Med 1994;69(10 Suppl):S66-S68.
13. Kelly WF, Papp KK, Torre D, Hemmer PA. How and why internal medicine clerkship directors use locally developed, faculty-written examinations: Results of a national survey. Acad Med 2012;87(7):924-930.
14. Norcini JJ, Diserens D, Day SC, et al. The scoring and reproducibility of an essay test of clinical judgment. Acad Med 1990;65(9 Suppl):S41-S42.
15. Day SC, Norcini JJ, Diserens D, et al. The validity of an essay test of clinical judgment. Acad Med 1990;65(9 Suppl):S39-S40.
16. Houston JE, Myford CM. Judges' perception of candidates' organization and communication in relation to oral certification examination ratings. Acad Med 2009;84(11):1603-1609.
17. van der Vleuten CPM, Swanson DB. Assessment of clinical skills with standardized patients: State of the art. Teach Learn Med 1990;2(2):58-76.
18. Elnicki DM, Shockcor WT, Morris DK, Halbritter KA. Creating an objective structured clinical examination for the internal medicine clerkship: Pitfalls and benefits. Am Med Sci 1993;306(2):94-97.
19. Ramsey PG, Shannon NF, Fleming L, et al. Use of objective examinations in medicine clerkships: Ten-year experience. Am J Med 1986;81(4):669-674.
20. Ainsworth MA, Roger LP, Markus JF, et al. Standardized patient encounters: A method for teaching and evaluation. JAMA 1991;266(10):1390-1396.
21. Rosebraugh CJ, Speer AJ, Solomon DJ., et al. Setting standards and defining quality of performance in the validation of a standardized-patient examination format. Acad Med 1997;72(11):1012-1014.
22. Kelly WF, Durning SJ, Denton GD. Comparing a script concordance examination to a multiple choice examination on a core internal medicine clerkship. Teach Learn Med 2012;24(3):187-193.
23. Fournier JP, Demeester A, Charlin B. Script concordance tests: Guidelines for construction. BMC Med Inform Decis Making 2008;8:18. <www.biomedcentral.

com/1472-6947/8/18>. Accessed May 14, 2015.
24. Charlin B, Roy L, Brailovsky C, et al. The script concordance test: A tool to assess the reflective clinician. Teach Learn Med 2000;12(4):189-195.
25. Goulet F, Jacques A, Gagnon R, et al. Poorly performing physicians: Does the script concordance test detect bad clinical reasoning? J Contin Educ Health Prof 2010;39(3):161-166.
26. Cuddy MM, Dillon GF, Clauser BE, et al. Assessing the validity of the USMLE Step 2 Clinical Knowledge examination through an evaluation of its clinical relevance. Acad Med 2004;79(10 Suppl):S43-S45.
27. Zahn CM, Saguil A, Artino AR, et al. Correlation of National Board of Medical Examiners scores with United States Medical Licensing Examination Step 1 and Step 2 scores. Acad Med 2012;87(10):1348-1354.
28. Jackson JR, Scott LK, Dismukes WE. The relationship between prior clerkship experience and student performance in medicine clerkships: Implications for grading. Med Educ 1982;16(3):133-136.
29. Baciewicz FA, Arent L, Weaver M, et al. Influence of clerkship structure and timing on individual student performance. Am J Surg 1990;159(2):265-268.
30. Kies SM, Roth V, Rowland M. Association of third-year medical students' first clerkship with overall clerkship performance and examination scores. JAMA 2010;304(11):1220-1226.
31. Nahum GG. Evaluating medical student obstetrics and gynecology clerkship performance: Which assessment tools are most reliable? Am J Obstet Gynecol 2004;191(5):1762-1771.
32. Lurie SJ, Mooney CJ. Assessing a method to limit influence of standardized tests on clerkship grades. Teach Learn Med 2012;24(4):287-291.
33. Holtzman KZ, Swanson DB, Ouyang W, et al. Use of multimedia on the Step 1 and Step 2 Clinical Knowledge components of USMLE: A controlled trial of the impact on item characteristics. Acad Med. 2009;84(10 Suppl):S90-S93.
34. Cuddy MM, Swanson DB, Dillon GF, et al. A multilevel analysis of the relationships between selected examinee characteristics and United States Medical Licensing Examination Step 2 Clinical Knowledge performance: Revisiting old findings and asking new questions. Acad Med 2006;81(10 Suppl):S103-S107.
35. Hemmer PA, Pangaro LN. The effectiveness of formal evaluation sessions during clinical clerkships in better identifying students with marginal funds of knowledge. Acad Med 1997;72(7):641-643.
36. Hemmer PA, Markert RJ, Wood V. Using in-clerkship tests to identify students with insufficient knowledge and assessing the effect of counseling on final examination performance. Acad Med. 1999;74(1):73-75.
37. Parenti CM. A process for identifying marginal performers among students in a clerkship. Acad Med. 1993;68(7):575-577.

Chapter 16
Writing Multiple Choice Questions

Ruth-Marie E. Fincher, M.D.
Robert R. Nesbit, Jr., M.D.

Many clerkship directors use locally constructed exams as part of their students' evaluations. Use of multiple choice questions is the most efficient way to create such exams. All faculty who write multiple choice questions (items) should master the principles of item-writing.[1,2] The purpose of this section is to help faculty to write multiple choice items that evaluate student knowledge and ability to apply knowledge to clinical situations.[3] We will emphasize the NBME multiple choice item formats, including extended matching questions, that enable item-writers to create items that simulate real clinical case decisions.

An excellent resource is *Constructing Written Test Questions for the Basic and Clinical Sciences* by Case and Swanson, available for download from the NBME at <www.nbme.org/publications/item-writing-manual.html>[4] (accessed May 8, 2015). The guidelines endorse only "one best answer" (Type A and matching) items. We discuss only these formats. We do not cover obsolete multiple choice item types such as K-type (1, 2 and 3 only, 1 and 3, etc.), multiple true/false, or "A-B-Both-Neither." Table 16 summarizes recommendations to avoid common mistakes that make questions less valid.

16.1. Multiple Choice, One-Best-Answer Items

Multiple choice, one-best-answer items require the student to select the single *best* response. A knowledgeable student should be able to determine the correct answer without looking at the option list. There are two types of one-best-answer items:
- *Single stem items* (Type A) have a single stem, the lead-in (actual question), and usually four or five response options.
- *Extended Matching* (Type R) items have a theme, a lead-in statement, and a set of two to ten stems and up to 26 options. Extended matching items are no longer used on USMLE Step 1 exams, but are used on USMLE Step 2 CK exams.

Both items types can test recall or application of clinical knowledge. We believe it is better to test application of knowledge than just information recall.

16.2. Recall vs. Application of Knowledge Examples
Example # 1: Recall

Which of the following is the most common physical finding in patients with pulmonary embolus? (The correct answer is indicated by the asterisk.*)

A. Jugular venous distension
B. Right ventricular heave
C. S3 gallop
D. Tachypnea*
E. Unilateral leg swelling

This question tests recall of an isolated fact. In contrast, the following item requires the student to apply knowledge to a clinical situation, rather than simply recall a fact.

Table 16. Item-Writing Recommendations (informed by Case and Swanson[4])

Guideline	Practical Suggestions
Address important concepts.	Follow an examination blueprint derived from the content and importance of the material to be assessed.
Write clinical vignettes whenever possible.	Present information in order: age and gender, history, physical examination, laboratory data.
Write a focussed question or lead-in statement.	Examinees should be able to propose an answer without reading options. Ask: "Can the question be answered without looking at the options?" E.g., "What is the most likely diagnosis?" or "The most likely cause is ..."
Write homogeneous options.	All diagnoses, all laboratory tests, all outcomes. It is easy to write homogeneous options if the lead-in is focussed.
Alphabetize options.	This addresses the tendency for a certain option to be correct more often than others.
Avoid ambiguous phrases.	E.g., may, usually, frequently, rarely. How often is usually? Frequently? Rarely?
Avoid absolute phrases.	E.g., always, never. These are almost always wrong answers.

Avoid implausible or inconsistent options.	Options should be:
	  Plausible and not deceptive.
	  Same length.
	  Same perspective (e.g., all positive or all negative).

Avoid overlapping numeric responses.	E.g., A. 10-25. B. 20-40.
Do not use "all of the above" or "none of the above."	Include more than one point in the same response if necessary. E.g., A. Murmur, Fever, Fatigue. Rather than: A. Murmur. B. Fever. C. Fatigue. D. All of the Above.
Avoid unnecessarily long or tricky options.	Test knowledge, not ability to interpret what item means.
All options should be the same relative length.	Correct answer is usually the longest.
Be sure options are grammatically correct with lead-in.	Grammatically incorrect responses are almost always incorrect.
Do not repeat a word from the lead-in in the options.	Cues the correct answer.

Example # 2: Application of Knowledge

A 66-year-old woman had abrupt onset of shortness of breath and left-sided pleuritic chest pain 1 hour ago. She had been recovering well since a colectomy for colon cancer 2 days ago. Blood pressure is 160/90 mm Hg, pulse is 120/min, and respirations are 32/min. She is diaphoretic. Breath sounds are audible bilaterally, but inspiratory effort is decreased, S1 and S2 are normal, and jugular veins are not distended. Which of the following is the most likely cause of her acute condition?

  A. Acute myocardial infarction
  B. Dissecting aortic aneurysm
  C. Pneumonia
  D. Pneumothorax
  E. Pulmonary embolus*

Example # 3: Application of Knowledge (Higher Order)

The following example tests higher order application of knowledge than the previous question.

A 66-year-old woman is brought to the emergency department because of dyspnea and pleuritic chest pain for 1 hour. Her blood pressure is 160/90 mm Hg, pulse is 120/min, and respirations are 30/min. Her lungs are clear to auscultation. S1 and S2 are normal, and no murmur or gallop is heard. Electrocardiogram shows sinus tachycardia and nonspecific ST and T wave changes. Portable chest x-ray shows poor inspiratory effort and clear lung fields. Laboratory studies show:

  WBC 12,000/mm^3
  Hematocrit 44%
  Arterial blood gas (room air) PO_2 62 mm Hg
    PCO_2 30 mm Hg
    pH 7.52

Which of the following is the most appropriate next diagnostic step?

  A. Cardiac catheterization
  B. CT angiogram of the chest*
  C. Echocardiogram
  D. Pulmonary arteriography
  E. Duplex venous scan of the lower extremities

The student must suspect the most probable diagnosis (pulmonary embolus) and determine the next appropriate diagnostic procedure.

Patients often present with signs and symptoms, not a diagnosis. Therefore, examination questions should strive to replicate the process of clinical problem solving. Questions such as "Which of the following is true about polymyalgia rheumatica?" or worse yet, "Which of the following is not true about polymyalgia rheumatica?" do not elicit clinical thinking. They are a series of true-false statements.

16.3. Constructing One-Best-Answer Items (Type A) in the NBME Format

16.3.1. The Stem and Lead-in Question

The stem should be a clinical vignette, whenever possible, and have some or all of the following, in this order:
- Patient's age and gender (be consistent about inclusion of race; either include it only if it is important to the question or include it in all items)
- Presenting symptom(s)
- Pertinent history (be sure time sequences are clear)
- Pertinent physical examination
- Pertinent laboratory findings

The lead-in question at the end of the stem should be clear and answerable without having read the options for the answer.

Examples of good lead-in questions are:
- Which of the following is the most likely diagnosis?
- Which of the following is the most appropriate next step in treatment?
- Which of the following is the most likely explanation for the patient's findings?
- Treatment with which of the following could have prevented the patient's condition?
- Which of the following put the patient at risk for this condition?

An example of a poor lead-in question is:
Which of the following statements about _____ is correct?

Lead-in questions such as the poor lead-in example are imprecise and nearly always contain heterogeneous options (e.g., mixture of diseases, laboratory data, mechanisms of disease, treatments, complications).

16.3.2. The Responses (Options for Answers)

The stem should be longer than any options, as demonstrated:

```
XXXXXXXXXXXXXXXXXXXXXXXXXXXXXX
XXXXXXXXXXXXXXXXXXXXXXXXXXXXXX
XXXXXXXXXXXXXXXXXXXXXXXXXXXXXX
XXXXXXXXXXXXXXXXXXXXXXXXXXXXXX

  A. XXXXXXXXXX
  B. XXXXXXXXXX
  C. XXXXXXXXXX
  D. XXXXXXXXXX
  E. XXXXXXXXXX
```

Good responses (options) should:
- Be homogeneous, i.e., responses should be all diagnoses, all tests, or all mechanisms of disease, etc. Do not mix categories of responses.
- Be approximately the same length.
- Have a grammatically correct ending to the lead-in statement or answer to the question.
- Not include "None of the above" or "all of the above."
- Not be tricky or picky questions. The goal is to assess knowledge and its application, not test-taking ability.[5]
- Be alphabetized. Item-writers have a tendency for the correct answer to be in one position more frequently than the others (e.g., "B").

Example # 4: Flawed One-Best-Answer Item

A 7-year-old girl is brought to a physician's office by her mother complaining of chronic abdominal pain, irritability and crankiness. Her mother also hints there may be family problems. Which of the following would be most helpful to aid understanding of this patient's problem?

A. Elicit further information about the family problems and other potential stressors.
B. Perform a physical examination.
C. Reassure the mother that it is a normal phase her daughter is going through.
D. Refer the girl to a gastroenterologist.
E. Refer parents for marital counseling.

The flaws in this item include:
- The clinical findings in the stem are inadequate.
- The stem does not pose a clear question.
- One cannot arrive at the correct answer without looking at the options.
- The options are heterogeneous.
- The distracters (wrong answers) are not of similar length or complexity.
- The wording in the stem is unclear. Who is complaining of pain, patient or mother?

Example # 5: Better Written One-Best-Answer Item

A 20-year-old woman, accompanied by her mother, comes to the emergency department because she has had chest pain for 2 hours. The pain began while she was sitting at home, and was accompanied by palpitations, lightheadedness, and difficulty breathing. Four months ago, while at a mall, she experienced the sudden onset of similar symptoms. She has had three similar attacks while shopping, each of which spontaneously resolved after 10 minutes. For the past month she has been afraid to leave the house because she feared recurrence of symptoms. Physical examination, blood glucose, and EKG are normal. Which of the following is the most likely diagnosis?

A. Generalized Anxiety Disorder
B. Hypochondriasis
C. Panic disorder*
D. Simple phobia
E. Unsocial phobia

16.4. Constructing Matching Items (Type R)

Matching items offer more options, are less suggestive, and therefore more closely resemble actual clinical situations than do other multiple choice item formats.[6] Consequently, matching items evaluate students' diagnostic and management skills more accurately. Because of the larger number of possible options (Examples 7 and 8), extended matching questions offer the opportunity to write items that cross disciplines. For example, an item about causes of altered mental status could have options that include cardiac, pulmonary, metabolic, psychiatric, and neurologic possibilities. This technique counters the tendency of students and faculty to compartmentalize knowledge by specialty.

Extended matching items require a computer-readable answer sheet that has more than the usual five choices (A-E). Some answer sheets allow up to 10 responses (A-J); others allow up to 26 options (A-Z).

Elements of a well-constructed extended matching set are:
1. Theme.
2. Lead-in statement.
3. Option list.
4. At least two item stems.

16.4.1. Theme

Each matching set needs a theme, e.g., chest pain, depressive symptoms, or abdominal pain. Identify the theme before writing a matching set.

16.4.2. Lead-in Statement

This statement tells the student the theme of the set and what to do. For example, "For each patient with chest pain, select the most likely diagnosis," or, "For each patient with fever, select the most appropriate next diagnostic test."

16.4.3. Considering a List of Options

Make a list of possible responses for your theme. There must be at least five responses, but the total number is limited only by the number of options on the computer scan sheet. Forcing students to choose from longer lists of possible options more closely simulates real clinical situations. The option list should include only one option type (e.g., diagnoses, drugs). Options that cross disciplines make the set more closely resemble real-life situations.

16.4.4. Item Stems

Clinical vignettes used in matching questions should be similar to those used in the stems of Type A questions. Each vignette in a set should contain the same amount and type of information. Most stems in R-type items are no more than five lines long. A knowledgeable student should be able to determine the correct response by reading the stem, without looking at the list of options.

Example # 6: Extended Matching Item Set

Theme: Fatigue.
Options:
- A. Cushing's disease
- B. Acute intermittent porphyria
- C. Congestive heart failure
- D. Major depression
- E. Epstein-Barr virus infection
- F. Folate deficiency
- G. Dysthymic disorder
- H. Hyperthyroidism
- I. Hypothyroidism
- J. Mitral valve prolapse
- K. Lyme disease
- L. Bipolar disorder
- M. Substance abuse
- N. Vitamin B12 deficiency

Lead-in: For each of the following patients with fatigue, select the most likely diagnosis.
Stems:
1. A 19-year-old woman has had fatigue, fever, and sore throat for 1 week. Her temperature is 38.3°C (101°F). Examination reveals cervical lymphadenopathy and splenomegaly. Leukocyte count is 5000/mm^3 (80% lymphocytes, many of which look atypical). Serum aspartate amino-transferase (AST, SGOT) is 200 IU/L. Serum bilirubin concentration and serum alkaline phosphatase are within the reference range. (Answer: E)
2. For the past 2 months, a 50-year-old woman has been fatigued and "lacked energy." She has gained 15 pounds in the same time interval. Physical exam reveals delayed deep tendon reflexes. (Answer: I)

Example # 7: Extended Matching Item Set

Theme: Chest Pain.
Options:
- A. Angina pectoris
- B. Aortic stenosis
- C. Costochondritis
- D. Dissecting aortic aneurysm
- E. Gastro-esophageal reflux
- F. Herpes zoster
- G. Mitral valve prolapse
- H. Myocardial infarction
- I. Panic disorder
- J. Pericarditis
- K. Pulmonary embolus

Lead-in: "For each patient with chest pain, select the most likely cause."
Stems:
1. For 1 hour, a 72-year-old man has had worsening chest pain that feels like "someone tearing my chest." The pain radiates to his back. Blood

pressure is 160/90 mm Hg in the right arm and 105/70 mm Hg in the left arm. A murmur of aortic regurgitation, not previously present, is heard. (Answer: D)
2. For 12 hours, a 28-year-old woman has had anterior chest pain made worse by deep breathing or lying supine. She has had systemic lupus erythematosus for 4 years. There is a friction rub over her left sternal border. (Answer: J)
3. A 48-year-old man has recurrent episodes of burning chest pain located at the level of the lower sternum. The episodes last 15 to 45 minutes and are frequently relieved by antacids. The pain is often precipitated by lying supine or eating a large meal. (Answer: E)
4. A 60-year-old woman has severe burning, left-sided chest pain that radiates from the mid-sternum around the left side of the chest to the back. Touching the skin over the involved area lightly with a Q-tip causes an unpleasant, burning sensation. Lung and cardiovascular examinations are normal. The skin over the affected area appears normal. Electrocardiogram is normal. (Answer: F)
5. A 22-year-old man has had persistent chest pain over and to the left of the upper sternum for 3 days. He describes it as a "nuisance ache," aggravated by lifting weights. Blood pressure, and cardiac and lung exams are normal. The pain is reproduced by pressure at the junction of the upper left thoracic ribs and the sternum. (Answer: C)

16.5. Constructing the Examination

Course, clerkship, and program directors are responsible for the quality of internally produced, faculty-written examinations, even if they do not themselves write most of the items. Ensure that the individual items are high-quality and that the overall examination assesses knowledge of important concepts. Topics that are easy to write examination questions for may not be the most important topics to assess on the examination. It is helpful to follow these steps when constructing an examination:

- Develop an examination blueprint. The blueprint should list the topics to be covered on the examination (e.g., chest pain, fatigue, prevalence, specificity, ectopic pregnancy) and the domain to be assessed (e.g., definition, diagnosis, management, interpretation of data).
- Teach faculty how to write multiple choice items consistent with the format used on the examination. Even 1-hour item-writing workshops are helpful.
- Ask faculty to submit items that follow the examination blueprint. Many of the items probably will be poorly written and will require considerable editing.
- Ideally you should select the items for the examination during a test construction meeting where the contributing authors read their items aloud, followed by discussion, questions, improvements, and an accept/reject decision. Faculty are likely to resist the process because

they must submit items far enough ahead of the administration date to allow time for review and editing, and because item-writing becomes a "public," rather than "private," process. Remind the group that the goal is to produce the highest quality items, not to defend one's submissions. The process is worth the effort and produces higher quality examinations.[7,8]

If this approach is not feasible, edit submitted items and return them to the author for further input or approval. After you are satisfied with the quality of the examination, ask a colleague to review the examination critically before its administration. Ask the colleague to read the examination through the eyes of a student. Reviewing the examination without the answer key helps to highlight ambiguities that might otherwise be missed.

16.6. Summary

Written examinations are an important way to assess clinical competence. While many medical schools use externally developed examinations, such as the NBME subject tests, some departments develop their own clerkship examinations. Examination items should cover important concepts and assess students' ability to apply knowledge to clinical situations or solve clinical problems. They should not test recall of factual information, and should minimize the likelihood that test-wise students will be able to answer items correctly without clinical knowledge or problem-solving skills.

References

1. Haladyna TM, Downing SM. A taxonomy of multiple choice item-writing rules. Appl Meas Educ 1989;2(1):37-50.
2. Boland RJ, Lester NA, Williams E. Writing multiple-choice questions. Acad Psych. 2010;34(4):310-316.
3. Hawkins RE, Swanson DB. Using written examinations to assess medical knowledge and its application. In: Holmboe ES, Hawkins RE, eds. Practical Guide to the Evaluation of Clinical Competence. Philadelphia: Mosby, 2008: 42-59.
4. Case SM, Swanson DB. Constructing Written Test Questions for the Basic and Clinical Sciences - third edition, revised - Philadelphia, National Board of Medical Examiners, 2003. <www.nbme.org/publications/item-writing-manual.html>. Accessed February 9, 2015.
5. Case SM, Downing SM. Performance of various multiple-choice item types on medical specialty examinations: Types a, b, c, k and x. Proceedings of Twenty-Eighth Annual Conference of Research in Medical Education. Washington, DC: AAMC, 1989: 167-172.
6. Case SM, Swanson DB. Extended matching items: A practical alternative to free-response questions. Teach Learn Med. 1993;5(2):107-115.
7. Wallach PM, Crespo LM, Holtzman KZ, et al. Use of a commttee review process to improve the quality of course examinations. Adv Health Sci Educ Theory Pract 2006;11(1):61-68.
8. Jozefowicz RF, Koeppen BM, Case S, et al. The quality of in-house medical school examinations. Acad Med. 2002;77(2):156-161.

Table 17.1. Assessment Limitations Addressed by Standardized Patients

Limitations of Assessment in a Clinical Setting	Potential Advantages of SP-Based Assessment
Evaluator Skill: Faculty who supervise students may not have the motivation, training, or skills for optimal evaluation.	SPs can be selected for interest and aptitude, and trained to predefined and measureable standards of accuracy.
Evaluator Time: Faculty who supervise students have other responsibilities which limit their opportunities for direct observation.	The sole focus of an SP encounter is clinical teaching and assessment.
Evaluator Standardization: Faculty observe a range of student behaviors, and have varying standards for student performance.	Skills to be assessed and standards for mastery can be defined in advance, and each SP portraying a case can be trained to the same standards.
Sampling of Challenges: The random clinical problems encountered by students may not match the problems they need to master.	Clerkship directors can select the range of problems an examinee encounters in an SP examination.

Table 17.2. Cost Components for SP-Based Assessment Exercises

Direct Costs	Indirect Costs
SP training SP portrayal Training materials: • Copying costs • Development of video training materials Consumables: • Patient gowns and sheets • Items used by the students during the examination, such as gloves, tongue blades, disposable tips for otoscopes Support of technology used by the SPs in rating students (computers, iPads) ; direct cost for video recording	Facility development, use, and maintenance (may be centralizable / shareable) • Capital building / development • Database management / retrieval Staff salaries (for recruitment and training of SPs) (may be centralizable / shareable) Technical support (for support of computer systems and audiovisual archiving software) (may be centralizable / shareable) Faculty time for: • Case development • Examination development, scoring, and interpretation • Direct observation during the examination • Student orientation and supervision during the exam

Chapter 17
Standardized Patient-Based Assessment of Clinical Skills in Clerkships

Michael Ainsworth, M.D.
Karen Szauter, M.D.

17.1. Standardized Patient Methodology in Health Care Education

Standardized patients are generally laypersons trained to simulate patient encounters accurately and consistently for teaching or evaluation purposes, and are used in virtually all U.S. medical schools for teaching or assessment. There are technical distinctions between "standardized" and "simulated" patients. The term "standardized patient (SP)" is used widely in the North American literature and is used consistently throughout this chapter.[1] The value of SPs arises from their ability to allow teaching and assessment of skills that range from basic data-gathering in the medical interview, to physical examination, to more complex communication or patient education skills.[1-4]

17.2. Standardized Patients for the Assessment of Clinical Skills

Clinical skills assessment presents different challenges from those encountered in medical knowledge assessment. Accurate and reliable assessment of students' medical knowledge depends on use of rigorously designed examinations. Such examinations supplement the less standardized assessment conducted by teachers in the clinical setting. Likewise, SP-based assessment of clinical skills provides a "quantified" ("objective") component that complements teachers' more subjective student assessments in the clinical setting. SP-based assessments require careful attention to examination blueprints, sampling of case challenges, and construction of scoring criteria. Evaluation of clinical skills often has limited correlation with measures of medical knowledge and problem solving, suggesting that these two skill domains encompass unique characteristics.[5] Traditional clinical skills assessment in the clinical setting relies heavily on random observations or inference, based on written records and oral presentations of patient encounters. SP-based activities also offer opportunity to provide objective observation and documentation of students' medical interviewing and physical examination abilities.[1]

SP-based systematic and direct observation of patient encounters overcomes four limitations of traditional assessment by clinical faculty (Table 17.1, above, p. 200).

17.3. Designing an SP-Based Assessment

Involving SPs in the assessment of learners requires careful planning. The use of any SP-based exercise requires a stepwise process of design and formatting. For clerkship-based examinations, these decisions should be based on the clerkship's goals and objectives, and should reflect the students' learning experiences.

A decision to implement SP-based assessment in a clinical skills course, clinical clerkship, or subinternship carries a commitment to decision making in the following examination design categories:

17.3.1. Blueprinting: Design of the Exam Should Parallel the Clerkship Objectives

Review the clerkship's content goals and objectives. Review the clerkship's *skill* goals and objectives. Ensure that students have sufficient opportunity to be exposed to the biomedical content, psychosocial challenges, or skills that will be evaluated (through patient encounters or supplementary activities) before inclusion in an assessment exercise, especially if the assessment is summative or for high stakes. Blueprints (see Chapter 7) draw attention to the mix of patients (age, gender, ethnicity) and examination content, ensuring that the challenges are clinically relevant and are aligned with the stated objectives of the course.[6,7]

17.3.2. Examination Construction

Determine, based on educational philosophy and practical constraints, whether to select a format that emphasizes a small number of relatively comprehensive patient encounters, often referred to as a clinical skills assessment (CSA), or a larger number of relatively focussed encounters, often called an OSCE. This labeling distinction is artificial, but reflects the trade-offs inherent in exam design.[8-10] The number of patient encounters should reflect the range of skills being assessed. Adequate sampling is essential to limit the effects of case specificity on examination reliability. The length of each patient encounter should reflect the complexity of the task. Examination formats can range from as brief as a few minutes ("Perform a history of present illness for this patient's chest pain"), to as long as an hour or more ("Complete a comprehensive interview, physical and neurologic examination on this new patient with hemiplegia, discuss the patient's most likely diagnoses with him, and conduct patient counseling on long-term care and lifestyle modification"). In practice, most SP-based exam encounters in clerkships tend to range from 10-15 minutes for problem-focussed encounters to 25-30 minutes for more comprehensive evaluations. Practical considerations, including student testing volume, testing space limitations, and financial support influence the format of a program.[11]

17.3.3. Checklists

The most common method of student assessment in SP exercises is checklist-based ratings completed by SPs after each encounter. Checklists must be created that are relevant to the case, of reasonable length, and include items that can be efficiently scored by the SPs. Long checklists (unless scored by a separate observer) or checklists requiring medical knowledge to complete, threaten the reliability and validity of SP-generated scores.[12-15] SPs may also be asked to complete checklist items which document a student's interpersonal skills. These checklist items are often adapted from existing rating instruments by an SP program, with the benefit that experienced SPs will have encountered these items during other assessments.

17.3.4. Encounter Enhancements and Post-Encounter Exercises

One of the limitations of SP-based encounters is the challenge of including abnormal physical examination (pathological) findings, which are often not found in the available SPs. Assessment of physical examination skills can include appropriate choice of maneuvers and the technical skill in performing the exam. However, to assess whether students would modify their exam based on an abnormal finding requires inclusion of actual physical findings. A well-trained SP can simulate a variety of physical findings.[16] SPs with stable physical findings (e.g., the abnormal joints of rheumatoid arthritis, hearing impairment) can also be recruited for a specific role. SPs can use make up, moulage, and wearable prostheses. With the advancement of technology-based simulation, SP encounters can be supplemented with tools, task trainers, or mannequins to introduce physical findings.[17-19]

The SP-based exam format lends itself to linking patient encounters with post-encounter exercises. Such exercises, typically 5-10 minutes immediately after the SP encounter, most commonly include written notes, oral presentations, or written responses to questions about the preceding case. The post-encounter exercise may introduce photographs of physical findings (e.g., optic fundus or a tympanic membrane), radiographic images, or laboratory results related to the case to challenge students' critical thinking.[20]

17.3.5. Faculty Involvement

Involvement of faculty is a critical component of SP-based assessments. This can include case writing, exam development, and participation in the assessment exercises themselves by directly observing and grading students during the encounters, or involvement in the post encounter activities through facilitating oral presentations, reviewing post-encounter patient notes, or scoring responses to questions during post-encounter exercises. Faculty gain valuable insight into the range of skills demonstrated by students, and feedback from faculty is valuable to ensure that the assessment adequately meets the intended goals and objectives.

17.4. Resource Requirements of SP-Based Assessment

The clerkship director and involved faculty form the nucleus for successful

SP-based assessments. Yet, successful integration of SP-based assessments into a clerkship requires resources that often exceed the capacity and budgets of individual courses or departments. A key component of an SP program involves professional staff who can assist with the creation of the patient script and checklist, recruit and train SPs, and guide the logistical challenges of exam administration. Space for the assessment should mirror the clinical setting. A dedicated simulation center with capacity for video recording is ideal because review of recorded encounters with students allows for personalized and high impact feedback.

17.5. Benefits and Limitations of SP-Based Assessments

SPs are in a unique position to rate student skills from the vantage point of a patient. They can be trained to score medical interview and physical examination performance accurately on dichotomous scales (done vs. not done). The technical correctness of examination maneuvers can also be scored by the SP, at times providing a more accurate account of the exam than can be observed through direct or video monitoring. One notable benefit derived from involving SPs in student assessment is their ability to assess interpersonal communication skills from the patient perspective. Nonverbal behaviors, and other nuances of the encounter, may be evident only to the SP.[21]

Subtle distinctions of student performance typically require the judgment of a physician rater. SPs should not be expected to evaluate students' clinical reasoning or problem-solving abilities. Reasoning and problem-solving assessments are best accomplished by direct student-faculty contact. Depending on the objectives of the assessment, SP-based ratings in combination with the expert judgment of clinical faculty may be required to optimize student evaluation. Although SP-based assessment is quantified and "objective," it cannot replace the judgment of clinical faculty in student evaluation.[22,23] Best practices in evaluation suggest that SPs should be used to *observe* and *record* student performance data; medical faculty are responsible to *judge* the data (see Chapter 2).

One noted limitation of SP-based assessments is the "artificial" nature of the patient encounter. Students may perform in a way that they believe is expected, often stating that this is not how they would act with a "real" patient. Actual physical findings may be ignored.[24] The examination setting also introduces anxiety which may interfere with a student's ability to focus on the case challenges.[25]

17.6. SP-Based Assessment Costs

SP-based assessments require considerable resources, including both direct and indirect costs (Table 17.2, above, p. 200). Time must be invested in case and checklist development, preparation of the SPs, examination administration, maintaining physical space, and data recording and retrieval infrastructure. Hourly payments to SPs vary widely across institutions, and within an institution costs will be influenced by the complexity of the tasks required. Published cost estimates have used various methods of cost calculations, and provide little generalizable information for estimating overall costs. Typical estimates of direct (SP) costs for exams range from $50-$200/student.[26-28]

17.7. SP-Based Assessment and the Research Literature

17.7.1. "Patient" Issues

17.7.1.a. Realism and Consistency

Well-trained SPs can simulate a clinical encounter so realistically that they cannot be distinguished from genuine patients, even when scheduled into the physician's practice unannounced.[29] SPs can consistently reproduce interview and examination findings more than 90% of the time.

17.7.1.b. Reliability in Checklist Ratings (Interrater Reliability)

Scoring reliability is influenced by checklist complexity, but within certain parameters (15-25 checklist items, < 4-5 hours of portrayal with breaks), SP reliability appears to match physician raters. Adding multiple observers to a case adds little to exam reliability.[30,31]

17.7.2. Examination Issues

17.7.2.a. Case-Specificity (Inter-Case Reliability)

A single patient encounter, whether genuine or SP-based, will not provide a reliable indicator of an examinee's skills. Four to six hours (or more) of total testing time is typically required to reach levels of reliability (generalizability) expected for Pass/Fail decisions on high-stakes examinations.[8] Exercises designed to assess less complex skills, or which focus on teaching and feedback are typically not as time-intensive.

17.7.2.b. Validity

Assessment of validity of SP-based examinations is a complex issue, influenced by the content and structure of the exam, and by the value placed on correlation between SP-based assessment and other performance measures. Correlations between SP-based assessment and MCQ examinations are only moderate, because these assessments measure skill sets that only partially overlap. Most measures of validity attempt to establish a relationship between SP exam performance and faculty clinical evaluations without a standard for that comparison. Learners at higher levels tend to perform better than their lower-level counterparts (fourth-year students compared to second-year students, or residents compared to students, for example). These studies do not establish a precise correlation between experience and performance (see Chapter 2 for definitions of validity and reliability).

Checklist-based assessments may not capture the subtlety of skills demonstrated by higher levels of learners.[32] This is one reason why the decision to have SPs rate students (using discrete checklist items) vs. having faculty observers rate them (often using global rating scales) is so challenging. Student perceptions of the scoring system may also influence performance, as students try to second-guess what is expected of them, rather than demonstrate actual skills.[33]

17.8. Incorporating SP-Based Assessment into a Comprehensive Evaluation

The success of a clerkship-based SP program can be substantially influenced by student exposure to SPs elsewhere in the curriculum. Students' acceptance of SP-based testing is enhanced when they have encountered SPs as teaching tools earlier in the curriculum. Use of SPs by multiple courses also strengthens the practicality of developing stable school-level resources, such as a dedicated SP testing center and a permanent professional staff for patient recruitment and training. Ideally, the skills upon which students are tested during clerkships are skills that have been stressed and reinforced through practice and testing in earlier courses.

The addition of an SP-based clinical skills component to the USMLE Step 2 examination (Step 2 CS) has contributed to the increased emphasis that individual medical schools now place on similar types of internal skills-based examinations.[26] Some schools have attempted to use internal SP-based examinations as predictors of Step 2 CS performance, but heterogeneity across schools makes generalizability of such studies difficult. It is hard to identify which, if any, factors would help to predict which students are likely to pass or fail this licensing examination.[34,35] What is essential at the school level is the recognition that a failing performance on an SP-based assessment may occur for several reasons. Careful review of individual student performance, and remediation tailored to the student's specific deficits, is essential to optimize student learning.[36,37]

An extensive list of articles relating to SPs in medical education is available at <www.utmb.edu/ocs/sp-bibliography.asp> (updated annually; last update June 2014; accessed May 10, 2015).

References

1. Cleland JA. Abe K. Rethans JJ. The use of simulated patients in medical education: AMEE guide no. 42. Med Teach 2009;31(6):477-486.

2. Teherani A, Hauer KE, O'Sullivan P. Can simulations measure empathy? Considerations on how to assess behavioral empathy via simulations. Pat Educ Couns 2008;71(2):148-152.
3. Allen SS, Miller J, Ratner E, Santilli J. The educational and financial impact of using patient educators to teach introductory physical exam skills. Med Teach 2011;33(11):911-918.
4. Gunderson AJ, Smith KM, Mayer DB, et al. Teaching medical students the art of medical error full disclosure: Evaluation of a new curriculum. Teach Learn Med 2009;21(3):229-232.
5. Harik P, Clauser BE, Grabovsky I, et al. Relationships among subcomponents of the USMLE Step 2 Clinical Skills examination, the Step 1, and the Step 2 Clinical Knowledge examinations. Acad Med 2006;81(10 Suppl):S21-S24.
6. Mookherjee S, Chang A, Boscardin CK, et al. How to develop a competency-based examination blueprint for longitudinal standardized patient clinical skills assessments. Med Teach 2013;35(11):883-890.
7. Kachur EK, Zabar S, Hanley K, et al. Organizing OSCEs (and other SP exercises) in ten steps. In: Zabar S, et al., eds. Objective Structured Clinical Examinations. New York: Springer, 2013: 7-34
8. Turner JL, Dankoski ME. Objective structured clinical exams: A critical review. Fam Med 2008;40(8):574-578.
9. Khan KZ, Gaunt K, Ramachandran S, Pushkar P. The objective structured clinical examination (OSCE): AMEE guide no. 81. Part II: Organisation & administration. Med Teach 2013;35(9):e1447-e1463.
10. Casey PM, Goepfert AR, Espey EL, et al. To the point: Reviews in medical education: The objective structured clinical examination. Am J Obstet Gynecol 2009;200(1):25-34.
11. Pell G, Fuller R, Homer M, Roberts T. How to measure the quality of the OSCE: A review of metrics: AMEE guide no. 49. Med Teach 2010;32(10):802-811.
12. Whelan GP, Boulet JR, McKinley DW, et al. Scoring standardized patient examinations: Lessons learned from the development and administration of the ECFMG clinical skills assessment (CSA). Med Teach 2005;27(3):200-206.
13. Hettinga AM, Denessen E, Postma CT. Checking the checklist: A content analysis of expert- and evidence-based case-specific checklist items. Med Educ 2010; 44(9):874-883.
14. McLaughlin K, Ainslie M, Coderre S, et al. The effect of differential rater function over time (DRIFT) on objective structured clinical examination ratings. Med Educ 2009;43(10):989-992.
15. Yudkowsky R, Park YS, Riddle J, et al. Clinically discriminating checklists versus thoroughness checklists: Improving the validity of performance test scores. Acad Med 2014;89(7):1057-1062.
16. Barrows HS. An overview of the uses of standardized patients for teaching and evaluating clinical skills. Acad Med. 1993;68(6):451-453.
17. Verma A, Bhatt H, Booton P, et al. The ventriloscope as an innovative tool for assessing clinical examination skills: Appraisal of a novel method of simulating auscultatory findings. Med Teach 2011;33(7):e388-e396.
18. Kneebone R, Nestel D, Yadollahi F, et al. Assessing procedural skills in context: Exploring the feasibility of an integrated procedural performance instrument (IPPI). Med Educ 2006;40(11):1105-1114.
19. Hernandez C, Mermelstein R, Robinson JK, et al. Assessing students' ability to detect melanomas using standardized patients and moulage. J Am Acad Derm 2013;68(3):e83-e88.

20. Walling A, Moser SE, Dickson G, et al. Are students less likely to report pertinent negatives in post-encounter notes? Fam Med 2012;44(1):22-25.
21. Fiscella K, Franks P, Srinivasan M, et al. Ratings of physician communication by real and standardized patients. Ann Fam Med 2007;5(2):151-158.
22. Durning SJ, Artino A, Boulet J, et al. Making use of contrasting participant views of the same encounter. Med. Educ 2010;44(10):953-961.
23. Brewster LP, Risucci DA, Joehl RJ, et al. Comparison of resident self-assessments with trained faculty and standardized patient assessments of clinical and technical skills in a structured educational module. Am J Surg 2008;195(1):1-4.
24. Szauter K, Ainsworth M. Use of standardised patients with actual findings. Med Educ 2006;40(11):1143-1144.
25. Hulsman RL, Pranger S, Koot S, et al. How stressful is doctor-patient communication? Physiological and psychological stress of medical students in simulated history taking and bad-news consultations. Int J Psychophysiol 2010;77(1):26-34.
26. Hauer KE, Hodgson CS, Kerr KM. A national study of medical student clinical skills assessment. Acad Med 2005;80(10 Suppl):S25-S29.
27. Patricio MF, Julião M, Fareleira F, et al. Is the OSCE a feasible tool to assess competencies in undergraduate medical education? Med Teach 2013;35(6):503-514.
28. Poenaru D, Morales D, Richards A, O'Connor HM. Running an objective structured clinical examination on a shoestring budget. Am J Surg 1997;173(6):538-541.
29. Rethans JJ, Gorter S, Bokken L, Morrison L. Unannounced standardised patients in real practice: A systematic literature review. Med Educ 2007;41(6):537-549.
30. McLaughlin K, Gregor L, Jones A, Coderre S. Can standardized patients replace physicians as OSCE examiners? BMC Med Educ 2006;6:12.
31. Swanson DB, van der Vleuten CPM. Assessment of clinical skills with standardized patients: State of the art revisited. Teach Learn Med 2013;25(Suppl 1):S17-S25.
32. Hodges B, Regehr G, McNaughton N, et al. OSCE checklists do not capture increasing levels of expertise. Acad Med. 1999;74(10):1120-1134.
33. McIlroy JH, Hodges B, McNaughton N, Regehr G. The effect of candidates' perceptions of the evaluation method on reliability of checklist and global rating scores in an objective structured clinical examination. Acad Med 2002;77(7): 725-728.
34. Berg K, Winward M, Clauser BE, et al. The relationship between performance on a medical school's clinical skills assessment and USMLE Step 2 CS. Acad Med 2008;83(10 Suppl):S37-S40.
35. Chang A, Boscardin C, Chou CL,et al. Predicting failing performance on a standardized patient clinical performance examination: The importance of communication and professionalism skills deficits. Acad Med 2009;84(10 Suppl):S101-S104.
36. Pell G, Fuller R, Homer M, Roberts T. Is short-term remediation after OSCE failure sustained? A retrospective analysis of the longitudinal attainment of underperforming students in OSCE assessments. Med Teach 2012;34(2):146-150.
37. Mavis BE, Wagner DP, Henry RC, et al. Documenting clinical performance problems among medical students: Feedback for learner remediation and curriculum enhancement. Med Educ Online 2013;18. <med-ed-online.net/index.php/meo/article/view/20598>. Accessed May 10, 2015.

Chapter 18
Assessment Using Simulation Technologies

Keith F. Muccino, S.J., M.D.
Viva Jo Siddall, M.S., M.S., R.R.T., R.C.P., C.C.M.E.-P.

18.1. The Educational Context

Successful clinical educators in today's complex health care environment are mindful of the paradigm shift that has taken place in education, particularly in professional education. The focus has shifted from *teaching*, to *learning*, to *competence*, and to the current emphasis on assessment of *performance*.[1-2] (See Chapter 2 for terminology of competence and performance.)

Effective educational programs must pay close attention to each and all of these constitutive elements - the need for effective teachers who can facilitate genuine learning; learning that generates desired competence; competence that can be demonstrated in performance; performance that is critically observed and objectively measured.[3]

Quality clinical education, the medical school clerkship being a representative example, is increasingly being defined as education that is confirmed in demonstrated and measurable performance. This evolving paradigm is consonant with the competency model articulated by Miller in 1990, with its stratified levels and developmental hierarchy of competence - *knows*, *knows how*, *shows how*, and *does*.[4]

Across the spectrum of medical education, from undergraduate to the maintenance of certification within the specialties, assessments and certifications are increasingly performance-based and practice-based, where learners are assessed as they *show how to*, and *do*, what is required for safe clinical practice. Such a performance-driven paradigm shift "ups the ante" for clerkship directors when developing their curricular blueprints, especially in the choices they make regarding assessment instruments.

18.1.1. Aligning Assessments with Learning Objectives

In developing learning objectives for an educational curriculum, clerkship directors must give proper forethought not only to the competencies that are desired in the learner and intended as part of the learning process, but also to the appropriate means by which those competencies will be effectively measured or evaluated in performance. Clerkship directors must assure that the assessment of a learner is properly aligned with the stated learning objectives (content validity) and that the assessment instruments and evaluation modalities chosen, optimally serve to assess competence manifested in measurable performance (construct validity).[5]

Clerkship directors are responsible for carefully deciding which among their curriculum's stated learning objectives warrant formal assessment of competence in learners, since not every educational objective that guides learning can be formally assessed. Clerkship directors must then judge whether those learning objectives, identified as warranting assessment, in fact allow for accurate assessment of competence (feasibility).[5,6]

This process calls for developing assessment activities that allow learner competence to be demonstrated transparently in performance and assessed with instruments or modalities that produce readily interpretable and applicable data. The notion of validity, attributed to measurement instruments or to the overall assessment process, is ultimately about the quality of interpretations made from the data generated by evaluative instruments that enable decisions to be made that allow required actions to be taken.[7,8]

With this notion serving as a guide, the clerkship director's responsibility is to select or design assessment instruments that can generate reliable performance data. These data, which typically take the form of scores, then become the supportive evidence for making necessary interpretations and allow judgments to be made about competence, as in the assignment of grades. This ultimately enables proper decisions to be made and appropriate actions to be taken in advancing, promoting, or remediating learners. Simulation-based evaluations are uniquely suited to the third level in Miller's pyramid ("shows how") where learners can be evaluated while demonstrating targeted areas of clinical ability.[4]

18.1.2. Advantages of Educational Technology

In 2007, the AAMC reflected on the use of educational technology (including simulation) in medical education and the unique advantages provided in the area of contextual learning. Table 18.1 lists these perceived advantages.

As listed among the advantages, simulation offers added value to competency assessment by providing clerkship directors with the ability to assess learners in controlled environments, using evaluations that can be carefully standardized. This allows assessments to be more consistent across all learners.[9-11]

Building upon what has been presented in preceding chapters, and mindful of the need to utilize effective assessment instruments in the educational process, this chapter: (1) briefly introduces clerkship directors to the wide variety of simulation technologies that have emerged in recent years; (2) provides a perspective on and rationale for their utilization in assessing learners in the setting of undergraduate medical education; (3) makes explicit the practical considerations that govern decisions to use simulation-based assessment activities; and (4) discusses forces influencing and reshaping clinical education and professional development.

The aim of the concluding discussion is to empower clerkship directors to use simulation technologies as creative and adaptive strategies in designing their assessment programs in a rapidly changing educational environment.

Table 18.1. Advantages of Educational Technology
(Copyright © 2007 Association of American Medical Colleges - Effective Use of Educational Technology in Medical Education. Used with permission)

Educational technologies are advantageous in providing:
- safe, controlled environments that eliminate risk to patients
- enhanced, realistic visualization
- authentic contexts for learning and assessment
- documentation of learner behavior and outcomes
- instruction tailored to individual or group needs
- learner control of the educational experience
- repetition and deliberate practice
- uncoupling of instruction from place and time
- standardization of instruction and assessment
- perpetual resources and new economies of scale

18.2. Expanding the Options - Assessment Using Simulation

Over time, a variety of measurement instruments have become the armamentarium from which clerkship directors can draw in assessing their learners. MCQs, global rating scale evaluation forms, SP encounters, and OSCEs are just a few among the many instruments to be considered in developing assessment plans for courses or clerkships.[10,12]

In addition to these commonly employed assessment tools, there is a continuously emerging host of simulators that aim at enhancing simulation-based training and performance assessment. These simulation technologies range from basic, procedure-oriented task trainers, to more advanced computer-enhanced human mannequins (CEMs), and virtual reality/environment (VR) simulators (see Table 18.2).[9,13] In addition to providing a general list of simulators available for consideration, Table 18.2 offers comments to help clerkship directors begin to identify the roles which simulation modalities might play when incorporated into an assessment plan for their learners.

Clinical educators now have, at their disposal, a seemingly daunting array of sophisticated technologies designed and marketed to aid in training and assessing a broad spectrum of learners. Among the merits and benefits that simulation offers to clerkship directors is the ability to create assessments targeting competencies that are either difficult to assess by other measures, or whose assessments by those traditional approaches (e.g., floor evaluations) may not be either as reliable as required for making necessary interpretations or sufficiently standardized across cohorts of learners.[14] Simulation offers an alternative modality for clerkship directors to draw upon in creating robust assessment blueprints for their learners, and when used discerningly, standardized simulation-based assessments can serve to generate highly reliable data to be used in the evaluation of learner performance.[15-18]

If your institution is just beginning to develop its simulation center, then you are encouraged to take advantage of the opportunity to learn from the experience of others who have already gone through the process. Helpful information is available in the literature[19,20] and is regularly provided at workshops offered by educators involved with simulation-based education, at meetings sponsored by a variety of organizations like the Society for Simulation in Healthcare or the American College of Surgery.

18.3. A Rationale for Simulation-Based Assessment

An adage, drawn from experience in clinical medicine, states, "Whenever there is a multiplicity of medications that can be prescribed for a given medical condition, it is reasonable to suspect that no one of them is singularly effective." This insight is applicable to educational assessment, where no one modality or assessment instrument is likely to succeed in measuring all of what one seeks to assess.[6,10,12] It reveals the challenge faced by medical educators in their need to assess proficiency across the broad spectrum of the six, soon to be eight, ACGME competencies.[21] Extending the analogy further, just as clinicians must often prescribe a combination of several antihypertensive drugs to address effectively the multiple physiologic pathways contributing to hypertension, educators must consider using a number of assessment instruments in order to evaluate competence in the learner effectively. This is where simulation can be an asset for clerkship directors, e.g., offering a multi-part exercise that includes an SP encounter to assess data gathering and communication skills, followed by a mannequin-based clinical scenario to assess diagnostic reasoning and crisis management skills, concluding with a partial task trainer activity to assess the learner's proficiency in performing essential clinical procedures like nasogastric tube placement or central line insertion.[5,9]

18.4. Form Follows Function [22]

This principle is no less applicable to educational design and should guide the process of developing appropriate simulation-based assessment activities and choosing the proper technologies to support learner assessment.[22] The anticipated purpose and desired function of an assessment activity must be carefully and clearly delineated at the outset of any educational planning process.

Table 18.2. Sample Listing of Simulation Technologies

Simulation Modalities	Type of Assessment	Targeted Learner	Suggestions for Implementation
Partial Task Trainers Central Venous Line Foley Catheter NG Tube Airway Venipuncture ABG Lumbar Puncture Thoracentesis Paracentesis Tube Thoracostomy	Formative or Summative	Clinical Clerks (MS-III) Subinterns (MS-IV)	Procedure training for clinical Clerkships. MS-III training: Beginning of year orientation or just-in-time training prior to each clerkship. Useful for deliberate practice learning. Can be also used for mastery learning activities.
Minimally Invasive Surgery (Laparoscopic) Box Trainers	Formative or Summative	Subinterns (MS IV)	Suitable for residency readiness boot camps.

Computer Enhanced Mannequins
Cardiac Auscultation Adult Mannequins Pediatric Mannequins
  Infant
  Adolescent
Birthing Mannequins
	Formative or Summative	Clinical Clerks (MS-III)
		
		Subinterns (MS-IV)
			Adaptable to all levels of learners with calibrated scenario development.

Procedure Trainers Endoscopy Upper/Lower Bronchoscopy Uro Mentor	Formative or Summative	Most appropriate for GME and fellowship training	May provide PGY-I readiness opportunities for MS-IV students applying to integrated surgical residency/fellowship.
Virtual Reality Surgical Trainers Lap Mentor Pelvic Mentor Percutaneous Mentor Hysteroscopy Sim Angio/Endovascular Trainer TURP Mentor Arthroscopy Mentor	Formative or Summative	Most appropriate for GME and fellowship training	May provide PGY-I readiness opportunities for MS-IV students applying to integrated surgical residency/fellowship.
Ultrasound/Echo Torso (with superimposed, real-time 3D anatomical representation)	Formative or Summative	Calibrates to wide spectrum of learners	Can be utilized horizontally throughout educational curriculum, reinforcing relevant anatomy in clinical contexts.
Virtual Cadaver	Formative or Summative	Calibrates to wide spectrum of learners	Can be used to instruct and assess, and to reinforce basic science for clinical application.
Virtual Patients in Computer Generated Environments	Formative or Summative	Typically scalable to wide spectrum of learners	Teaches patient care skills, correlates basic science with clinical medicine.
Robotic Surgery Simulation Trainers	Formative or Summative	Most appropriate for fellowship training, GME, and MOC - CME	May provide residency readiness for MS-IV applying to integrated surgical residency/fellowship.

The process of constructing an effective assessment activity can be aided by taking the time, early in the planning process, to ask very practical questions of the intended function of the assessment:
- Is the assessment meant to be summative or formative?
- Which competencies will I be seeking to evaluate in my assessment?
- Have I properly calibrated my assessment to the level of the learner?
- Is it my intention to assess individuals or teams?
- Will the assessment be determinative of mastery with respect to a given competency or skill?

The answers to these types of questions are what allow form to follow function in educational planning and can help clerkship directors, working together with their institution's simulation education staff, to construct assessments that are rationally designed and properly aligned with their educational goals and purposes.[6,10] For instance, the decision to create a summative assessment is an important initial distinction to be made. It should lead clerkship directors to design an assessment activity that can succeed in eliciting the observable performance of targeted competencies and provide interpretable measurements of the performance of those competencies in such a way that can be translated into a score or grade.

"High-stakes" or summative assessments make fidelity to relevant aspects of the environment and assigned tasks a greater priority and place greater demands on the rating scales, checklists, and performance metrics selected for the assessment.[14]

With competencies related to interprofessional collaboration now being incorporated into health care education, team-related assessment activities are increasingly being required as part of educational programs. Clerkship directors need to be mindful of the unique challenges posed in framing simulation-based assessment activities that are intended to evaluate the performance of teams and team dynamics. Attention must be paid not only to creating clinical cases that can succeed in eliciting behaviors appropriate to team-delivered care, but in creating the proper checklists to capture quality data related to team performance. Rigor in this assessment process also requires that raters be properly trained to assure the reliability of the data collected.[23,24]

Mastery learning, an outcomes-based instructional approach that requires learners to demonstrate their achievement of desired levels of proficiency, is drawing attention in medical education. Evidence, thus far, has shown it to be superior to traditional, time-based, non-mastery learning, particularly when incorporated into simulation-based medical education.[25-32] Clerkship directors will have opportunities to explore the role and benefits of mastery learning in helping medical students to achieve proficiency in high-priority areas of clinical competency, such as communication (e.g., delivering bad news, securing informed consent, performing hand-offs), patient management (e.g., cardiopulmonary resuscitation) and procedural skills (e.g., placing a Foley catheter using sterile technique, inserting a central venous catheter using ultrasound guidance). In these instances, the development of one's assessment instrument requires that careful attention be given to setting standards, including the minimum passing level (MPL) for the determination of mastery.[10,33]

The decision to use simulation for more formative assessment activities should lead clerkship directors to consider factors related to delivering constructive feedback to the learner such as:
- Who will provide the feedback, and are they properly trained to do so?
- Will the feedback be delivered in a timely fashion so as to benefit the learner going forward?
- Will opportunities for deliberative practice, and the correction of errors, based on feedback, be allowed?

Providing constructive feedback in real time during a simulation-based assessment activity requires trained facilitators or confederates, working closely with the learners, who can skillfully redirect the learners and assure that tolerance of errors or the unintended reinforcement of poor performance does not occur.

18.5. Feasibility

Good ideas do not guarantee success. The best laid plans can fail to deliver. The image of the luxury cruise ship, *Costa Concordia*, lying on its side, having run aground off the coast of Italy on January 13, 2012, is a vivid reminder that things don't always go as planned.[34] It is, therefore, important that clerkship directors take into account the many variables that can potentially cause a seemingly well-constructed simulation-based assessment to run aground. *Reliability* and *validity* (see Chapter 2) are essential considerations with respect to assessment instruments and evaluative activities. Clerkship directors can, if necessary, enlist the help of statisticians or psychometricians to assure reliability and validity in designing their assessment activities.

The important area that clerkship directors must take personal responsibility for, however, is in discerning and assuring the *feasibility* of the assessment that they have constructed. Can it be successfully implemented and easily sustained?

Feasibility relates to whether or not something is possible. Feasibility requires that clerkship directors give proper consideration to those critical factors that can support or thwart their planned activities, such as:
- Resources - facilities, equipment, personnel (tech support, trained evaluators).
- Scheduling - space, learners, faculty.
- Costs - budgeting, allocation of expenses.
- Logistics - sequencing, put-through (of the learners).

18.5.1. Needed Resources

The following is a sampling of resources to consider:
- Space.
- Equipment.
- Support personnel, including clinical faculty who may require protected time for their involvement with education.

Educators who are just beginning to incorporate simulation as an educational or assessment strategy are encouraged to begin slowly and build progressively with respect to space, equipment, and personnel. Simple activities should be piloted first. Benefits should be carefully determined and convincingly communicated to key educational stakeholders. Early sentinel successes can serve to generate enthusiasm and build confidence among educators seeking to use simulation-based modalities resourcefully.

Clerkship directors should begin this process by building strong and collaborative working alliances with simulation-based educators and experts in their institution who can help to:
- Assure the availability of appropriate space.
- Stage the activity (set-up and take-down) properly.
- Acquire, program, maintain, and troubleshoot the needed simulators.
- Determine the necessary support personnel.

Included among the support personnel must be individuals who are not simply assigned to be part of an assessment activity, but properly trained to be effective facilitators and reliable evaluators. Evidence exists that evaluators who are neither faculty members nor physicians (EMS personnel, SPs, etc.) are not inferior to physicians in the reliability of their evaluations.[35,36] This finding frees clerkship directors from the need to rely solely upon busy clinical faculty to serve as evaluators or raters. It is, however, important to remember that, although reliable performance data can be generated by non-clinician raters, it remains the responsibility of clerkship directors or their delegated clinician-educators to interpret the data and to make appropriate judgments and decisions about a learner's performance in summative assessments.

18.5.2. Scheduling

Clinical education is a time-sensitive undertaking. Adding simulation to the curricular calendar, if it is to be feasible, requires commitment and careful coordination:
- Commitment: to valuing the contribution that simulation-based experiences can make to clinical learning and assessment.
- Coordination: so that simulation education activities interface harmoniously with the other components of the learners' clinical education and evaluation.

Clerkship directors must coordinate with their simulation center and its staff to identify optimal dates and times within the clerkship calendar for simulation education and assessment activities. They must likewise be cooperative in releasing the learners from other required responsibilities in order to allow them to participate freely and effectively in complementary simulation-based educational experiences and competency assessments.

18.5.3. Costs

Incorporating simulation technologies into educational activities and assessment programs can be a costly undertaking. As institutional budgets are increasingly stretched to provide needed services, the cost of simulation-based education can be perceived as a real barrier. However, evidence is beginning to emerge in the literature which demonstrates the downstream cost and safety benefits and favorable return on investment of simulation-based training.[27,37-39] That said, clerkship directors must show themselves to be not only knowledgeable users of simulation technologies to promote quality education and assessment, but also responsible stewards of the financial resources within their institution.

Accordingly, clerkship directors, in designing educational blueprints that incorporate advanced simulation technologies for performance assessment, will likely find it necessary to collaborate with, and obtain approvals from, not only curriculum management representatives, but also stakeholders from the institution's finance and budgeting offices.

18.5.4. Logistics

Simulation-based education and performance assessment can ultimately only be successful when a critical eye has been given to the timing and flow of the planned activity. In other words, one must be able to guarantee that the cohort of learners assigned to an educational session or assessment activity can move, as intended, through the exercise in the allotted times, at the designated spaces, with everyone - including evaluators and support staff - able to be where they need to be, when they need to be there. In addition, if one's assessment activity includes multiple parts that require being carried out in a preferred order, one must make certain that the flow of the activity sequences properly for all participants.

Conducting a piloted run-through of an exercise prior to the formal activity is highly recommended, for it allows you and your staff to correct any unforeseen problems before going live with the event. Only when attention is given to logistics can you assure the feasibility, sustainability, and resource effectiveness of your simulation-based education and assessment. Accordingly, again, clerkship directors are wise to ally themselves with simulation personnel.

18.6. Novel Driving Forces

The early driving forces behind that revolution and the growth in popularity of simulation-based education and assessment are, by now, well-known, and their benefits have been cited in the scientific literature.[7,41] Perhaps the best known and most obvious factors supporting the introduction and utilization of simulation have been the ability of educators to replace or amplify real experiences that evoke or replicate substantial aspects of the real world in a fully interactive manner.[11,42]

Medical educators no longer have to rely on engaging populations of patients in the hospital or clinic as the sole or necessary substrate for educational experiences and training. Neither is the learners' education limited solely to the conditions, illnesses, or circumstances represented in those populations. Simulation now provides medical educators with a vast array of effective, complementary alternatives and highly programmable options. One of the most compelling factors that has promoted the use of simulation is the perceived social mandate to mitigate risk and better assure patient safety.[43]

Training for complex skills, including procedural skills (e.g., endoscopic,[44] endovascular[45]) and surgical skills (e.g., arthroscopic,[46] laparoscopic,[47] robotic[15]) can now be accomplished, using simulation, without exposing patients to inconvenience or risk of harm.

In addition to the classic, historical, forces that spurred the use of simulation, there are several novel forces adding impetus to this movement:
- Accountability within health care training.
- Flexibility in providing learners with educational experience and skill acquisition aligned to specific fields of practice.

18.7. Readiness for Residency

Medical schools and residency programs are increasingly challenged to demonstrate that their graduates have the skills appropriate to the level of care that they are allowed to provide to patients.[49] Residency program directors have increasingly expressed concern that medical school graduates, despite impressive academic credentials, are not as optimally prepared to begin residency as they could be.[50-52] When and how to provide some of what they need for just-in-time training is not clear - it can be in the final year or just prior to the start of the PGY-1 year. Fourth-year clerkship directors should give careful consideration to using simulation-based activities that can provide opportunities for deliberate practice and mastery training for skills identified as being critical to the transition from medical school to residency.

In the push to strengthen the final year of undergraduate medical education, particularly following National Residency Match Program (NRMP) Match Day, one can envision the month of April in the final year being targeted as the designated month for intensive, "readiness for residency" education and assessment activities, supported by simulation.

18.8. The Milestones Project and Entrustable Professional Activities

Finally, clerkship directors need to be aware of the impact on undergraduate medical education as a result of a transformation taking place in graduate medical education. In 1999, ACGME introduced the six domains of clinical competency to the profession, and in 2009, it began a multiyear process of restructuring its accreditation system to be based on educational outcomes in these competencies. The result of this effort is the NAS, which began a phased implementation in July 2013.[21,57]

This new system changes the focus for accreditation of residency training programs from process and structure to outcomes.[57] Competency-based graduate medical education is being transformed and held accountable by rigorous performance-assessment requirements.[58] Program accreditation will now be based on performance-related outcomes that document whether or not trainees have achieved desired levels of competency appropriate to their level of training and related to specified dimensions of practice.

"A lack of understanding of how the knowledge, skills, and attitudes needed to perform complex tasks develop over time, ultimately led to the introduction of milestones - that seek to further deconstruct the competencies into subcompetencies and developmental levels of entrustable activity connected to real life practice."[58] As a result, the Milestones Project allows the various specialties to identify competency-based behaviors and attributes, with attention given to specifying performance standards and expectations connected to the level of residency training.

Figure 18.1 is a template for a milestone-based evaluation form as developed by the ACGME.

Showing this form with specialty-relevant content included, Figure 18.2 is an illustration of a milestone-based evaluation form to assess the subcompetency of data-gathering within the domain of patient care. Not only are the various levels criterion-based, but they also specify observable behaviors appropriate to developmental levels of learning. In this particular form, developed for the specialty of internal medicine, the five levels are intended to represent the following developmental levels:
- Critical Deficiencies.
- Early Learner.
- Advancing or Improving Learner.
- Ready for Unsupervised Practice.
- Aspirational (i.e., Master or Expert).

Figure 18.1. Milestone Template (used with permission)

Milestone Template:

Milestone Description: Template				
Level 1	Level 2	Level 3	Level 4	Level 5
What are the expectations for a beginning resident?	What are the milestones for a resident who has advanced over entry, but is performing at a lower level than expected at mid-residency?	What are the key developmental milestones mid-residency? What should they be able to do well in the realm of the specialty at this point?	What does a graduating resident look like? What additional knowledge, skills & attitudes have they obtained? Are they ready for certification?	Stretch Goals – Exceeds expectations

Comments:

© 2014 Accreditation Council for Graduate Medical Education

Figure 18.2. Milestones-Based Evaluation Form (Internal Medicine)
(Copyright © 2012 the Accreditation Council for Graduate Medical Education and the American Board of Internal Medicine. Used with permission.)

1. Gathers and synthesizes essential and accurate information to define each patient's clinical problem(s). (PC1)				
Critical Deficiencies			Ready for unsupervised practice	Aspirational
Does not collect accurate historical data Does not use physical exam to confirm history Relies exclusively on documentation of others to generate own database or differential diagnosis Fails to recognize patient's central clinical problems Fails to recognize potentially life threatening problems	Inconsistently able to acquire accurate historical information in an organized fashion Does not perform an appropriately thorough physical exam or misses key physical exam findings Does not seek or is overly reliant on secondary data Inconsistently recognizes patients' central clinical problem or develops limited differential diagnoses	Consistently acquires accurate and relevant histories from patients Seeks and obtains data from secondary sources when needed Consistently performs accurate and appropriately thorough physical exams Uses collected data to define a patient's central clinical problem(s)	Acquires accurate histories from patients in an efficient, prioritized, and hypothesis-driven fashion Performs accurate physical exams that are targeted to the patient's complaints Synthesizes data to generate a prioritized differential diagnosis and problem list Effectively uses history and physical examination skills to minimize the need for further diagnostic testing	Obtains relevant historical subtleties, including sensitive information that informs the differential diagnosis Identifies subtle or unusual physical exam findings Efficiently utilizes all sources of secondary data to inform differential diagnosis Role models and teaches the effective use of history and physical examination skills to minimize the need for further diagnostic testing

Comments:

Different specialties vary slightly in their designation of the developmental levels of skill acquisition.

Figure 18.3 shows a comparable milestones-based form for evaluating the subcompetency of data gathering in pediatrics.

For the specialty of pediatrics, the five developmental levels designated in this form are intended to correspond to the levels of skill acquisition put forth by Dreyfus:[59]
- Novice (Level 1).
- Advanced Beginner (Level 2).
- Competence (Level 3).
- Proficiency (Level 4).
- Mastery (Level 5).

Figure 18.3. Milestones-Based Evaluation Form (Pediatrics)
(Copyright © 2012 the Accreditation Council for Graduate Medical Education and the American Board of Pediatrics. All rights reserved. The copyright owners grant third parties the right to use the Pediatrics Milestones on a non-exclusive basis for educational purposes.)

PC1. Gather essential and accurate information about the patient					
Not yet Assessable	Level 1	Level 2	Level 3	Level 4	Level 5
	Either gathers too little information or exhaustively gathers information following a template regardless of the patient's chief complaint, with each piece of information gathered seeming as important as the next. Recalls clinical information in the order elicited, with the ability to gather, filter, prioritize, and connect pieces of information being limited by and dependent upon analytic reasoning through basic pathophysiology alone	Clinical experience allows linkage of signs and symptoms of a current patient to those encountered in previous patients. Still relies primarily on analytic reasoning through basic pathophysiology to gather information, but has the ability to link current findings to prior clinical encounters allows information to be filtered, prioritized, and synthesized into pertinent positives and negatives, as well as broad diagnostic categories	Demonstrates an advanced development of pattern recognition that leads to the creation of illness scripts, which allow information to be gathered while simultaneously filtered, prioritized, and synthesized into specific diagnostic considerations. Data gathering is driven by real-time development of a differential diagnosis early in the information-gathering process	Creates well-developed illness scripts that allow essential and accurate information to be gathered and precise diagnoses to be reached with ease and efficiency when presented with most pediatric problems, but still relies on analytic reasoning through basic pathophysiology to gather information when presented with complex or uncommon problems	Creates robust illness scripts and instance scripts (where the specific features of individual patients are remembered and used in future clinical reasoning) that lead to unconscious gathering of essential and accurate information in a targeted and efficient manner when presented with all but the most complex or rare clinical problems. These illness and instance scripts are robust enough to enable discrimination among diagnoses with subtle distinguishing features
Comments:					

Although the milestones introduced into the process of outcomes-based assessment were discernible stages in the development of specific competencies, there remained a need to translate this theoretical framework into the world of "real life" clinical practice. In an effort to facilitate this translation, the concept of EPAs was conceived, and groups of behaviors specific to daily practice were outlined.[56]

"Entrustable Professional Activities represent the core clinical activities of a specialist, subspecialist, resident, or medical student, appropriately scaled to level of experience. Performing these core clinical activities requires the individual to integrate the competencies and subcompetencies in their behavior, and provides a construct to help educators and program directors better define the requirements at key transition points in medical education (i.e., college to medical school, medical school to residency, and residency to practice or fellowship)."[56]

Figure 18.4 is an illustration from Carraccio that seeks to show how the EPAs, competencies, subcompetencies, and milestones are related to one another.

Figure 18.4. Entrustable Professional Activities: The Competencies and Milestones in Context (Carraccio[60])

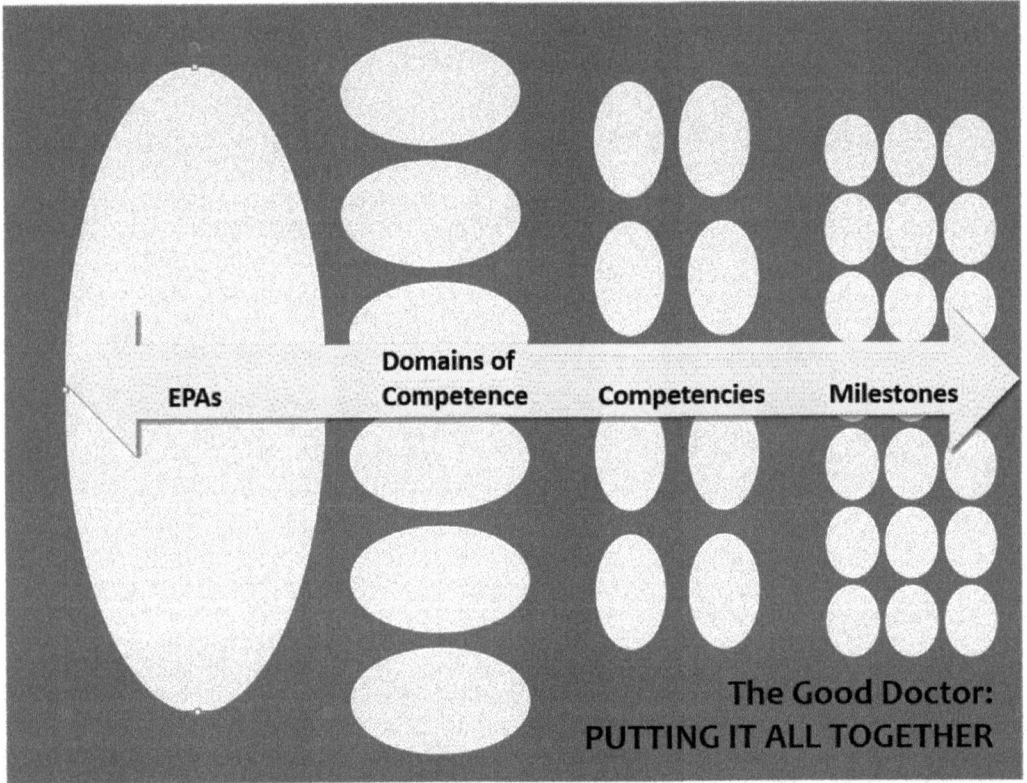

The illustration above can be expanded upon (Figure 18.5) to include the relevant elements in each of the four categories. As shown, there are six competency domains from which subcompetencies can be determined for purposes of assessment. The milestones add the developmental dimension, which seeks to assess and thereby determine where the trainee is in their skill acquisition. The EPAs provide a link to activities relevant to real practice behaviors which can be tailored to the unique activities within a discipline or specialty.

According to Carraccio (personal communication, April 28, 2014), "the use of Entrustable Professional Activities (EPAs) and Competencies defined by Milestones will allow for a comprehensive assessment of learners." The EPAs provide a holistic assessment of a learner based on the safe and effective outcome of a learner engaged in a professional activity that involves care

delivery. The competencies and their milestones provide a granular assessment of a learner's ability to perform the complex task specified by a given competency. The narrative behaviors described in the milestones are critical for formative feedback and remediation of the individual learner. Together, EPAs, competencies, and milestones provide tracking of performance:
- At the individual learner level, to inform decisions regarding promotion and readiness for independent practice.
- In the aggregate, to guide curriculum development.

Figure 18.5. Entrustable Professional Activities: The Competencies and Milestones in Context (adapted from Holmboe and Carraccio[60]) Key: EL = early learner; A, I = advancing or improving learner; UP = unsupervised practice

Core EPAER's

EPA 1: H & P
EPA 2: Differential diagnosis
EPA 3: Interpret common diagnostic and screening tests
EPA 4: Enter and discuss orders/prescriptions
EPA 5: Document a clinical encounter in the patient record
EPA 6: Provide an oral presentation of a clinical encounter
EPA 7: Form clinical questions and retrieve evidence to advance patient care
EPA 8: Give or receive a patient handover to transition care responsibility
EPA 9: Collaborate as a member of an interprofessional team
EPA 10: Recognize a patient requiring urgent or emergent care, and initiate evaluation and management
EPA 11: Obtain informed consent for tests and/or procedures
EPA 12: Perform general procedures of a physician
EPA 13: Identify system failures and contribute to a culture of safety and improvement

Domains of Competence: Knowledge, Communication, Professionalism, Patient Care, Practice-based Learning & Improvement, Systems-based practice

Competencies / Milestones (each rated EL, A,I, UP):
- Clinical Knowledge Testing & Procedures
- Communicates Well with Patient, Family
- Accepts Responsibility, Follows Through
- Gathers information / Performs procedures / Manages patients
- Responds to Feedback / Monitors Care to Improve
- Cost Effective Care

The Good Doctor: PUTTING IT ALL TOGETHER

To delineate those professional activities that all entering PGY-1 residents should be expected to perform on day one of residency without direct supervision, regardless of specialty, the Core Entrustable Professional Activities for Entering Residency (CEPAER) were developed in February 2014.[56] The EPAs embedded in Table 18.3 illustrate the CEPAER.

These core behaviors in Table 18.3, are suggested as integrated activities that should be expected of all medical school graduates. As such, this construct is relevant to medical school educators and clerkship directors who bear responsibility for assuring learner competence in these core professional activities.

Table 18.3. Proposed Core Entrustable Professional Activities for Entering Residency (CEPAER)[56]

EPA 1: Gather a history and perform a physical examination.
EPA 2: Develop a prioritized differential diagnosis and select a working diagnosis following a patient encounter.
EPA 3: Recommend and interpret common diagnostic and screening tests.
EPA 4: Enter and discuss patient orders / prescriptions.
EPA 5: Provide documentation of a clinical encounter in written or electronic format.
EPA 6: Provide an oral presentation / summary of a patient.
EPA 7: Form clinical questions and retrieve evidence to advance patient care.
EPA 8: Give or receive a patient handover to transition care responsibility to another health care provider or team.
EPA 9: Participate as a contributing and integrated member of an interprofessional team.
EPA 10: Recognize a patient requiring urgent or emergent care, initiate evaluation and treatment, and seek help.
EPA 11: Obtain informed consent for tests and/or procedures that the day one intern is expected to perform or order without supervision.
EPA 12: Perform general procedures of a physician.
EPA 13: Identify system failures and contribute to a culture.

The adoption by medical schools of the CEPAER will likely serve as a driving force, calling forth targeted measures of assessment that focus on whether or not graduating medical students are ready to begin year one of residency and be entrusted to perform professional activities appropriate to their level of experience.

Effective methods for assessing the subcompetencies within the various EPAs are necessary. Developing and employing the necessary assessments allows educators to take the first step in verifying whether students, about to begin residency, have acquired the desired skill sets. While it remains a priority to situate, whenever possible, the evaluation of trainees within the traditional context of real-time delivery of care to patients in the hospital or outpatient clinic, an important and, in certain instances, preferable role exists for simulation-based assessment.

Effective assessment activities using simulation, created for the evaluation of competence in graduate medical education, have the potential to become a shared resource, which, with proper calibration to the level of the learner, can be utilized for the assessment of medical students. Allied to this process is the shared need that both clerkship directors and residency program directors have to assure that clinical faculty, who are involved in learner assessment, are properly trained to serve as effective facilitators and evaluators within this newly evolving system - one which will likely draw upon simulation-based assessment activities.

References

1. Frank JR, Snell LS, ten Cate O, et al. Competency-based medical education: Theory to practice. Med Teach 2010;32(8):638-645.
2. Carraccio C, Wolfsthal SD, Englander R, et al. Shifting paradigms: From Flexner to competencies. Acad Med 2002;77(5):361-367.
3. Kern DE, Thomas PA, Hughes MT, eds. Curriculum Development for Medical Education: A Six-Step Approach - second edition - Baltimore: Johns Hopkins University Press, 2009.
4. Miller GE. The assessment of clinical skills/competence/performance. Acad Med 1990;65(9 Suppl):S63-S67.
5. Swanwick T, ed. Understanding Medical Education Evidence, Theory and Practice - second edition - London: Wiley Blackwell, 2013.
6. Norcini JJ, Anderson B, Bollela V, et al. Criteria for good assessment: Consensus statement and recommendations from the Ottawa 2010 conference. Med Teach 2011;33(3):206-214.
7. McGaghie WC, Issenberg SB, Petrusa ER, Scalese RJ. A critical review of simulation-based medical education research: 2003-2009. Med Educ 2010; 44(1):50-63.
8. Linn RL, ed. Educational Measurement, sponsored jointly by National Council on Measurement in Education and American Council on Education - third edition - Phoenix, AZ: Oryx, 1993.
9. Scalese RJ, Obeso VT, Issenberg SB. Simulation technology for skills training and competency assessment in medical education. J Gen Intern Med 2008;23(Suppl 1):S46-S49.
10. Downing SM, Yudkowsky R, eds. Assessment in Health Professions Education. New York: Routledge, 2009.
11. Dent JA, Harden RM, eds. A Practical Guide for Medical Teachers - fourth edition - London: Churchill Livingstone Elsevier, 2013.
12. Epstein RM. Assessment in medical education. N Engl J Med 2007;356(4):387-396.
13. Acton RD, Denmark TK, Clark A, et al. Simulation in medical student education. In: ACE Guidebook for Clerkship Directors - fourth edition - North Syracuse, NY: Gegensatz Press, 2012: 265-276.
14. Pugh CM. Simulation and high stakes testing. In: Kyle RR, Murray WB, eds. Clinical Simulation: Operations, Engineering, and Management. London: Elsevier, 2008: 655-666.
15. Abboudi H, Khan MS, Aboumarzouk O, et al. Current status of validation for robotic surgery simulators: A systematic review. BJU Int 2013;111(2):194-205.
16. Todsen T, Henriksen MV, Kromann CB, et al. Short- and long-term transfer of urethral catheterization skills from simulation training to performance on patients. BMC Med Educ 2013;13:29.
17. Blum RH, Boulet JR, Cooper JB, Muret-Wagstaff SL, Harvard Assessment of Anesthesia Resident Performance Research Group. Simulation-based assessment to identify critical gaps in safe anesthesia resident performance. Anesthesiology 2014;120(1):129-141.
18. Issa N, Salud L, Kwan C, et al. Validity and reliability of a sensor-enabled intubation trainer: A focus on patient-centered data. J Surg Res 2012;177(1):27-32.
19. Palaganas JC, Maxworthy JC, Epps CA, Mancini ME. Defining Excellence in Simulation Programs. Philadelphia: Wolters-Kluwer, 2015.
20. Kyle RR, Murray WB, eds. Clinical Simulation: Operations, Engineering, and Management. London: Elsevier, 2008.

21. ACGME Outcome Project. <dconnect.acgme.org/outcome/comp/compHome.asp>. Accessed February 5, 2015; not reachable April 6, 2015, but see <www.acgme.org/acgmeweb/tabid/435/ProgramandInstitutionalAccreditation/NextAccreditationSystem.aspx>, accessed April 6, 2015.
22. Sullivan L. The tall office building artistically considered. Lippincott's Magazine. March 1896;57:403-409.
23. Rosen MA, Salas E, Silvestri S, et al. A measurement tool for simulation-based training in emergency medicine: The simulation module for assessment of resident targeted event responses (SMARTER) approach. Simul Healthc 2008;3(3):170-179.
24. Rosen MA, Salas E, Wilson KA, et al. Measuring team performance in simulation-based training: Adopting best practices for healthcare. Simul Healthc 2008;3(1):33-41.
25. Wayne DB, Butter J, Siddall VJ, et al. Mastery learning of advanced cardiac life support skills by internal medicine residents using simulation technology and deliberate practice. J Gen Intern Med 2006;21(3):251-256.
26. Wayne DB, Fudala MJ, Butter J, et al. Comparison of two standard-setting methods for advanced cardiac life support training. Acad Med 2005;80(10 Suppl):S63-S66.
27. Barsuk JH, McGaghie WC, Cohen ER, et al. Simulation-based mastery learning reduces complications during central venous catheter insertion in a medical intensive care unit. Crit Care Med 2009;37(10):2697-2701.
28. McGaghie WC, Issenberg SB, Cohen ER, et al. Does simulation-based education with deliberate practice yield better results than traditional clinical education? A meta-analytic comparative review of the evidence. Acad Med 2011;86(6):706-711.
29. Barsuk JH, Ahya SN, Cohen ER, et al. Mastery learning of temporary hemodialysis catheter insertion by nephrology fellows using simulation technology and deliberate practice. Am J Kidney Dis 2009;54(1):70-76.
30. Barsuk JH, Cohen ER, Caprio T, et al. Simulation-based education with mastery learning improves residents' lumbar puncture skills. Neurology 2012;79(2):132-137.
31. Butter J, McGaghie WC, Cohen ER, et al. Simulation-based mastery learning improves cardiac auscultation skills in medical students. J Gen Intern Med 2010;25(8):780-785.
32. Wayne DB, Barsuk JH, O'Leary KJ, et al. Mastery learning of thoracentesis skills by internal medicine residents using simulation technology and deliberate practice. J Hosp Med 2008;3(1):48-54.
33. McGaghie WC, Siddall VJ, Mazmanian PE, et al. Lessons for continuing medical education from simulation research in undergraduate and graduate medical education: Effectiveness of continuing medical education: American College of Chest Physicians evidence-based educational guidelines. Chest 2009;135(3 Suppl):62S-68S.
34. BBC News Europe. Costa Concordia: What happened? <www.bbc.com/news/world-europe-16563562> Accessed July 14, 2015.
35. Adler MD, Trainor JL, Siddall VJ, McGaghie WC. Development and evaluation of high-fidelity simulation case scenarios for pediatric resident education. Ambul Pediatr 2007;7(2):182-186.
36. McEvoy MD, Smalley JC, Nietert PJ, et al. Validation of a detailed scoring checklist for use during advanced cardiac life support certification. Simul Healthc 2012;7(4):222-235.
37. Cohen ER, Feinglass J, Barsuk JH, et al. Cost savings from reduced catheter-related bloodstream infection after simulation-based education for residents in a medical intensive care unit. Simul Healthc 2010;5(2):98-102.
38. Wayne DB, Didwania A, Feinglass J, et al. Simulation-based education improves quality of care during cardiac arrest team responses at an academic teaching hospital: A case-control study. Chest 2008;133(1):56-61.
39. McGaghie WC, Draycott TJ, Dunn WF, et al. Evaluating the impact of simulation

on translational patient outcomes. Simul Healthc 2011;(6 Suppl):S42-S47.
40. Satava RM. Emerging trends that herald the future of surgical simulation. Surg Clin North Am 2010;90(3):623-633.
41. Issenberg SB, McGaghie WC, Petrusa ER, et al. Features and uses of high-fidelity medical simulations that lead to effective learning: A BEME systematic review. Med Teach 2005;27(1):10-28.
42. Gaba DM. The future vision of simulation in health care. Qual Saf Health Care 2004;13(Suppl 1):2-10.
43. Homsted L. Institute of medicine report: To err is human: Building a safer health care system. Fla Nurse 2000;48(1):6.
44. Van Sickle KR, Buck L, Willis R, et al. A multicenter, simulation-based skills training collaborative using shared GI mentor II systems: Results from the Texas Association of Surgical Skills Laboratories (TASSL) flexible endoscopy curriculum. Surg Endosc 2011;25(9):2980-2986.
45. Naughton PA, Aggarwal R, Wang TT, et al. Skills training after night shift work enables acquisition of endovascular technical skills on a virtual reality simulator. J Vasc Surg 2011;53(3):858-866.
46. Koehler RJ, Nicandri GT. Using the arthroscopic surgery skill evaluation tool as a pass-fail examination. J Bone Joint Surg Am 2013;95(23):e1871-e1876.
47. Nguyen T, Braga LH, Hoogenes J, Matsumoto ED. Commercial video laparoscopic trainers versus less expensive, simple laparoscopic trainers: A systematic review and meta-analysis. J Urol 2013;190(3):894-899.
48. Loyd GE, Lake CL, Greenberg RB, eds. Practical Health Care Simulations. Philadelphia: Elsevier Mosby, 2004.
49. Cohen ER, Barsuk JH, Moazed F, et al. Making July safer: Simulation-based mastery learning during intern boot camp. Acad Med 2013;88(2):233-239.
50. Lyss-Lerman P, Teherani A, Aagaard E, et al. What training is needed in the fourth year of medical school? Views of residency program directors. Acad Med 2009;84(7):823-829.
51. Naylor RA, Hollett LA, Castellvi A, et al. Preparing medical students to enter surgery residencies. Am J Surg 2010;199(1):105-109.
52. Okusanya OT, Kornfield ZN, Reinke CE, et al. The effect and durability of a pregraduation boot camp on the confidence of senior medical student entering surgical residencies. J Surg Educ 2012;69(4):536-543.
53. Haller G, Myles PS, Taffé P, et al. Rate of undesirable events at beginning of academic year: Retrospective cohort study. BMJ 2009;339:b3974.
54. Phillips DP, Barker GE. A July spike in fatal medication errors: A possible effect of new medical residents. J Gen Intern Med 2010;25(8):774-779.
55. Esterl RM,Jr, Henzi DL, Cohn SM. Senior medical student "boot camp" can result in increased self-confidence before starting surgery internships. Curr Surg 2006; 63(4):264-268.
56. AAMC. Core Entrustable Professional Activities for Entering Residency. <www.mededportal.org/icollaborative/resource/887>. Accessed February 7, 2015.
57. Nasca TJ, Philibert I, Brigham T, Flynn TC. The next GME accreditation system: Rationale and benefits. N Engl J Med 2012;366(11):1051-1056.
58. Carraccio C, Burke AE. Beyond competencies and milestones: Adding meaning through context. J Grad Med Educ 2010;2(3):419-422.
59. Dreyfus SE, Dreyfus HL. A Five-Stage Model of the Mental Activities Involved in Directed Skill Acquisition. Berkeley: Operations Research Center, 1980.
60. Holmboe ES, Carraccio C. The Horizon in Medical Education: From Milestones to EPAs to a New Accreditation System, 2014. <bhpr.hrsa.gov/grants/medicine/technicalassistance/medicaleducation.pdf>. Accessed May 17, 2015.

Table 19.1. Pros and Cons of Different Testing Formats

Test Type	Pros	Cons
Locally Developed MCQ	- Well accepted format. - Can be adapted to the local content of the clerkship. - No "direct" purchase cost. - Easily keyed and graded. - Straightforward to administer.	- Very difficult to produce sufficient number of MCQs measuring higher order function without professional test writing, editing, and vetting. - Difficult to keep the question pool from getting out to the students.
NBME Subject Test	- Well accepted format. - Good psychometric information available. - Graded for you (2 week lag). - Constantly changing question pool. - Helps to prepare student for NBME Step 2 written exam. - Straightforward to administer.	- Cost (around $43 per student). - May not reflect the local curriculum.
Locally Developed Constructed Response - Written	- Accepted format. - Easier to develop items to measure higher order function. - Well suited to subspecialty elective rotations.	- Time-consuming to grade (recommend typed into to computer to alleviate handwriting issues ...). - Difficult to key incorrect aspects of an answer.
Locally Developed Constructed Response - Oral	- Accepted format. - Easier to develop items to measure higher order function. - Prepares student for some ABMS-style oral examinations. - Well suited to subspecialty elective rotations.	- Hard to corral sufficient faculty to administer for large clerkship. - Hard to uniformly grade (interrater problems).
Objective Structured Clinical Exercise (OSCE)	- an accepted format on the clerkship level. - Prepares student for NBME Step 2 Clinical Skills Exam. - Can be used in formative and summative testing situations. - Can test higher order function.	- Requires appropriate facility and expertise to develop questions, train patients, etc. - Developing checklists (keys) to favor higher order function can be difficult. - Expensive to produce - more so for summative than formative testing. - Difficult to get the reliability of an MCQ test.

Chapter 19
Designing and Setting Standards in Clerkship Examinations

Julia Corcoran, M.D., M.H.P.E.

Clerkship examinations serve several purposes - motivators for student study, assessments of student knowledge, objective contributions to grade assignment, and tools for evaluating clerkships. Nearly all clinical clerkships rely heavily on faculty appraisals of student performance for grade assignments; most also add a testing component. This chapter describes the strategy and related processes for blueprinting examinations, the practicalities of constructing and administering tests, and for determining passing standards for examinations in light of their quality (reliability and validity). It complements discussions of available testing methods (Chapter 15) and focusses on how *individual* exams are graded. This discussion is extended in Chapter 20 to how grades of specific examinations are *combined* with teachers' grades into a summary clerkship grade.

19.1. Testing vs. Performance Appraisal

Testing by means of examinations can be more "objective" or "quantified" than performance appraisals in a clinical clerkship, in which a personal teacher-student dimension is present. Tests lack the "halo effect" that an energetic, youthful student can generate. They can also more efficiently sample a larger portion of the knowledge domain, allowing the student to demonstrate breadth as well as depth.

Performance appraisals by medical faculty, notoriously, may have a limited range of responses, tend to be skewed toward the upper end of the scale, and often lack specific descriptors or examples of the student's clinical performance.[1] Even when the appraisal form is well constructed, more than seven faculty evaluations are necessary to balance so-called doves, hawks, and indifferent appraisers.[2] Furthermore, it is often difficult to obtain from numerical scales a critique that can be used for feedback, and written comments may be vague. "The best student I have ever worked with" does not help students constructively any more than the lack of negative critique for struggling students. For some dimensions of performance, clerkship tests can be used to distinguish good from poor student performance, and to offer a basis for feedback that may not be forthcoming from faculty appraisals. (For a contrasting discussion about teachers' evaluations, see Chapter 8.)

19.2. Reliability and Validity

For tests to serve the purposes noted in the introductory paragraph they must produce reliable scores that can be used for valid decision making.

Reliability refers to the accuracy and reproducibility of assessment data or scores over time or occasions and is a quality of test data.[3] Reliable tests perform consistently (whether scores are high or low) within and between groups of students. They correctly classify students who are achieving at, above, and below an accepted level. Statistical models can help to assess the reliability of tests (KR-20 and 21), test items (p), and evaluators (interrater reliability). These statistical models help to determine how much of the variance in scores is related to student knowledge of the subject as opposed to test flaws and other unexplained sources (see Chapter 2).

Validity is not a quality of the test score but of the meaning, decisions, and inferences drawn from that score. Prior concepts of validity concentrated on validity of content (representation of the subject area), construct validity (the test proper for the skill, e.g., an essay to judge writing), and criterion validity (whether the information correlates with other findings). The current concept of validity is that of a unified hypothesis supported by data available from a current test. Validating a test is the process of collecting empirical data and logical arguments to support that our inferences (grades assigned) are correct.[4] Ultimately, validity is achieved when grades correspond accurately to a certain level of skill or knowledge in the clerkship domain. Validating requires correlations and corroborations rather than straightforward statistical analysis. Kerfoot *et al.* present a flowchart for the iterative process of validating a test for students on a urology rotation.[5] An example of corroborative evidence for validity of a pediatrics final examination is provided in a correlation study by Hijazi *et al.*[6]

19.3. Testing Options: What, When, If, and How?

Tests should be appropriate to the purpose and situation (clerkship lengths, number of students, etc.); several examples follow. In a two or four-week elective clerkship on a subspecialty service with a single student involved, it would be difficult to develop and validate a long MCQ examination. In that setting, a collection of short essays or an oral examination (constructed responses [CR]) may be more useful at the end of the rotation (summative). In an 8-12 week rotation, however, it might be quite possible to develop and validate local MCQ exams, administer an NMBE subject test (shelf exam), or create an OSCE with SPs or a structured oral examination with faculty (see Chapters 16 and 17). During longer clerkships, even formative testing early in a clerkship with exams of lower, but acceptable, reliability, can be useful to identify students at risk of failing the clerkship final examination. This approach has been studied in medicine and surgery clerkships.[7-9] Table 19.1 (above, p. 228) summarizes the pros and cons of the commonly used test formats.

19.4. Planning the Test: Blueprinting

Tests should be planned to reflect the course curriculum, including knowledge, skills, and professional behaviors and attitudes. Documentation that specifies the content areas to be tested is referred to as the test blueprint (see also Chapter 7). This documentation also serves to indicate sources of evidence to establish the validity of the test.

To develop a blueprint, the faculty must establish which knowledge content is important, which skills are important, which domains are to be examined (e.g., book knowledge, clinical skills, technical skills, communication skills, professionalism), the level of cognition demanded (recall, application, problem solving, etc.), and the relative importance of each element. The content of the examination should be linked directly to the curriculum of the clerkship. For example, asking random pediatric questions on an obstetrics/gynecology examination detracts from the validity and reliability of the ob/gyn on factors other than knowledge about ob/gyn. Blueprints should be developed for *all* tests, whether MCQ, CR, or OSCE.

An example of a blueprint for a third-year surgery clerkship summative OSCE is found in Table 19.2. Knowledge objectives were surveyed in each of the subspecialty domains to determine where they fell on the Bloom's taxonomy of mastery of knowledge: recall (remembrance or recitation of facts), application (ability to apply knowledge such as interpretation of tables, etc.), or problem solving (using knowledge in a novel situation to solve the problem, also called synthesis).[10] The objectives focus knowledge questions at this level. Course objectives state whether students are expected to be able to diagnose, triage, or manage any given surgical problem. Patient care questions are limited by the extent of the objective. The number of stations or questions for each surgical specialty is based on the percentage of student-hours which that specialty represents for the average student in the clerkship. Competencies are schoolwide and reported back to the students on a central dashboard for feedback on their development in each area. Scoring of the exam is done by checklists and answer key.

Systems considerations are important. Once the blueprint is developed, it should be disseminated to the departmental curriculum committee to confirm that it reflects the intentions of the curriculum design. The faculty should review the blueprint for instructional design and item development. Most importantly, students should see the blueprint at the start of the rotation, so that they understand the expectations of the clerkship examinations. If they know that they will be held responsible for physical exam material and patient counseling material, hopefully they will study in these contexts.

Giving the blueprint to the students is not equivalent to handing them the specific content of the examination. In the example above (see Table 19.2), the students are given the blueprint (general surgery, orthopedics, etc.), but without the subject matter (acute abdomen, fracture, etc.). They are told that subject matter comes directly from the objectives. This decreases the amount of variance in student scores due to factors surrounding content of the examination and increases the validity of the using the test scores in grading broad acquisition of knowledge.

Table 19.2. Sample Test Blueprint: 12-Station OSCE in Third-Year Surgery Clerkship, Northwestern University Feinberg School of Medicine

Specialty Domain	Subject Matter	Format	Skill	Competency
General Surgery	Acute Abdomen	SP	Abdominal Exam	Physical Exam
General Surgery	Acute Abdomen	Constructed Response	Order Set	Patient Care; Written Communication
General Surgery	Breast	SP	History - Verbal	Communication - Listening
General Surgery	Breast	SP	Breast Self-Exam	Communication - Counseling
Orthopedics	Fracture	SP	Extremity Exam	Physical Exam
Orthopedics	Fracture	Constructed Response	Radiographs Management	Patient Care
Urology	Scrotal Mass	SP	Genital / Groin Exam	Physical Exam; Communication - Uncomfortable Exam
Urology	Scrotal Mass	Constructed Response	Differential Diagnostic Work-Up	Differential Patient Care
ENT	Neck Mass	SP	Oral / Neck Exam	Physical Exam; History
ENT	Neck Mass	Constructed Response	Chart Entry	Medical Knowledge; Written Communication
Ophthalmology	Red Eye	Constructed Response	Case-Based Written Scenario	Medical Knowledge
Neurosurgery	Changing ICP	Constructed Response	Case-Based Written Scenario	Medical Knowledge

19.5. Constructing the Test

Once the blueprint has been approved, developing items and assembling them into a test is the next task. This administrative work includes setting a timeline and assigning topics to the subject matter experts - i.e., your faculty - and collecting the items. (Busy clinicians can be hard to pin down, but persistence pays off.) The specifics of how to write good multiple choice items and develop SP cases and OSCEs are covered in Chapters 16 and 17.

Concise instructions help the faculty members develop items that fit into the blueprint. A letter of intent outlining the subjects to be covered, the format to be used, a copy of the pertinent course objectives, and a similar item in another domain which can be used as a template is one approach. Lead time is essential; start almost six months in advance. Routine follow-up with electronic correspondence and contact with office assistants is helpful. Visiting the faculty in their offices, operating room, or clinic can also be important.

Editing begins once the items have been submitted. The first round of editing includes checking that items match the blueprint and course objectives. The phrasing must be clear, without double negatives, *double entendre*, or red herrings. Item flaws, such as colloquial language, misspellings, and grammatical errors must be eliminated.[10] Medical transcriptionists make good copyeditors in this situation - they have heard the vocabulary but cannot read into the meaning.

The test items should then be put in order of administration and an answer key / checklist developed. Piloting the test, using the core faculty to check both the items and the key is optimal; but using residents may risk the confidentiality of test contents.

These steps for collecting, editing, assembling, and keying a test are the same regardless of the test format. Documentation of each of the events also feeds into the validity evidence.

19.6. Administration and Security

Cheating, clearly, decreases the variance in scores and must be discouraged vigilantly. Cheating takes many forms - advance copies of examinations, direct copying of answers from an unwitting student, or even cooperative cheating among a group of students. The best solution to this problem is prevention.

Once assembled, paper tests and examination documents should be kept under lock and key. If possible, use a computer that is off the network, so that accidental dissemination is less likely; otherwise, computers should be password protected. Other electronic copies of the test are kept on an external drive under lock and key. Constructed response and SP situations are less likely to be affected than MCQ tests by advance leaks of test content, but content should be protected.

When administering pencil and paper examinations, students should be seated in a well-lighted room with ample space between students. Tests should be numbered and counted at the end of the test to assure that no copies leave the room. Students should be oriented to the examination in a context of professionalism. They should be informed that "passing questions on" does not help either themselves or future students, and that this type of behavior in NBME and ABMS examinations is also considered a serious breach, as well as a copyright violation.

Test scores should be reviewed promptly. A quick look at the descriptive statistics, including the low score, high score, distribution of scores, and mean will tell the test administrator a lot about irregularities. Scores should reflect the range of student abilities. Clustering of scores at a certain number, an unusually high number of students achieving high or low grades, or a sudden change in the range of scores, can each indicate irregularities. If such irregular scores show up, then the test should be reviewed for any errors in the answer key, the test itself, or its assembly. If all is well with test and key, then the possibility of cheating must be considered. Misadministration also can cause irregularities, which should be documented by the exam proctor. Examples include pairing the wrong key with a test, loss of power during testing with projected or audio stems, attrition of an SP, loss of a student's response sheet, or loss of data entered into a computer system.

The next step in testing is to record the scores and submit them for inclusion in the grading process. Scores should be reported to the students and to the faculty. Grades, and sometimes scores, should be reported to the dean's office. Grading spreadsheets should be considered privileged data and kept under lock and key as well. Much like patient information, student information is considered protected personal data.

19.7. Psychometric Evaluation of the Test

Different tests require different evaluations. As mentioned above, a quick glance at the descriptive statistics surrounding any test will give a rough guide to its performance as an instrument for discriminating among students' achievement levels. The broader distribution curves will accent differences between students, as long as the source of that variance is the test itself and not irregularities. Statistical reliability analysis can shed more light on the examination's performance.[3,10]

The Kuder-Richardson formulae (KR-20 and 21) are reliability analyses suitable for multiple choice examinations and larger OSCE examinations. KR-20 and 21 are indexes of how well the test assesses a single body of information. The equivalent reliability index for rating scale data is Cronbach's *alpha*. The exam is tested against itself, internally - essentially broken in half and the halves compared with as many combinations of questions as possible. The math is complex, but can be done by computer programs such as SAS or PASW (formerly SPSS). If locally developed exams are used, then these statistics may be provided by the school's computer center when they score exams, as when Scantron "bubble sheets" are used. The NBME score reports provide statistical analyses. Clerkship directors should review available statistical support and formats for reporting examinations with their institution's own computer scoring center.

An acceptable KR-20 or 21 for end of clerkship MCQ tests is in the range of 0.7 to 0.8. Reliability coefficients for high-stakes examinations, such as the USMLE, run around 0.9. One way to increase the reliability of the test is to increase the number of items on the examination, rather than extensively rewrite the questions themselves. With fewer samples of a student's ability, *alpha* for OSCEs tend to be lower, in the range of 0.6, for a twelve-station format.

Another way of considering evaluation of an OSCE is factor analysis. While KR-20 and 21 are used to assess whether a test covers a cohesive unit of knowledge, factor analysis can help to determine whether multiple scales (e.g., skills in an OSCE) are being sampled. Through a data-reduction statistical method, factor analysis determines which items act similarly, i.e., test a single skill (load on a single axis, in statistical parlance). Chesser *et al.* reported analyzing a high-stakes OSCE with factor analysis to help the faculty to determine the Pass/Fail cut point.[11]

As an example, in this chapter author's first two years of administering a summative OSCE examination in a multidisciplinary surgery clerkship, it took us a while to build the checklists and clinical stations. The reliability coefficients that we calculated were consistently low, in the range of 0.48 to 0.53. Factor analysis subsequently revealed that we had four axes which grouped around skills in (1) physical examination, (2) clinical problem management, (3) communication skills, and (4) motor skills. Knowing these qualities of the items, we felt that we could comment on the students' mastery of the skills. Using the function of "reliability if this item were excluded," we identified stations of higher unreliability and concentrated our editing efforts on those items, which, over time, increased the reliability of the exam as a whole.

Another test evaluation method is item analysis. The performance of the item is measured grossly by its difficulty, "p," which is the percentage of students who correctly answer the examination. Items with $p < 0.3$ are items which students may be guessing randomly. Items with $p > 0.8$ are mastery items or easy items that most students know. Items between these extremes are the items that help to discriminate between students of varying knowledge. The point biserial (p-bis) is a discrimination index reflecting which students correctly answer the questions, those in the upper, middle, or lower third. A p-bis of > 0.20 indicates that a question discriminates well between high, middle, and low performers. Items that are too easy, too hard, or non-discriminating add noise to the variance. If a test is purely to mark achievement, then it can be composed of pure mastery questions with a $p > 0.8$. But if we are to use the test for assigning ranks (i.e., grades), then discrimination should be sought.

19.8. Determining Pass/Fail Cutoff - Setting a Standard

Several methods to determine Pass/Fail points are available. Historically, norm-referenced Pass/Fail schemes were commonplace - that is, grading "on the curve." A problem with norm referencing is that it does not require a prior decision about what should be known and must be known. Criterion-referenced schemas develop an absolute numerical Pass/Fail point, and depend upon judgments about what constitutes sufficient mastery. Different schemas produce different cutoff points.

When developing long, high-stakes tests, these rigorous methods for setting cut points are worth the investment of time, energy, and money. In the classroom, some simplified combination methods are available - the Hofstee method and the direct borderline method (an Angoff variant).

19.8.1. The Hofstee Method

The Hofstee method requires the faculty to choose a minimum percentage correct, so that, even if everyone achieved this score, it would be acceptable for all students to pass; and the maximum percentage correct, so that, even if everyone achieved this score, all should fail. The lowest and highest number of failures acceptable are plotted. The cumulative distribution curve is plotted against these points to determine the cutoff point. This schema has elements of relative and absolute design and seems well-understood by faculty and students. Cusimano and Rothman applied this technique and compared it to other schemas on a fourth-year summative OSCE.[12] They found that it gave consistent and acceptable statistical and real data. We have used this method on our clerkship's composite score to determine the Pass/Fail cut point for our clerkship.[13]

19.8.2. The Direct Borderline Method

The direct borderline method is very useful in clerkship examinations. Downing and colleagues compared this method to the Nedelsky, Hofstee, and Ebel methods in establishing Pass/Fail cutoffs for two basic science MCQ examinations and found that it performs favorably, compared with the more established methods.[14] In the direct borderline method, for each item, the clerkship director asks whether the borderline failing/passing student would get the question correct - yes or no. The affirmative responses are added for the cutoff score. Unlike the Angoff method, probabilities and panels are not used making the direct borderline method achievable for the course director. Because the direct borderline method relies on a single or small number of faculty, it is quite feasible. At the same time that the faculty review the test and check the answer key, the question can be rated for the Pass/Fail point of a borderline student. Having worked with our faculty, I have found the direct borderline method useful in establishing cut points to develop certifying checklists for procedures and for individual OSCE stations.

19.9. Item Banking

Item banking refers to keeping track of test items in an orderly format. After going to the trouble of developing high-quality test items, keeping track of them only makes sense. In addition to storing each item itself, statistical information about the item performance (p and p-bis), when the item was used (clerkship, quarter, year), qualities of the question (subject matter, level of knowledge mastery, type of question: MCQ, CR, OSCE), and tagging the item to competency, can be done for future reference. Item banking can be as simple as an Excel spreadsheet or as complicated as a database set up by the school's department of education or IT services.

There are several benefits to this kind of organization of data about test items. By examining the performance of an item over time, outdated items can be removed and poorly performing items can be culled as better ones are developed, increasing the overall quality of the test items in the bank. With a sufficiently large item bank, we might create parallel exam forms, in which different sets of questions taken from the bank yield comparable reliability and validity. Using a test blueprint and an item bank, we would select different questions of similar difficulty and subject matter, but which have not been used in the past two clerkship iterations. This type of item rotation increases the security of the test because tests for subsequent clerkships will be different, yet are considered equivalent because item statistics produce comparable reliability. While this concept is appealing, it can be difficult to create parallel forms of an exam on the clerkship level that perform similarly enough to grade across groups of students, and equivalence of the exams should be demonstrated, rather than assumed.

If multiple clerkship directors, regionally or nationally, keep data about items in a similar manner, items could be traded between institutions, so that local faculty need not come up with fresh items every year.

19.10. Summary

Objective, quantified testing is an important component in assigning grades to clinical clerks. Attention to detail of the test content, test format, and test administration contributes to valid decisions about students. Evaluation of the test with the goal of continual improvement can decrease random variance, increasing reliability and adding validity evidence. The inferences that we can draw in order to grade our students can only be as good as the tests that we base them upon.

Each step outlined above can provide evidence for the validity hypothesis. Clear information about the expectations and objectives in the clerkship, the competencies and skills that will be encountered, what will be tested, and how it will be tested establish a strong syllabus. Developing appropriate, well-constructed tests reflecting the local curriculum and faculty values that are linked to the established syllabus allows faculty to set standards, so that grading decisions are fair, not capricious, and can be explained to students and the educational community at large.

Additional Resources

Waugh CK, Gronlund NE. Assessment of Student Achievement - tenth edition - Boston: Pearson, 2013.

Haladyna TM. Developing and Validating Multiple Choice Test Items - second edition - Mahwah, NJ: Erlbaum, 1999.

References

1. Williams RG, Klamen DA, McGaghie WC. Cognitive, social, and environmental sources of bias in clinical performance ratings. Teach Learn Med 2003;15(4): 270-292.
2. Carline JD, Paauw DS, Thiede KW, Ramsey PG. Factors affecting the reliability of ratings of students' clinical skills in a medicine clerkship. J Gen Intern Med 1992; 7(5):506-510.
3. Downing SM. Reliability: On the reproducibility of assessment data. Med Educ 2004;38(9):1006-1012.
4. Kane MT. Validation. In: Brennan RL, ed. Educational Measurement - fourth edition - Westport, CT: Praeger, 2006: 17-64.
5. Kerfoot BP, Baker H, Valkan K, et al. Development of a validated instrument to measure medical student learning in clinical urology: A step toward evidence based education. J Urol 2004;172(1):282-285.
6. Hijazi Z, Premadasa IG, Moussa MA. Performance of students in the final examination in paediatrics: Importance of the "short cases." Arch Dis Child 2002;86(1):57-58.
7. Hemmer PA, Pangaro LN. The effectiveness of formal evaluation sessions during clinical clerkships in better identifying students with marginal funds of knowledge. Acad Med 1997;72(7):641-643.
8. Denton GD, Durning SJ, Wimmer AP, et al. Is a faculty developed pretest equivalent to pre-third year GPA or USMLE Step 1 as a predictor of third-year internal medicine clerkship outcomes? Teach Learn Med 2004;16(4):329-332.
9. Corcoran J, Halverson AL, Schindler N. A formative midterm test increases accuracy of identifying students at risk of failing a third year surgery clerkship. Am J Surg 2014;207(2):260-262.
10. Linn RL, Gronlund NE. Measurement and Evaluation in Teaching - eighth editon - Upper Saddle River, NJ: Merrill, 2000.
11. Chesser AM, Laing MR, Miedzybrodzka ZH, et al. Factor analysis can be a useful standard setting tool in a high stakes OSCE assessment. Med Educ 2004;38(8): 825-831.
12. Cusimano MD, Rothman AI. Consistency of standards and stability of pass/fail decisions with examinee-based standard-setting methods in a small-scale objective structured clinical examination. Acad Med 2004;79(10 Suppl):S25-S27.
13. Schindler N, Corcoran J, DaRosa D. Description and impact of using a standard-setting method for determining pass/fail scores in a surgery clerkship. Am J Surg 2007;193(2):252-257.
14. Downing SM, Lieska NG, Raible MD. Establishing passing standards for classroom achievement tests in medical education: A comparative study of four methods. Acad Med 2003;78(10 Suppl):S85-S87.

Chapter 20
Converting Evaluations into Grades

Michael Battistone, M.D.

The clinical performance of students on clerkship rotations involves a constellation of attributes and behaviors. These attributes and behaviors are not physical properties (e.g., height, weight) that can be measured directly. Rather, clinical performance can be considered a psychological construct, or a theoretical concept, which offers a framework for interpreting and discussing the meaning of specific observations of performance within their defined context. Another example of a psychological construct is "emotional intelligence." This is difficult to measure directly, yet is accepted in popular culture and recognized in academic settings. Clinical performance is a construct in which knowledge, skills, attitudes, and values can be discussed, with these specific domains serving as frames of reference, which focus observations and guide reflection.

This chapter considers how teachers' judgment about students' performance in the workplace, in either skill or attitudes or case-specific knowledge considered discretely, or in their progress in the RIME framework, may be combined with quantified assessments to yield summative grades to be submitted to the school's registrar. We consider the decisions that must be made about whether students should be compared against each other at a time in the academic year, and whether criteria should be applied consistently throughout the year. Our approach here is not prescriptive, as general policies on grading must be decided by each school's or department's education (curriculum) committee functioning as a planning committee; and decisions about specific students are made by a specifically constituted progress committee, or by an education committee functioning as a grading or advancement committee in clerkship-level decisions about students' progress[1] or as a competency committee, as is now required for residency programs in the U.S.[2]

20.1. Evaluations and Grades

In considering the issues involved in deriving grades from evaluations, it is important to reiterate the distinction between evaluation and grading (see Chapter 2). Evaluation of the performance of an individual (student, teacher) or program (course, curriculum) involves critical reflection on observations made during the period of evaluation - reflection that considers these observations within the framework of the expectations of the evaluators. (Ideally, these expectations are congruent with those of the program.) Evaluations of student performance are strengthened when specific observations are reported in detail and interpreted with reference to course requirements.

Grading, on the other hand, involves the assignment of rank to a set of evaluations; often the performances are classified across ordinal categories (Honors, High Pass, Pass, Low Pass, Fail, or A-B-C-D-F), or expressed quantitatively as points or percentages.

Policies on the framework (Pass/Fail, A-B-C-D-F, etc.) in which grades are reported to the registrar's office are typically set by the institution, not by departments or clerkship directors. While there is heterogeneity in grading practices and in the number of students receiving the top grades across U.S. medical schools,[3] 90% of American schools use a system of three to five rankings[4] (see Table 20.1).

Table 20.1. The Number of Possible Scores Used in U.S. Medical School Grading Systems, after Takayama et al. (2006)[4]

# of scores	% of schools
2	5
3	28
4	31
5	19
6	1
7	3
8	1
11	1
Continuous numbering	1
Not classifiable	10

20.2. Methods of Converting Evaluations into Grades

There are many reasonable methods by which evaluations may be converted into grades, and each institution and clerkship has specific needs that require unique solutions. To assist those responsible for developing solutions in the form of policy, some common questions are identified below and discussed dialectally ("point-counterpoint"). Specifically, these are: (1) whether those who evaluate students should also grade them, (2) whether evaluations of performances later in a clerkship or later in the clinical year should count more toward a student's final grade, and (3), whether normative (population-based) or criterion-referenced (fixed standard) approaches should be used in determining Honors. Examples and descriptions of how these issues are addressed at one institution (the University of Utah School of Medicine) are included. Finally, there is a review of several approaches used in computing the final grade, and a brief discussion of some of the issues involved in grades that may be considered "Low Pass" or "Fail."

20.2.1. Links Between Evaluators and Graders - Should Teachers Grade?

Question for clerkship directors: Should teachers grade or simply evaluate?

20.2.1.a. Point: Those Who Evaluate Should Be Those Who Grade

At many institutions, evaluators (faculty, and often house staff) are expected to submit both evaluations and grades, which are often documented in a single instrument (see Chapter 8). There is "face validity" to this method (i.e., it seems reasonable and consistent with the assumption that teachers know their students);[5] and though students may dispute a grade, their complaints often appeal to issues of communication or observation (e.g., unclear expectations or infrequent or inadequate sampling of performance), rather than to an argument that this approach is fundamentally unfair. Similarly, faculty and residents have traditionally accepted the responsibility to grade students who have been assigned to work with them on clinical rotations. If this model is chosen, the clerkship director and departmental education committee determine the percentage of each student's grade to be allocated to each level of teacher (resident, attending), and the final grade will primarily be a calculation of input from the graders.

20.2.1.b. Counterpoint: Those Who Evaluate Should Not Be Those Who Grade

The rationale for this approach is based on the view that the relationship between the trainee and the evaluator introduces bias, and thereby poses a substantial threat to validity.[6,7]

20.2.1.c. Managing Variance Between Teachers

A recent study found that 60% of the variance in student performance ratings was attributable to the interaction between rater and student, and the dependability of individual ratings was very low (4%).[8] In deciding how to incorporate the recommendations of individual teachers into a final summative grade, the clerkship director must weigh the experience of the teacher, the kind and amount of contact with the student, and how much confidence there is in the individual assessments themselves. This last factor involves dealing with variance in teacher behaviors, and can be difficult to quantify. Some faculty may feel pressure to "inflate" grades, particularly in settings where they are giving feedback to students directly ("face-to-face").[9] Even though not all evaluators succumb to the pressures to inflate grades, there is variance across the range of raters. On the other hand, some instructors may defend their practice of rarely, if ever, awarding a perfect score with the comment, "No medical student is perfect"; while others may typically give high marks because they are afraid of discouraging students if they do otherwise. Under these conditions, grades tell us less about the performance of the individual student than they do about the operational constructs and philosophy of the rater. This is a very serious problem, and must be addressed if the validity of evaluations is to be preserved.

We recommend two approaches to consider in a system in which the evaluators also grade: (1) Include a systematic and ongoing method of training raters (ideally in "real time") to use your evaluation and grading techniques.[10,11]

(2) Develop mechanisms to detect, identify, and modulate the extent of rater leniency or severity. With the growth of electronic and online evaluation, some computer programs may assist in this task, and it may be possible to adapt currently available software to use in your existing evaluation method.

Some clerkships have addressed these threats to validity by separating the processes of evaluation from grading. In these systems, evaluators are instructed to focus their efforts on producing detailed written documentation of their observations of student performance. All student evaluations are then reviewed by a grading committee, which may include the clerkship director. This method seeks to protect the evaluators from the pressures of grade inflation, and to preserve the ability of the clerkship director to serve as student advocate.

Following is an example of one method, then a discussion of it:

Regardless of whether evaluators are charged with the responsibility of grading, the links between evaluation and grading should be strong, and the process of converting evaluations to grades should be systematized under the auspices of the department. In some schools the dean's office provides guidelines to ensure interdepartmental equivalence. Resources should be directed to ensure both adequate periods for faculty and residents to observe students and the timely collection of valid evaluations. The clerkship director may want to identify a minimum time of exposure (e.g., two weeks) that is required before a rater can be expected to submit an evaluation. However, the length of the assigned tour of duty may not be the most significant factor in determining whether a given evaluation is credible. Valid evaluations of clinical performance are predicated on valid observations of clinical performance. There may be substantial variance across raters regarding their efficiency and effectiveness in observing their students - it may be that one rater can submit a credible evaluation after a period of only one week, while another rater may not be able to do this despite having been assigned three weeks with the team. If there have been several changes in evaluators over a given period of observation (for example, a change in supervising residents), then it may be reasonable for the raters to submit a single evaluation that represents their shared opinion. Since some students may contest how clinical grades are calculated, we recommend that the clerkship's handbook should only indicate their consideration in grade calculation, and that the department will allocate grading with input based on student performance evaluations (see Chapter 21).

When teachers "grade," it is especially important to guide their observations. As a method for achieving consistent input from teachers, the internal medicine clerkship at the University of Utah used formal evaluation sessions, held every three weeks during inpatient rotations (see Chapter 8), moderated by the clerkship director (or assistant clerkship director) and attended by ward residents (PGY-2 and PGY-3) and faculty on service. Interns were not required to attend the sessions or to submit evaluations; their impressions were communicated through their supervising residents. Each evaluator verbally described the students' performance using the RIME construct,[12] and provided specific observations to substantiate the rating. Evaluators were directed to conclude their critiques by identifying specific "next steps" to which students' future efforts should be directed. The vocabulary terms identified and discussed at the evaluation session were converted to numerical ratings; this is discussed in more detail below.

Immediately after the evaluation session, the students met individually with the clerkship director to review the written evaluations, as well as the verbal comments. Each student appointment was scheduled for fifteen minutes, and strategies for achieving the prescribed "next step" were discussed.

20.2.2. Considering Student Progress Within the Course - Should Later Evaluations Count More?

Question for clerkship directors: should later evaluations count more?

20.2.2.a. Point: The Final Grade of Clinical Performance Should Be One in Which Each Individual Evaluation (Grade) Is Weighted Equally

Each observer has something to offer in the evaluation of a student. Not counting each evaluation toward the final grade risks diminishing the importance of each individual period of observation, in the eyes of both the students and the instructors. In addition, the dependability of the final evaluation increases with the number of ratings - the more evaluations included, the more dependable the grade will be.

20.2.2.b. Counterpoint: The Final Grade Should Emphasize Student Performance at the End of the Clerkship

In many cases, student performance is seen to improve over the course of a clinical rotation. It may be that the trajectory of student growth (the learning curve) may be more predictive of future performance than any individual point on the line. Students who start strong, but do not progress, may be at greater risk for future marginal performance than students who struggle initially, then "get it" and demonstrate rapid improvement. Certainly students who demonstrate declining performance raise concern. If each individual evaluation is graded and given equal weight, valuable information about student development may not be captured or reflected in the final grade.

20.2.2.c. Examples and Discussion

This topic actually includes two separate issues; the slope of the learning curve, and the final level of performance. In addressing the first, it is important to know whether the specific evaluation system being used is responsive to student growth. In comparing a global numeric rating system with the RIME descriptive vocabulary,[13,14] we found that the descriptive method was superior to the numeric system in demonstrating student progress through the nine-week inpatient portion of the clerkship. If any given evaluation method were relatively unresponsive to student growth, it would lack construct validity for the premise that students do in fact improve, this issue would be moot, and it would be important to include as many ratings as possible (assuming valid methods of observation and evaluation) to ensure adequate dependability.

In addressing the final level of performance that the student achieves, the clerkship director must also consider whether the same grading standard should be applied uniformly across the year. Data suggest that, particularly for the NBME examinations, students who are assessed later in the clinical year perform better than students who are tested earlier.[15,16] However, this effect may not hold for all forms of assessment; a 2000 report describing an OSCE with case content linked to learning objectives in an ambulatory care clerkship did not demonstrate any effect linked to student maturation.[17]

20.2.2.d. Question for Clerkship Directors

Should the same grading standard for clinical performance evaluations apply in the first half of the clerkship year as in the second half?

Dynamic, or progressive, grading criteria (a system in which adjustments are made over the course of the year) require a different approach than static criteria. For example, at the University of Utah, in converting the RIME descriptors to numeric grades, adjustments were made to account for the level of experience the student had in the clerkship year to that point (Table 20.2). By the end of our clerkship rotation, a student's performance must consistently have been rated at the level of reporter in order to receive a grade of "Pass." Since we do not currently award grades of "Low Pass" or "Marginal Pass," there is no numerical equivalent for sub-reporter work (identified as the "observer" rank in our system) for the final period of evaluation. If performance in the final three weeks (which is always taken in the second semester) is judged to be at the reporter level, then a grade of 2.5 (out of a possible 4.0) is given. If the same performance is seen in the first semester, the score is slightly higher (2.75). As shown in Table 20.2, similar adjustments are made for each of the descriptors. For a grade of Honors, a rating of "manager" is required. This converts to 3.5 (the numeric criterion for Honors) for the second semester ("meets expectations for Honors"), and 3.75 in the first semester ("exceeds expectations for Honors").

Table 20.2 illustrates how a criterion-based (fixed standard) framework can still be used to equilibrate grades based on the time of the academic year.

The table lists the numeric equivalents for a given descriptive rating for the first and second semesters of the internal medicine clerkship. Intermediate steps between descriptors (e.g., reporter/interpreter) are used when student performance is deemed to be in transition between vocabulary terms.

Table 20.2. Adjusting Grading Criteria for Late in the Clerkship Year

Descriptor	Numeric Equivalent (4.0 possible points)			
	First Semester		Second Semester	
Observer	0	"PASS"	0	"FAIL"
Observer/Reporter	2.0		0	
Reporter	2.75	"HIGH PASS"	2.5	"PASS"
Reporter/Interpreter	3.0		2.75	
Interpreter	3.25	"HONORS"	3.0	"HIGH PASS"
Interpreter/Manager	3.5		3.25	
Manager	3.75		3.5	"HONORS"
Manager/Educator	4.0		3.75	
Educator	4.0		4.0	

20.2.3. Normative vs. Criterion-Based (Fixed Standard) Approaches

Question: Should clerkship directors compare students to each other or to fixed standards?

20.2.3.a. Point: Honors Grades Should Be Normative, Reflecting the Top, Predetermined Percent of Medical Student Performances for Any Given Year, Irrespective of How Strong Their Performances Are

This approach is often favored by certain "consumers" of the evaluation and grading process - the deans who write summary letters and the residency program directors who review them. Normative grading indicates where students rank in relation to their peers, although the confidence one places in this information should not exceed their confidence in the validity of the methods used to derive the ranking (see Chapter 2). Takayama *et al.* found that the number of students receiving the highest grade when three or more were available (i.e., not Pass/Fail) ranged from 27% to 35% across specialty of clerkships (highest for psychiatry and family medicine, lowest for surgery), but with significant variation across schools.[4]

Students may also favor this method, if the evaluation and grading schemes are strict. If the top 20% of the class receives Honors regardless of individual scores, this may include more students than under a criterion-based system.

20.2.3.b. Counterpoint: Honors Grades Should Indicate the Number of Students Who Meet the Stated Requirements for Honors (Criterion-Based, Fixed Standard)

Students endorse this practice when the Honors criteria are believed to be attainable. It promotes an atmosphere of collaboration instead of competition, and may be more motivating. Criterion-based systems focus attention on course goals, and facilitate teachers and course directors in working as student advocates. If the criteria and standards are too "easy" and do not challenge the students sufficiently, or if student performance relative to the criteria is not rigorously assessed, there is a risk that so many Honors ratings may be distributed that the distinction of this grade would be lost.

Many schools use nationally normed subject examinations from the NBME (shelf exams). Although these tests are scored and reported normatively, their contribution to the individual student's grade often is criterion-referenced. Here are some examples of policies based on this approach: "In order to be eligible for an Honors rating in the clerkship, the student's score on the NBME pediatrics subject exam must be in the top quartile." "Students whose score on the NBME psychiatry subject exam is within the bottom decile will be considered to have failed the examination, and will receive a grade of "Incomplete" for this clerkship. Their grade will remain Incomplete until they have repeated the exam and scored above the bottom decile."

20.2.3.c. Example and Discussion

Grading systems may combine normative and criterion-based approaches, seeking to capture the strengths of each. In the internal medicine clerkship at the University of Utah, we prefer criterion-referenced methods in grading individual components of the overall grade (e.g., clinical performance evaluations, the NBME medicine subject examination, and formal case presentation). This provides a context for evaluators to assess and describe student performance relative to department goals, facilitates meaningful feedback to students, and primes the process of strategic planning with students as they consider how they will work toward achieving the prescribed "next steps."

At the University of Utah, a student's final grade is computed as follows:

Clinical evaluations:	70%
OSCE:	10%
NBME medicine subject exam:	20%
Formal Case Presentation:	Pass/Fail
TOTAL:	100%

The clinical performance evaluations are provided by faculty and residents who have worked with the student during the evaluation period, as described above. RIME descriptors are generated in formal evaluation sessions and transformed to the numerical scale shown in Table 20.2. We use a normative approach in retrospective (end-of-year) evaluation of the clerkship itself. We consider the percentage of students receiving Honors (for each component of the course, as well as for the final clerkship grade) to be a useful and meaningful measure of the robustness of our combination of evaluation methods. We have confidence in awarding Honors for an overall grade if 20%-30% of students each year achieve this, as defined by their performance across the array of criterion-referenced assessment tools. If less than 20% receive Honors, we retroactively adjust to a normative approach to identify *additional* students, so that no less than 20% of the class will receive Honors (though this will also trigger a comprehensive course evaluation process). If more than 30% receive Honors, methods of observation, evaluation, and grading are reviewed, and new assessment tools and techniques are considered for the following year.

20.3. ACE Groups' Use of Methods and Examinations

Clerkship directors may find some guidance from colleagues in other clerkship groups in the Alliance for Clinical Education (ACE) about how to calculate grades from data provided by clerkship directors' groups. These were summarized from the reports of different groups by Hemmer and colleagues[14] and are seen in Table 20.3.

Table 20.3. Use of Teacher Evaluations, NBME Subject Exam, and OSCE Across Clerkships (NR = not reported)

	Medicine	Pediatrics	Surgery	Psychiatry	Family Med	Ob/Gyn
Teacher Evals (Use %)	98	100	NR	89.3	100	92
Teacher Evals (% Contribution to Grade)	63.5	55	NR	NR	61	45
Prevalance of Use of NBME (%)	85	67	91	69	14.3	74
NBME Mean Contribution to Final Grade (%)	24.4	20.4	33.9	31	25	24
OSCE (Use %)	33.3	8.3	NR	NR	22	22
OSCE (% Contribution)	11.8	2.4	NR	NR	17	3

Clerkship directors must decide how much different types of final examinations will contribute to a student's grade calculation, and this may depend upon their satisfaction with the method. In a 1999 survey, the CDIM Evaluation and Research Committee queried clerkship directors as to the types of quantifiable examinations they used, their satisfaction with each approach, and the weight they gave each method when calculating the final grade (Table 20.4). The response rate for this survey was 89%, and it showed that most clerkship directors used the NBME medicine subject exam and stipulated a minimum score. Satisfaction was measured using a five-point modified Likert scale (1 = very satisfied, 2 = moderately satisfied, 3 = satisfied, 4 = moderately dissatisfied, 5 = very dissatisfied). These data were presented at CDIM's Tenth Annual Meeting.

Table 20.4. Internal Medicine Clerkship Final Examination Methods

	NBME	Faculty Written Exam	OSCE
% of Clerkships Using this Method (n)	83 (90)	27 (29)	28 (30)
% of Clerkships Requiring Minimum Score to Pass	80 (72)	66 (19)	63 (19)
Minimum Score Required to Pass (Mean +/- SD)	59 (2.21)	66 (15.3)	69
% of the Final Grade (Mean (+/- SD, Range)	24 (10.3, 0-50)	22 (10.2, 7.5-50)	15 (10.5, 0-33)
Clerkship Director Satisfaction with Method	2.1	2.0	1.9

In addition to CDIM, national organizations of directors of other clerkships have studied the issue of use of in-house, faculty written examinations. Table 20.5 presents the results of a 2003 survey of the Association of Directors of Medical Student Education in Psychiatry (ADMSEP), which sought to identify the primary methods of student assessment in psychiatry clerkship programs at 141 accredited U.S. and Canadian allopathic medical schools.[18]

Table 20.5. Psychiatry Clerkship Grading Methods

Evaluation Method	% of Schools	Mean % of Grade (Range %)
Teachers' Evaluations	99	54 (10-100)
NBME Subject Exam	75	31 (0-100)
Departmental Exam	37	22 (0-50)

The duration of a clerkship may influence the selection of evaluation methods. The recent survey of 150 U.S. and Canadian clerkship directors in psychiatry (Table 20.6) showed that shorter clerkships were more likely to use the NBME subject test, and less likely to incorporate oral examinations.[18]

Table 20.6. Psychiatry Clerkship Grading Methods in Relation to Clerkship Length

Grading Method (% using)	Clerkship Length		
	Four Weeks	Six Weeks	Eight Weeks
NBME	77	74	83
OSCEs	14	20	14
Direct Observation	14	29	10
Oral Examination	5	24	42
Logbooks	14	18	29

Finally, the use of the NBME subject examination has also been studied in the context of the surgical clerkship. The results of a survey of surgery clerkship directors were presented at the 2004 Annual Meeting of the Association for Surgical Education (ASE[19]) and are included in Table 20.7.

Table 20.7. Minimal Passing Scores for NBME Subject Exam Across Clerkships

	Surgery	Medicine	Psychiatry
Prevalance of use of NBME test (%)	91	83	75
Prevalance of minimum score requirement (%)	88	80	N/A
Minimum passing score (mean, raw)	58	59	59

20.4. Failing Grades

The criteria for failing either a component of the clerkship or the clerkship in its entirety should be clearly stated. This is unambiguous when the criteria can be quantified (e.g., a score on the NBME subject examination of less than or equal to 58, a cumulative score from clinical performance evaluations of less than 50% of the total possible points, etc.). In addition, careful descriptive evaluations (e.g., "This student was consistently unprepared, unreliable, and interacted poorly with patients and with the other members of the team.") can serve to trigger administrative action that can lead to a summary judgment of failure by an appropriate supervisory body (e.g., a departmental committee), even without requiring formal calculation of a grade.

20.5. Conclusion

Key issues in converting evaluations to grades include deciding who should evaluate and who should grade, how to account for student progress within the course, and what role normative or criterion-referenced approaches should play.

The assessment, evaluation, and grading of performance has been described in the context of the classical sequence: "observation-reflection-action." The process of converting evaluations into grades is the process of transitioning from reflection into action. Each institution and clerkship will develop individualized methods that best serve their specific needs, although assuring that good observations of students are made by faculty, residents, or any other evaluator, is essential. Valid grades can only be derived from valid evaluations; valid evaluations must be based on valid observations. Ensuring that valid observations are made is perhaps the most important factor - and also the greatest challenge.

References

1. Gaglione MM, Moores L, Pangaro LN, Hemmer PA. Does group discussion of student clerkship performance at an education committee affect an individual committee member's decisions? Acad Med 2005;80(10 Suppl):S55-S58.
2. ACGME. Frequently Asked Questions: Clinical Competency Committee and Program Evaluation Committee. Common Program Requirements. <www.acgme.org/acgmeweb/Portals/0/PDFs/FAQ/CCC_PEC_FAQs.pdf>. Accessed May 13, 2015.

3. Alexander EK, Osman NY, Walling JL, Mitchell VG. Variation and imprecision of clerkship grading in U.S. medical schools. Acad Med 2012;87(8):1070-1076.
4. Takayama H, Grinsell R, Brock D, et al. Is it appropriate to use core clerkship grades in the selection of residents? Curr Surg 2006;63(6):391-396.
5. Crocker L, Algina J. Introduction to Classical and Modern Test Theory. Mason, Ohio: Cengage Learning, 2009.
6. Downing SM, Haladyna TM. Validity threats: Overcoming interference with proposed interpretations of assessment data. Med Educ 2004;38(3):327-333.
7. Williams RG, Klamen DA, McGaghie WC. Cognitive, social, and environmental sources of bias in clinical performance ratings. Teach Learn Med 2003;15(4):270-292.
8. van Barneveld C. The dependability of medical students' performance ratings as documented on in-training evaluations. Acad Med 2005;80(3):309-312.
9. Coletti LM. Difficulty with negative feedback: Face-to-face evaluation of junior medical student clinical performance results in grade inflation. J Surg Res 2000;90(1):82-87.
10. Durning SJ, Pangaro LN, Denton GD, et al. Intersite consistency as a measurement of programmatic evaluation in a medicine clerkship with multiple, geographically separated sites. Acad Med. 2003;78(10 Suppl):S36-S38.
11. Battistone MJ, Milne C, Sande MA, et al. The feasibility and acceptability of implementing formal evaluation sessions and using descriptive vocabulary to assess student performance on a clinical clerkship. Teach Learn Med 2002;14(1):5-10.
12. Pangaro LN. A new vocabulary and other innovations for improving descriptive in-training evaluations. Acad Med 1999;74(11):1203-1207.
13. Battistone MJ, Pendleton B, Milne C, et al. Global descriptive evaluations are more responsive than global numeric ratings in detecting students' progress during the inpatient portion of an internal medicine clerkship. Acad Med 2001;76(10 Suppl):S105-S107.
14. Hemmer PA, Papp KK, Mechaber AJ, Durning SJ. Evaluation, grading, and use of the RIME vocabulary on internal medicine clerkships: Results of a national survey and comparison to other clinical clerkships. Teach Learn Med 2008;20(2):118-126.
15. Reteguiz JA, Crosson J. Clerkship order and performance on family medicine and internal medicine National Board of Medical Examiners exams. Fam Med 2002;34(8):604-608.
16. Baciewicz FA, Arent L, Weaver M, et al. Influence of clerkship structure and timing on individual student performance. Am J Surg 1990;159(2):265-268.
17. Thomas PA, Shatzer JH. Standardized patient assessment of ambulatory clerks: Effect of timing and order of the clerkship. Teach Learn Med 2000;12(4):183-188.
18. Rosenthal RH, Levine RE, Carlson DL, et al. The "shrinking" clerkship: Characteristics and length of clerkships in psychiatry undergraduate education. Acad Psychiatry 2005;29(1):47-51.
19. Alliance for Clinical Education. Abstracts from the Proceedings of the 2004 Annual Meeting of the Association of Surgical Education (ASE). Teach Learn Med 2005;17(3):297-303.

Chapter 21
Legal Aspects of Assigning Failing Grades

Thomas Jamieson, M.D., J.D.
Paul Hemmer, M.D., M.P.H.
Louis N. Pangaro, M.D.

The challenge of formally evaluating learners is a distinguishing, solemn responsibility for medical school faculty and institutional departments. Medical educators' duty to society is accountability for its "finished product." Clerkship directors oversee the last major step in *standardization* for producing physicians ready to begin supervised practice, since, after the clerkship, there is more flexibility and allowance for individualization in the curriculum. Therefore, clerkship grading decisions at the Pass/Fail threshold are especially important. While distinctions among higher grades may have consequences for students, such as selection by residency programs, the core interest of society at large resides in those departmental grading decisions which may affect a medical student's promotion, remediation, demotion, or disenrollment. The notion of institutional accountability for a "finished product," whether imposed by courts or fashioned as an expectation of society, is placing an even greater burden on clerkship directors and clinical faculty to identify those who are not ready for the level of independence expected of a new graduate upon entering the internship year.[1] This chapter will emphasize the legal implications of grading in clerkships, though its principles apply to all courses in the curriculum.

The reluctance of an individual teacher to judge a student as deficient "on the record" may create a tension with an institution's larger responsibility to maintain acceptable standards in its graduates and, ultimately, to protect the public.[2] Students may, of course, threaten legal action if they receive failing grades in clerkship rotations, and institutions need to recognize their obligations to struggling learners. While adequate "notice and hearing" requirements must be met, and the process must be fair and reasonable, the courts, relying on the U.S. Supreme Court, have held in Michigan v. Ewing, and *reiterated*, that judicial review of academic decision making is narrow in scope,[3] and therefore courts will grant academic deference to faculty decisions, under a presumption of academic freedom. Judicial holdings have consistently avoided imposing judicial fiat on medical schools or other institutions of higher learning in matters of evaluative process and outcomes. Of critical importance is that administrators and faculty members have a duty (i.e., requirement) to exercise professional judgment, and to avoid arbitrary (without a clear institutional expectation, and so up to a subjective "arbiter") and capricious (applying expectations without consistency across students) actions in qualitatively assessing a learner's performance and promotion.[4]

This chapter reviews principles applicable in assigning failing grades, the decision most likely to provoke litigation, and emphasizes an institution's duty and a learner's expectations at the Pass/Fail threshold in the context of the American legal system. The focus here is on "dichotomous" assignment of grades (Pass/Fail), rather than on "scalar" grading, which would include High Pass and Honors designations (see Chapter 2). Whether the general principles of substantive and procedural due process also apply to distinctions between higher grade assignment remains speculative and lacks judicial history at this time.

21.1. Legal Concepts

A well-worn aphorism in the American legal system is that "ignorance of the law is no defense." Whether informed or not, medical educators owe a particular legal duty, mainly constitutional protections, to their students and house officers in training. The Fourteenth Amendment to the U.S. Constitution expressly says, "... [no state] shall deprive any person of life, liberty, or property without due process of law; nor deny to any person within its jurisdiction the equal protection of the law ..."[5] The Supreme Court has spoken clearly and directly on the extent of the basic constitutional rights of learners enrolled in publicly supported institutions, and has specifically articulated a standard for medical learners of procedural and substantive due process that we will now address.

21.1.1. Procedural and Substantive Due Process

Due process of law has two distinct forms: 1. "Procedural due process" is a constitutional guarantee of procedural fairness, which, at a minimum, entitles an affected party the guarantee of "notice," and, in some circumstances, the opportunity of a "hearing." 2. "Substantive due process" is a constitutional guarantee of protection from arbitrary and unreasonable action. Perhaps it is convenient to think of due process conceptually as "why" measures are being taken against a student (substantive due process) and "how" those measures are being imposed (procedural due process). Clinical educators in America should be aware of two landmark Supreme Court cases that continue to define "the process due" a medical learner, and that necessarily shape a department's approach to assigning failing grades.

21.1.1.a. Michigan v. Ewing: Looking at a Student's Entire Record

In Regents of the University of Michigan v. Ewing (1985) the Supreme Court accepted a medical student litigant's premise to "assume the existence of a constitutionally protected property right in [a medical student's] continued enrollment."[3] The case was brought by a student who had been dismissed from medical school after failing USMLE Step 1 and was not permitted a retake of the examination. As noted in Ewing, the medical school's own promotional pamphlet stated: "Everything possible is done to keep qualified medical students in the medical school. This even extends to taking and passing National Board Exams. Should a student fail either part of the National Boards, an opportunity is provided to make up the failure in a second exam."

In Michigan v. Ewing, the Supreme Court held that, while denial of an opportunity to retake the examination (a historic precedent for an institution that had permitted thirty-nine students with prior examination failures a retake) "may constitute evidence of arbitrariness," it was not in itself confirmatory but, rather, it was only a single fact, among other facts, for the jury to consider. In supporting the school in their final ruling, the Supreme Court noted that the medical school considered the student's *entire record* in reaching the decision to dismiss, not merely the results of a single examination.[4,5] Thus, clerkship directors and their departments not only are entitled to consider the *entirety* of the student's clerkship record in making a grading decision, but also *should* do so as part of a deliberate, and deliberative, process. Importantly, we recommend that it should be expressly stated in any document about the process of assigning a student a low grade that such a review of the "entirety of the record" was conducted. The Supreme Court also held that *reasoned decision making* in academic matters is, *per se*, not arbitrary or capricious. Moreover, the burden of proof is on the student to show that a decision was not factually based and was made irrationally. Unless there is evidence that a case was arbitrary or capricious, courts, viewing themselves as inappropriate mediators in academic matters, will not overturn faculty decisions. Therefore, in meeting the obligations set forth as part of the Michigan v. Ewing case, we *strongly* recommend that departments charge a committee to review all potentially failing grading outcomes, and that all available sources of information, i.e., the entirety of the student's clerkship record, be considered and be the stated basis in determining a final grade.

21.1.1.b. Missouri v. Horowitz: Judicial Deference to Academic Process

The ruling in the Ewing case reaffirmed the Supreme Court's prior holding in University of Missouri v. Horowitz (1978) that enrollment in medical school is a basis for students to invoke constitutional protections of due process, while the Court also reinforced the principle of judicial restraint in academically based decisions.[6] In Horowitz, the student was dismissed from medical school in her final year, after receiving negative evaluations in multiple third and fourth year rotations. The medical school's Council on Evaluation (progress or promotions committee) had reviewed the entirety of the student's performance throughout the final two years of medical school, had previously taken action to place her on academic probation, and had issued her notice prior to the decision for disenrollment. The Court held that the medical school had adequately met, and even exceeded, the constitutional requirements of the Fourteenth Amendment for procedural due process. The Court noted that school officials had notified the student of her academic deficiencies and had identified potential adverse outcomes, including dismissal. The Horowitz court also cited the school's careful and deliberate review of the student's academic performance.

21.1.1.c. Academic vs. Disciplinary Issues

Importantly, the Court's Horowitz decision held that the procedural due process requirements owed students for *academic* dismissals are less than those for *disciplinary* dismissals. The Court noted that academically dismissed students must be afforded "the opportunity to characterize (their performance) and put it in what he/she deems the proper context."[7] Though not always constitutionally required (in academic dismissals), as seen in Flaim v. Medical College of Ohio, it is always wise to produce some sort of record of proceedings."[7] In other words, for matters that are considered by an institution to be academic, which may include issues of professional behavior, the burden of proof is on the student to show that due process has been violated. Whereas, if the institution considers that a student's problem is disciplinary, rather than academic, then the burden of proof is on the institution. We recommend that performance problems that are considered part of professionalism (such as multiple, unexcused absences or, even, cheating) be expressly considered as academic issues. Describing the student as "competent but with a disciplinary problem" may cause confusion in the presumption of judicial non-interference in the medical school's judgment about what constitutes acceptable academic performance.

Indeed, student-perceived inequities, such as alleging that testing and grading policies are unfair, or an allegation that dismissal is premised on an instructor's incompetence, face a very challenging legal standard. Courts appear to regard the grading of in-house examinations as a matter of academic discretion and typically do not apply or impose a formalistic standard. However, if a student can demonstrate that a usual grading process was not followed, then a court may hold that an institution acted capriciously, i.e., that due process was denied.

21.1.2. Process: How Much Is Due?

Courts have not attached extensive procedural requirements to failing and/or disenrolling a medical student. While students may request, or even demand, such accommodations as an open hearing, the presence of personal legal counsel, recorded proceedings, or a written record of promotions (progress) committee deliberations, such procedural amenities have not been held in court decisions to be due. In fact, courts have consistently been wary of the "undue judicialization" of an administrative hearing in the academic environment.[8] There may be exceptions, of course, if an institution has codified its own policy of procedural measures (i.e., stating that such academic hearings are routinely recorded), or in the uncommon circumstance where a student is also facing criminal charges stemming from the incident in question.[9] Though a *formal* hearing before a school's decision making body is not a constitutional requisite in an academic dismissal, institutions would be wise to provide some form of hearing, even informal, to allow students facing potential adverse academic action (e.g., probation, deceleration, or dismissal) an opportunity to offer their own perspective. U.S. Supreme Court Justice Byron White observed in Gorman v. University of Rhode Island that in an academic dismissal "the Due Process Clause requires, 'not an elaborate hearing before a neutral party,' but simply 'an informal give-and-take between student and disciplinarian' which gives the student 'an opportunity to explain his version of the facts'."[9]

When a non-cognitive disciplinary issue is the basis for a student's failure, or a component factor, courts have imposed a slightly higher standard of due process (Goss v. Lopez), i.e., the requirement for a hearing.[10] It is not difficult to envision a disenrollment circumstance where the academic vs. disciplinary distinction may be arguable, blurred, or confusing. The most pragmatic approach for institutions may be to consider any distinction an abstraction, and to allow aggrieved learners not only written notice of the charges against them, but also explanations of the evidence and an opportunity to present their side of the story.

21.1.3. Breach of Contract

Though a theoretical possibility, courts have seldom considered contract-related arguments when public institutions adhere to procedural requirements and defined institutional policies. However, contract claims have been more frequently the subject of actions brought against private institutions. Although lacking the formality of an expressed written contract, the "promise" between an institution and a student conceivably could be enforced under the theory of implied contract. The provisions expressed, or implied, between the institution and the student derive mainly from the official documents as defined by the school. Courts may carefully examine student and faculty handbooks, policy statements, rules and regulations. Therefore, *please recognize that courts may bind you to what you write down in your clerkship handbook*. If a learner can demonstrate that an institution did not comply with its own articulated process and policy, then the benefit of traditional academic deference may be lost as the court will never reach it, to the obvious disadvantage of the institution. Also, importantly, an institution may be bound by the procedures afforded students in previous cases, even if the procedures are unwritten, and even if the facts of the cases are somewhat dissimilar.[11] Thus concessions to the preferences or requests of an aggrieved student, if allowed by promotion (progress) committees or institutional attorneys, might - even though not so initially - become future requirements.

21.1.4. Importance of the Student Handbook

For their part, students agree to follow a school's rules and to risk penalty, including suspension or dismissal if they do not. Clerkships should be explicit in their expectation that students read and follow policies and procedures that are written in a student guidebook. The institution, in exchange for the student's tuition payment, implicitly agrees to provide the academic programs and support services reasonably necessary for students to perform successfully. Contract theory, as a possible cause-of-action, serves to underscore the need for departments and clerkship directors to audit periodically those written materials that outline policies, rules, and regulations; and departments and schools should be sure that they do what they say they will do. We would recommend that such a periodic review occur at least annually, and be subject to departmental review and approval by key stakeholders (e.g., the clerkship director, site directors, and the department chair). In short, every director of an academic program must "read the document" of promulgated policies; this means that the clerkship director must be familiar with institutional grading policy and other procedural documents. The occasional failed student who prevails against an institution in court may do so by exposing the school for breaching its own stated procedural guarantees.[11]

21.2. Shifting Legal Issues and Possible Trends

21.2.1. Educational Malpractice

The time-honored traditional cause of action, a denial of basic constitutional due process rights, may now be only one of several legal theories advanced by a failed student as plaintiff.[12] The notion of "educational malpractice," alleging that a school, or program, wrongfully graduated a student whom they had reason to judge less than competent, likely derives from an increasing public expectation of accountability by educators as guarantors of their graduates' collective competence. Such legal actions are based on a different premise than a student's claim of "wrongful dismissal," and might be brought by patients or their families; i.e., those who feel that they have been injured by an institution's "wrongful graduation" of a student (or resident). However, whether this sentiment will ultimately translate into viability for the negligence-based tort claim of educational malpractice is not yet clear. Presently, there remains a judicial reluctance to engage claims of educational malpractice and nearly all have been summarily dismissed. Courts persist in an underlying belief that they not intrude on the "educational expertise" of teaching institutions.

A 1979 New York Court of Appeals case, Donahue v. Copiague, was the first instance of a court using the term "educational malpractice."[13] Donahue remains, even now, the leading case as to the judicial rationale for courts not recognizing educational malpractice as actionable. Perhaps of some promise to prospective plaintiffs, however, was the Donahue court's acknowledging that elements of negligence conceivably *could be* established even while ruling that public policy considerations remained a basis to deny plaintiff recovery. Ironically, the lack of specific, measurable teaching and learning standards has been problematic in defining, or imposing, a duty (i.e., precise standard-of-care) on educators and institutions.

However, as standards and curricular goals become less amorphous and more universally defined - such as with the implementation of milestones - courts may have less reluctance in considering educational malpractice as a cause of action. Also, if judicial viewpoint should redefine public policy to favor institutional accountability as being in the public interest then educational malpractice actions may become viable.

21.2.2. Assigning a Grade

A failing student may insist that a single evaluator unduly influenced a grade outcome. In settings where a faculty member (or house officer) is acting as the university's proxy, the faculty member fulfills one of the functions involved in an academy's "four essential freedoms." Universities have the "freedom" to decide "who to teach, what may be taught, how it shall be taught, and who may be admitted to study."[14] As grading is a pedagogic practice, the assignment of a grade is incorporated under the university's freedom to determine how a course is to be taught.[15] Therefore, a student should understand that individual faculty members may *recommend* a grade, but that the responsibility for final grade *determination* rightfully (and legally) rests with the university (and, by proxy, the clinical department). At the Uniformed Services University of the Health Sciences we inform and summarize the issue in our third year internal medicine clerkship handbook by noting: "We guide the faculty and housestaff in assessing how well you have met clerkship goals. Their role is evaluation; final responsibility for grading rests with the department."[16]

As noted, those who are involved with evaluating a medical student's performance during clinical clerkships are doing so as a proxy of the medical school (clinical department). As a result, teachers, be they housestaff, fellows, or attending physicians, should have faculty appointments within the medical school.

Faculty may be wary of recommending low grades for reasons that may include a fear of litigation.[3] Faculty can be encouraged to be candid in their evaluations by being reminded that departmental process is responsible for assigning grades, and that their own recommendation is precisely that, a *recommendation*. Moreover, if it is the "entirety" of the record,[4] which will be used by the department to determine the final grade, then the observation of an individual faculty member is less likely to be the basis of the final decision, unless the comments clearly document a compelling deficiency. Thus, faculty should be encouraged to convey their observations to clerkship directors, even if they feel that they have had limited time with students; and faculty should feel that their observations will not be over-interpreted in isolation, but may contribute to the overall pattern of a student's success (or deficiency).

Recent years have seen an expanding role for electronic communications in the evaluative process of students. Faculty must be aware that e-mail entries are not necessarily confidential conversations. In fact, just as with other entries in a student's file, e-mail is viewed as a "written document" and, therefore, may be "discoverable" in litigation. "Discovery" is a pre-trial process whereby one party can obtain facts and information about a case from the other party to assist in trial preparation. Importantly, institutions should not foster a culture of editorialized, informal discussion in evaluative e-mails but rather promote an expectation of honest and professionally worded responses.

21.3. Family Educational Rights and Privacy Act (FERPA)

FERPA is a federal law that protects the privacy of student education records.[17] The law applies to all schools that receive funds under an applicable program of the U.S. Department of Education. In the case of medical schools, FERPA confers upon students the right to inspect and review their education records as maintained by the school. Students have the right to request that an institution correct records which they believe to be inaccurate or misleading. If the school makes a decision not to amend the record, then the student has the right to a formal hearing. If the institution decides that no amending of the record is indicated after a hearing, then the student has the right to place a statement in the record setting forth the student's view as to the contested content. In general, a student must grant written permission to a school to allow release of any information from her/his education record. However, FERPA allows schools to disclose students' records without consent, pursuant to the following conditions or parties:

- School officials with legitimate educational interest.
- Other schools to which a student is transferring.
- Specified officials for audit or evaluation purposes.
- Appropriate parties in connection with financial aid to a student.
- Organizations conducting certain studies for, or on behalf of, the school.

- Accrediting organizations.
- To comply with a judicial order or lawfully issued subpoena.
- Appropriate officials in cases of health and safety emergencies.

Schools may disclose, without consent, "directory" information such as a student's name, address, telephone number, date and place of birth, honors, awards, and dates of attendance. However, schools must tell students about directory information and allow students a reasonable amount of time to request that the school not disclose directory information about them. Schools must notify students annually of their rights under FERPA. The actual means of notification is left to the discretion of each school.

The question of whether and how departments, or clerkship directors as their surrogates, communicate with other departments (clerkship directors) about individual students, especially those with academic difficulties, has benefits and risks[18] and is discussed above in Chapter 4. The concept is legally consistent with each school's prerogatives in setting its academic policies, but a school is expected to follow its own policies.

21.4. Recommendations

While courts have generally deferred to institutions in their reasoned judgments as to the fitness of students to continue in their training (academic deference), students do have a realistic expectation of both substantive and procedural due process. As clerkship directors, this impacts grading policies and procedures, which should be transparent to students, teachers, and the institution. The following are offered as general guidance:

21.4.1. Institutional Policies

General policies and procedures at the level of the institution are often implicit in the curriculum in the initial, pre-clinical years. For instance, students in their first year are instructed about the ethical behavior and professionalism expected in relationships with patients. Policies on cheating and plagiarism are, likewise, introduced early in the curriculum. These need not be repeated in detail in orienting clerkship students, but we do recommend a general statement during each orientation, and in the student handbook, reinforcing that ethical and professional conduct is expected, and suggest providing students with a reference to the existing policies at the medical school.

21.4.2. Consistency in Orientation; Course Handbooks for Students

The clerkship's handbook is an important tool for informing students about the processes to be followed in their evaluation and grading. Both the content of these handbooks and the orientations that students attend at the start of each rotation (or, if relevant, at each clerkship site) constitute portions of the due process to which students are entitled.[19,20] We recommend that all orientation materials, including handbooks, be reviewed and endorsed by a departmental committee (which includes the department chair) and also accepted by clerkship directors at each educational site, who may be responsible for dissemination of content. The clerkship director should also consider ways to monitor the orientations provided at any remote sites.[21]

21.4.3. Clerkship-Specific Expectations

Clerkship directors need to be explicit about expectations specific to their own rotations. In the pre-clerkship timeframe, for instance, lecture attendance may not be mandatory, but in the clerkship year it typically is mandatory for student-specific sessions, and this should be made explicit. Other examples may include: expectations for taking night call on the inpatient rotation, the number and timeliness requirement for submitting written histories and physicals, and the rapidity with which basic textbook material should be considered and understood.

21.4.4. Working with Teachers

As part of the faculty development process,[22] teachers should learn how to apply departmental expectations to the evaluation of individual students, and we advocate ongoing calibration of teachers' use of the school's evaluation framework, so that formative and summative assessment criteria are the same[23] (see Chapter 8). This will avoid the concern of a student that the evaluation was an arbitrary exercise. As much as possible, summative evaluation should be based on multiple teachers (or, in the case of private practice rotations with a single physician, on multiple, documented observations). As a quality improvement process to calibrate assessment, faculty should subsequently learn how their evaluations contributed to, rather than determined, a final summative grade by the department, so that they will not withhold from the department any observations of concern about the student.

21.4.5. Reviewing the Entirety of the Record

Clerkships benefit from having a regular education or competency committee to review the records of performance for students who are in jeopardy of receiving a failing grade.[24-26] We recommend that a group decision, reviewing the *entirety* of an individual student's clerkship performance, be an established practice. Engaging such practice will help to meet the necessary process expectations of the learner as a matter of routine. This process has been common for many years, and is now becoming standard at the graduate medical education level in the U.S. through the ACGME adoption of this process as a requirement for a "competency committee."[27] Clerkships are allowed to decide what materials are to be the basis for these decisions, and this may include evaluations ("recommended grades") from teachers, examination scores, and evaluations from nurses and others. Consistency is strongly recommended, since once a department has established an expectation for what materials are to be reviewed, this may constitute the precedent for judgment about other students in the future.

21.5. Summary Points

1. In the grading process, medical students are owed "due process" that is both *procedural* (*how* one will go about the decision making process grading) and *substantive* (*why* the decision is being made, related to the educational goals).
2. When assigning a failing grade, it is important that the *entirety* of the student's clerkship record be reviewed and considered and that an explanatory statement to that effect be part of the student's record.
3. Clerkship directors must know and follow any institutional policies and procedures, not just those relating to departmental grade determination.
4. Those overseeing evaluation and grading must follow their own defined expectations and procedures; i.e., "Say what you will do and do what you say." If there is a justifiable reason to deviate from "usual practice," you should clearly establish the reasons for doing so.
5. Create consistency in the orientation, evaluation, and grading processes. All students and teachers, irrespective of clerkship site location, must be aware of clerkship policies and procedures. A clerkship handbook is one element that can be effective.
6. Consider using a committee process that invests multiple stakeholders - the site directors, the chair, and pre-clerkship and post-clerkship (e.g., GME) directors - in the ultimate grading decisions for students. Be consistent in the use of the committee and the materials reviewed.

References

1. AAMC Data Book. <www.aamc.org/data/databook/>. Accessed February 9, 2015.
2. Williams RG, Klamen DA, McGaghie WC. Cognitive, social and environmental sources of bias in clinical performance ratings. Teach Learn Med 2003;15(4);270-292.
3. Univ. of Michigan v. Ewing, 474 U.S. 214 (1985). <supreme.justia.com/cases/federal/us/474/214/>. Accessed February 9, 2015.
4. Irby DM, Fantel JI, Milam SD, Schwarz MR. Legal guidelines for evaluating and dismissing medical students. N Engl J Med 1981;304(3):180-184.
5. Constitution of the United States of America. Amendments 11-27. <www.archives.gov/exhibits/charters/constitution_amendments_11-27.html>. Accessed February 5, 2015.
6. Board of Curators, Univ. of Missouri v. Horowitz, 435 U.S. 78 (1978). <supreme.justia.com/cases/federal/us/435/78/>. Accessed February 9, 2015.
7. Flaim v. Medical College of Ohio, 418 F.3d 629 (6th Cir. 2005). <law.justia.com/cases/federal/appellate-courts/F3/418/629/544508/>. Accessed February 9, 2015.
8. Wozniak v. Conry, 236 F.3d 888 (7th Cir. 2001). <law.justia.com/cases/federal/appellate-courts/F3/236/888/511096/>. Accessed February 9, 2015.

9. Gorman v. University of Rhode Island, 837 F.2d 7 (1st Cir. 1988). <law.justia.com/cases/federal/appellate-courts/F2/837/7/157750/>. Accessed February 9, 2015.
10. Goss v. Lopez, U.S. Supreme Court, 419 U.S. 565 (1975). <supreme.justia.com/cases/federal/us/419/565/case.html>. Accessed February 8, 2015.
11. Bergstrom v. Buettner, 697 F. Supp. 1098 (D.N.D. 1987). <law.justia.com/cases/federal/district-courts/FSupp/697/1098/2127602/>. Accessed February 9, 2015.
12. Schaer v. Brandeis University, 432 Mass. 474 (May 1 - September 25, 2000). <law.justia.com/cases/massachusetts/supreme-court/volumes/432/432mass474.html>. Accessed February 9, 2015.
13. Donohue v.Copiague UFSD, 47 N.Y.2d 440 (1979). <www.leagle.com/decision/197948747NY2d440_1440.xml/DONOHUE%20v.%20COPIAGUE%20UFSD>. Accessed February 9, 2015.
14. Helms LB, Helms CM. Forty years of litigation involving medical students, and their education. Acad Med 1991;66(2):1-7.
15. Sweezy v. New Hampshire, 354 U.S. 234 (1957). <supreme.justia.com/cases/federal/us/354/234/case.html>. Accessed February 9, 2015.
16. USU Internal Medicine Clerkship, Official Handbook for Students, Class of 2016. <www.usuhs.edu/med/clerkship/pdf/ClerkshipHandbook13DEC2013.pdf>. Accessed February 9, 2015.
17. Family Educational Rights and Privacy Act (FERPA), 20 U.S.C. § 1232g; 34 CFR Part 99. <www2.ed.gov/policy/gen/guid/fpco/ferpa/index.html>. Accessed February 5, 2015.
18. Pangaro LN. "Forward feeding" about students' progress: More information will enable better policy. Acad Med 2008;83(9):802-803.
19. Hicks P, Frazier S, Goepfert AR. Working with students with difficulties: Academic and non-academic. In: ACE Guidebook for Clerkship Directors - fourth edition - North Syracuse, NY: Gegensatz Press, 2012: 381-412.
20. Greenberg L, Ottolini, M. The clerkship orientation. In: ACE Guidebook for Clerkship Directors - fourth edition - North Syracuse, NY: Gegensatz Press, 2012: 31-42.
21. Hemmer PA. Directing a clerkship over geographically remote sites. In: ACE Guidebook for Clerkship Directors - fourth edition - North Syracuse, NY: Gegensatz Press, 2012: 489-516.
22. DaRosa DA, Simpson D, Roberts N, et al. Faculty development. In: ACE Guidebook for Clerkship Directors - fourth edition - North Syracuse, NY: Gegensatz Press, 2012: 531-566.
23. Pangaro LN. A new vocabulary and other innovations for improving descriptive in-training evaluations. Acad Med 1999;74(11):1203-1207.
24. Hemmer PA, Hawkins R, Jackson JL, Pangaro LN. Assessing how well three evaluation methods detect deficiencies in medical students' professionalism in two settings of an internal medicine clerkship. Acad Med. 2000;75(2):167-173.
25. Parenti C. A process for identifying marginal performers among students in a clerkship. Acad Med 1993;68(7):575-577.
26. Gaglione MM, Moores L, Pangaro LN, Hemmer PA. Does group discussion of student clerkship performance at an education committee affect an individual committee member's decisions? Acad Med 2005;80(10 Suppl):S55-S58.
27. ACGME. Frequently Asked Questions: Clinical Competency Committee and Program Evaluation Committee: Common Program Requirements. <www.acgme.org/acgmeweb/Portals/0/PDFs/FAQ/CCC_PEC_FAQs.pdf>. Accessed February 5, 2015.

Chapter 22
Conclusions

William C. McGaghie, Ph.D.
Louis N. Pangaro, M.D.

This is a coda to an integrated volume on medical student evaluation and assessment. We use the musical term, "coda," because it is a fitting description of a coming together, a wrap-up, a statement that closes a long professional journey. We take this occasion, not only to reflect on what unites the previous twenty-one chapters in this volume, but also to anticipate new directions from conceptual thinking, research advancements, new technologies, and contextual conditions. We hope to indicate areas of uncertainty, even controversy, and some opportunities for advancement. The critical concepts for consideration are:

- Conceptual Thinking: When and how do we know that an individual learner is successful (competent)? How do we know when an educational program is successful? How do we know when a health care system is successful in supporting its educational mission?
- Advancements in Educational Research: How do we develop and implement new assessment methods and how do we know that the methods are successful?
- New Technologies: How do new technologies support instruction and assessment methods and allow us to mine outcomes data within a health care system to support new conceptual thinking?
- Educational Context Conditions: How are the workplace assessments and structured assessments described in this *Handbook* used in a sampling plan that includes specific skills and "competencies" applied not only across clinical diagnoses and disciplines but also across the many settings in which physicians must practice?

We will discuss these for each section of the *Handbook* and then summarize the themes.

The unity of this book derives from its three sections that address (1) definitions and systems, (2) integrating medical student assessment methods, and (3) structured assessments for clerkships. Together these three sections and their member chapters depict medical student evaluation and assessment as a broad enterprise with many moving parts. Medical education deans and clerkship directors need to be ever mindful about the importance of student evaluation goals and tools, reliable data and valid (accurate) decisions, and the academic and professional consequences of medical student evaluation programs. All agree that this is serious, high-stakes business for students, schools, and patients. Its quality depends on medical educators' knowledge and skill about student evaluation practices and on the commitment to provide sufficient resources to meet the expected standard of fairness to patients and society, students, and teachers.

Section One lays a conceptual foundation (covering definitions and systems in Chapters 1, 2 and 3) and argues for a practical curriculum-wide approach, placing the clerkship in the context of curriculum phases. Readers learn about system approaches to student assessment (Chapter 3) and discover new ways to visualize a successful educational system. Sharing student information across courses and clerkships (Chapter 4), using pre-clerkship variables to identify high-risk students (Chapter 5), and assessment in the post-clerkship year (Chapter 6) round out Section One. The intent of these early chapters is to inform readers that medical student education and assessment are one woven cloth, seamless in purpose yet separate in appearance. Our job as medical educators is to unify student instruction and assessment, to make plain that medical student advancement depends on clear plans and rigorous data.

But in describing how three phases of the medical curriculum (pre-clerkship, clerkship, and post-clerkship) fit together, we invite readers to ask whether their schools have adequate conceptualizations (theory) - shared by faculty - about how each phase fits into a seamless whole, and whether we have the tools needed to describe professional development and progressive mastery of skills.

Section Two reviews available methods to assess student progress and addresses integrating medical student assessment methods (Chapter 7). Chapter 8 starts the discussion on descriptive and clinical performance evaluation in the workplace. Chapter 9 continues with discussion about time honored approaches to direct observations of students' clinical skills. Assessment of students' procedural skills and their transfer to bedside practices is covered in Chapter 10, while Chapter 11 explores methods to assess student clinical reasoning. Evaluation of medical student professionalism on a developmental arc is the focus of Chapter 12. Feedback, its purpose, form, substance, style, and impact, is the theme of Chapter 13. All chapters in Section Two remind readers that medical student assessment is done both **for learning** (formative) and **of learning** (summative). Separation of these evaluation goals is often very difficult in educational practice. We invite readers to discuss with the fellow clerkship directors or associate deans whether there are sufficient resources to have a systematic approach to observation, feedback, and grading that is consistent and fair to society, students, and teachers.

Section Three is a pragmatic approach to structured, quantified assessments that are typically used to determine final grades. We planned this section with a "hands on" approach and feel. Here readers learn about clerkship examinations (Chapter 15), how to write MCQs (Chapter 16), SP-based clerkship evaluations (Chapter 17), and student assessment using simulation technologies (Chapter 18). Practical advice about setting clerkship performance standards is given in Chapter 19, while issues of converting evaluations into school grades and legal issues in grading are covered in Chapters 20 and 21, respectively.

Readers should be aware that this book is a snapshot of medical student evaluation policies and practices that are in effect in the U.S. and western countries in early 2015. While many methods have been refined over decades and may be said to have stood the test of time, being alert to new developments is as important in education as in clinical medicine. The policies and practices are grounded in the modern medical education history that originated in the late nineteenth century[1] and advances to the present.[2] Let us ask, "What new directions can we anticipate about the education and evaluation of future generations of doctors and other health professionals?" Also, "What medical education challenges appear on the horizon that we must recognize and solve?"

22.1. Future Challenges

Four sets of new directions in medical education and personnel evaluation will shape future challenges. These address advancements in (a) conceptual thinking, (b) educational research advancements, (c) new technologies, and (d) educational context conditions.

22.2. Conceptual Thinking

Basic conceptual ideas about the structure and outcomes of medical education are undergoing profound change. Since the late 1970s, western medical education has evolved slowly from the idea that curricula must be time-based toward being outcomes-based.[3] This addresses the distinction between simply experiencing educational events like lectures and examinations and performing "good enough" on tests and other evaluations vs. mastering educational objectives. We are not saying that course, clerkship, and GME program directors were naively allowing trainees to advance without any thoughts about passing standards. Instead, there is now more of a focus on using assessments that have been validated with the same rigor that clinicians have always expected of tests for their patients. Nor are we saying that a comprehensive set of quantitative outcome measures is now available at all training sites. The issue is a cultural shift from what the teacher does to what the student learns. This parallels the shift toward patient-centered care and outcomes in clinical practice. The shift is driven by a desire for quality in service of the public, and quality control in the interest of the profession, which has almost universally moved to a more business-oriented model.

At this writing, medical education thought leaders, professional boards, and regulatory agencies argue that measured educational outcomes expressed as personal competencies or units of work, such as EPAs, should be the goal of medical education.[4] This idea holds, not only for measured learning outcomes from undergraduate medical education, but also for postgraduate medical learners[5] and physicians throughout their careers. Initial formation of medical competence, certified by rigorous measures, will be extended to the maintenance of measured clinical competence throughout each doctor's career.[6] The continuum of evaluation and assessment for medical professionals will match and even describe physicians' career trajectories.

In this concluding chapter we wish to emphasize that such a competency approach remains in development, that the theoretical idea of milestones and EPAs are still not widely understood, much less used, by the thousands of clerkship and program directors in the country. More importantly, the funding to support the research needed to operationalize these concepts, and the faculty time needed to train teachers to use them, are still woefully lacking.

Such outcomes-based thinking is a large departure from customary approaches to physician certification, licensure, relicensure, and maintenance of professional competence. At a minimum, these concepts mean that rigorous evaluation and assessment of professional competence will be a career-long reality for physicians, just like for other highly skilled professionals, such as commercial airline pilots and nuclear power plant operators. No doubt these concepts of lifelong physician evaluation and assessment will be met with resistance from many sources, yet public pressure for accountability and patient safety will prevail. What is not clear is how continuing education for physicians in practice will be funded. Will it be funded centrally by the government as bill payer (e.g., through tax deductions), through dedicated training time (as in the industries cited), or by patients and third party payers using the concept of billable hours?

22.3. Educational Research Advancements

Medical education research advancements will complement conceptual developments. We know, for example, that physicians in training and practice can acquire and maintain key clinical skills from rigorous education grounded in deliberate practice, formative evaluation, feedback, and improvement to mastery learning standards.[7] There is no longer any doubt that powerful educational interventions work more effectively than traditional teacher-based medical education, if learning goals are clinical skill acquisition[8] or maintenance of competence.[9,10] The question is how to implement such mastery methods systematically and to study the best techniques for this implementation.

The mastery learning model, coupled with deliberate practice embedded in medical simulation technology, embodies a form of educational engineering. The goal is to set conditions for knowledge and skill acquisition, deliberate practice, rigorous measurement, feedback, and continuous learner improvement to a mastery learning standard. The mastery approach to medical education has produced impressive results, not only under controlled, laboratory conditions, but also as translational (downstream) outcomes expressed as improved patient care practices and better patient outcomes.[7,11] As an engineering model, however, the approach expects that consistency in its implementation will be achieved and that studies will be funded to implement best practices on a broad scale. This, too, is analogous to the evidence-based standards for patient care which require wide-scale, multisite studies, firmly rooted in educational epidemiology. In addition to funding, infrastructure will be needed, expressed as diverse educational research teams, academic managers in clinical education (i.e., course, clerkship, and program directors), and clinical teams of physicians, nurses, and other health professionals.

The power and utility of mastery learning as a medical education intervention also questions the need for control groups in outcomes research to determine the efficacy of instructional methods. New research designs involving single-case (group) intervention research have recently been introduced.[12] These and other methodological advancements will continue to enrich and refresh medical education research. Since the balance of benefit and risk plus cost is as important in education as in clinical care, comparative methods with historical, if not concurrent, controls will be needed, and some demonstration of generalizability of instructional methods across settings will be sought.

Widespread acknowledgment that health care is now a "team sport"[13] means that team training will be a growth industry in health professions education. In particular, interprofessional education grounded in core competencies for health care teams will account for a much larger portion of curriculum and evaluation space.[14] Research on the outcomes of interprofessional education, measured rigorously, is a priority item on the scholarly agenda.

22.4. New Technologies

New and rapidly changing technologies are now part of everyday life and clinical practice. The technologies range from smart phones and tablets to low and high fidelity patient simulations, computer-based case presentations and assessments, electronic health records (EHRs), and many more. Data capturing and database management technologies are also a growing feature of student evaluation and assessment systems at most medical schools. The question is no longer, "Should we use new technologies for medical student evaluation and assessment?" Instead, the question now is, "What is the best way to integrate new technologies into medical student assessment programs?" This, too, should evolve from expert opinion, based on best available practice, to more systematic study of implementation.

We anticipate that the relatively new discipline of implementation science will soon become much more prominent in medical and health care education. In medical education, implementation science seeks to identify, isolate, and remove cultural habits, sources of inertia, financial disincentives, and other barriers that prevent evidence-based innovations from becoming part of routine instruction and assessment.[15,16] Adoption of innovations grounded in science has been very slow in medical education and needs to be accelerated.

Amin and colleagues recently addressed these questions in writing about technology-enabled assessment of health professions education.[17] Cook et al. have also recently reported a systematic review and meta-analysis on technology-enhanced simulation for health professions education.[18] While these works differ in purpose and methodological approach, they share at least four educational themes. First, evaluation goals must dictate the use of evaluation tools, whether or not the tools embody new technologies. Second, evaluation and assessment technologies must produce reliable data that can be used to reach valid (i.e., accurate) decisions about medical student advancement and promotion. Third, technologies used for medical student assessment should conform to students' real life experiences. Fourth, technology-based assessments must be integrated into a larger student and curriculum evaluation plan. Individual assessments, in sequence, should be collected, tracked, judged, and managed within an overall scheme that provides a comprehensive and coherent portrait of medical student achievement.

22.5. Educational Context Conditions

Medical education and learner assessment take place in a complex clinical, professional, institutional, and social context with many moving parts, priorities, and responsibilities. These context conditions compete every day and can affect the character and quality of medical education and assessment, especially as they shape and drive faculty behavior. Faculty are often torn between meeting (or exceeding) relative value unit (RVU) expectations and fulfilling teaching and student assessment responsibilities. Competing demands on faculty time and energy, together with the inertia which is embedded in any human system, conspire to make even maintenance of existing student evaluation systems challenging. Innovation and change under such contextual conditions is very difficult.

Since competence is usually situation-specific, newer methods of educational assessment must be tried out in the different settings in which competence would be expected, as trainees move toward higher levels of independent practice. These might include: acute emergency department care, acute ambulatory consultation, follow-up ambulatory care, intensive care unit or specialty unit care, acute and chronic hospitalized care, home visit care, and perhaps care in the setting of mass casualties and natural disasters. Many of these can only be achieved with close attention to the different educational contexts and thoughtful use of evaluation technologies.

All medical schools face these problems. They are not new. There are no easy answers, much less solutions. Leadership from deans, department chairs, division chiefs, and influential faculty is needed to address and redress the roadblocks and disincentives. Greater attention to medical faculty development as a means to boost faculty skills and morale is also a priority.[19] Fast answers or quick victories to persistent contextual issues simply do not exist. Faculty and administrative commitment and hard work have always been, and will continue to be needed to advance the medical education and student evaluation agenda.[20]

References

1. Osler W. The hospital as a college [1903]. In: Aequanimitas, with Other Addresses to Medical Students. Philadelphia: P. Blakiston's Son, 1932: 311-326.
2. Issenberg SB, McGaghie WC. Looking to the future. In: McGaghie WC, ed. International Best Practices for Evaluation in the Health Professions. London: Radcliffe, 2013: 341-360.
3. McGaghie WC, Miller GE, Sajid A, Telder TV. Competency-Based Curriculum Development in Medical Education: An Introduction. Public Health Paper No. 68. Geneva, Switzerland: World Health Organization, 1978.
4. Englander R, Carraccio C. From theory to practice: Making entrustable professional activities come to life in the context of milestones. Acad Med 2014;89(10):1321-1323.
5. Nasca TJ, Philibert I, Brigham T, Flynn TC. The next GME accreditation system: Rationale and benefits. N Engl J Med 2012;366(11):1051-1056.
6. Hawkins RE, Lipner RS, Ham HP, et al. American Board of Medical Specialties maintenance of certification: Theory and evidence regarding the current framework. J Contin Educ Health Prof 2013;33(Suppl 1):S7-S19.
7. McGaghie WC, Issenberg SB, Barsuk JH, Wayne DB. A critical review of simulation-based mastery learning with translational outcomes. Med Educ 2014;48(4):375-385.
8. McGaghie WC, Issenberg SB, Cohen ER, et al. Does simulation-based education with deliberate practice yield better results than traditional clinical education? A meta-analytic comparative review of the evidence. Acad Med 2011;86(6):706-711.
9. Wayne DB, Siddall VJ, Butter J, et al. A longitudinal study of internal medicine residents' retention of advanced cardiac life support skills. Acad Med 2006;81(10 Suppl):S9-S12.
10. Moazed F, Cohen ER, Furiasse N, et al. Retention of critical care skills after simulation-based mastery learning. J Grad Med Educ 2013;5(3):458-463.
11. Brydges R, Hatala R, Zendejas B, et al. Linking simulation-based educational

assessments and patient-related outcomes: A systematic review and meta-analysis. Acad Med 2015;90(2):246-256.
12. Kratochwill TR, Levin JR, eds. Single-Case Intervention Research: Methodological and Statistical Advances. Washington, DC: American Psychological Association, 2014.
13. Rosen MA, Salas E, Wu TS, et al. Promoting teamwork: An event-based approach to simulation-based teamwork training for emergency medicine residents. Acad Emer Med 2008;15(11):1190-1198.
14. Interprofessional Education Collaborative. Core Competencies for Interprofessional Collaborative Practice: Report of an Expert Panel. May 2011. <www.aacn.nche.edu/education-resources/ipecreport.pdf>. Accessed May 11, 2015.
15. Bonham AC, Solomon MZ. Moving comparative effectiveness research into practice: Implementation science and the role of academic medicine. Health Aff (Millwood) 2010;29(10):1901-1905.
16. McGaghie WC. Implementation science: Addressing complexity in medical education. Med Teach 2011;33(2):97-98.
17. Amin Z, Boulet JR, Cook DA, et al. Technology-enabled assessment of health professions education. In: McGaghie WC, ed. International Best Practices for Evaluation in the Health Professions. London: Radcliffe, 2013: 45-58.
18. Cook DA, Hatala R, Brydges R, et al. Technology-enhanced simulation for health professions education: A systematic review and meta-analysis. JAMA 2011; 306(9):978-988.
19. Steinert Y, Mann K, Centendo A, et al. A systematic review of faculty development initiatives designed to improve teaching effectiveness in medical education: BEME guide no. 8. Med Teach 2006;28(6):497-526.
20. Ludmerer KM. Let Me Heal: The Opportunity to Preserve Excellence in American Medicine. New York: Oxford University Press, 2015.

Index

360 degree assessment, 153, 155, 157
360 degree evaluation, 8
academic process, 253-254
academic versus disciplinary, 254-255
accreditation, 1-2, 4, 22, 29, 33, 35, 37-38, 147, 219-221, 248, 259
Accreditation Council for Graduate Medical Education (ACGME), 4, 20, 22, 32-33, 37, 62-63, 68, 72, 88, 90, 148, 212, 219-221, 260
administration of tests, 23, 89, 119, 140, 178-179, 181-184, 188, 198-199, 204-205, 228-230, 233-235, 237
admissions, 31, 49, 51-52, 257
aligning assessments, 30, 39-40, 209-210, 214
American Board of Internal Medicine (ABIM), 54, 85, 99, 121, 130, 148, 220
American Board of Medical Specialties (ABMS), 22, 228, 233
American Board of Pediatrics, 221
American College of Surgery (ACS), 212
analytic frameworks/models/approaches, 13, 19-21, 32, 72, 75, 87
Angoff, William H., 120, 179, 236
Angoff method, 120, 179, 236
angry learners, 170-171
application questions, 178, 181, 191, 193-195
Aristotle, 15
Arnold, Louise, 152-153, 156
assessment as learning, vii
assessment (as opposed to evaluation), 13-15
assessment by health care professionals, 157
assessment by peers, 79, 155-156
assessment by standardized patients (SPs), 46, 97, 176, 183, 200-206
assessment by supervisors, 8, 82, 153, 155, 157
assessment for learning, vii
assessment of clinical reasoning, 72, 127-142, 184, 204, 264
assessment of clinical skills, x, 7, 19, 34, 43, 45, 51, 53, 64, 83, 85, 97-108, 113, 119, 152, 176-177, 183-184, 201-206, 228, 264
assessment of professionalism, x, 5, 54, 62, 79, 147-160, 264
assigning grades, vii, xi, 1, 3, 13, 16-17, 81-82, 210, 229-230, 235, 237, 240, 251-261
Association for Surgical Education (ASE), 248
Association of American Medical Colleges (AAMC), 22, 59, 63, 97-99, 113-114, 118, 148-149, 176, 210-211
Association of Directors of Medical Student Education in Psychiatry (ADMSEP), 248
attitudes-skills-knowledge (ASK), 19-22, 61-62, 72-73, 77, 83, 87-88, 103, 219, 231, 239
bad news, 64, 81, 113, 119, 121-123, 167
Baile, Walter F., 121
baseline measurements, 13, 16, 34, 55, 119-121
Battistone, Michael J., xi, 87
Beckman, Thomas J., 24
behavioral observation training (BOT), 101, 104, 108
bias in evaluations, 6, 43, 45-47, 55, 77, 100, 154, 241
Bloom's taxonomy, 231
blueprints, 9, 25, 71-75, 192, 198, 201-202, 209, 212, 217, 229-232, 237
Boehler, Margaret L., 173
boot camp, 66, 213
Bordage, Georges, 98, 132
Branch, William T., 167-168
Braun, Ursula K., 154
breach of contract, 255-256
Brown University, 154
Buchanan, Robin G., 80
Calgary-Cambridge checklist, 107
Canada, 4, 20, 32, 72, 79, 88, 99, 137, 168, 248
Canadian CanMEDs Physician Competency Framework, 4, 20, 32, 72, 88
Canadian Qualifying Examination, 137
CanMEDs, 4, 20, 32, 72, 88

capstone, 66-68
Carraccio, Carol, 222-223
case context specificity, 129-130, 134-135, 141
Case, Susan M., 142, 191-192
Charcot, Martin, 135
Charlin, Bernard, 135, 142
chart stimulated recall (CSR), 139
checklists, 7, 99, 101, 107, 115-116, 119-123, 140, 142, 152, 155, 159, 202-206, 214, 228, 231, 233, 235-236
Chesser, Alistair M.S., 235
Chou, Calvin L., 166
Cizek, Gregory J., 24
clerkship assessments, 16, 61-62, 182
Clerkship Directors in Internal Medicine (CDIM), 18, 24, 53, 180, 247-248
clerkship examinations, x-xi, 23, 53, 175, 177-188, 199, 229-237, 264
clinical examination exercise (CEX), 99
clinical interpretive puzzle (CIP), 137, 139, 142
clinical reasoning, vii, x, 6, 14, 49, 53-54, 64, 72, 127-142, 184, 204, 264
clinical skills, x, 3, 7, 19, 21, 34, 37, 43, 45, 49-51, 53, 55, 64, 72-73, 83, 85, 97-108, 113, 117, 119, 152, 176-177, 180-181, 183-184, 201-206, 228, 231, 264, 266
clinical skills assessment (CSA), x, 7, 19, 34, 43, 45, 51, 53, 64, 83, 85, 97-108, 113, 119, 152, 176-177, 183-184, 201-206, 228, 264
cognitive load theory (CLT), 131-133, 135, 141
communication/conversation/dialogue, 4-5, 19-20, 27-28, 32-40, 44-47, 50, 53, 61, 64, 66, 80, 83-84, 86, 89, 91, 97, 99, 102, 106, 113-116, 118-123, 147-148, 155-156, 164, 168, 170, 172, 177, 201, 204, 212, 214, 216, 231-232, 235, 241, 243, 258-259
compensatory evaluation, 13, 18
competence, vii, 1-2, 8, 13, 18, 20-23, 35, 39, 45, 47, 49-50, 52, 55, 59-60, 63, 66, 71-73, 78, 83, 85, 99-100, 102-105, 108, 114-115, 117-118, 122, 132, 134, 141, 147, 149, 155, 177, 183-185, 199, 209-210, 212, 221, 223-224, 256, 266, 268
competence assessment, 1-2, 35, 60, 66, 71, 78, 83, 85, 99, 108, 115, 117, 122, 141, 184-185, 199, 210, 212, 224
competencies, vii, 4, 13, 20-24, 32-33, 35-37, 39, 43, 47, 51, 59-60, 62-63, 72, 77-79, 83, 88, 90, 97, 101-103, 108, 114-116, 118-119, 122, 147, 149, 152, 154, 156, 158, 169, 172, 177, 180, 184-185, 209-210, 212, 214, 217, 219, 221-223, 231-232, 237, 239, 260, 263, 266-267
competency-based approach, vii, 20, 43, 114, 219, 266
competency-based assessment, vii, 43, 101, 119, 122, 210, 214, 217, 224
competency framework, 4, 32-33, 36, 90
comprehensive integrative puzzle (CIP), 137, 139, 142
Comprehensive Osteopathic Medical Licensing Examination of the United States (COMLEX), 60
computer-enhanced human mannequins (CEMs), 211-213
conceptual thinking, 263, 265-266
confidentiality, 55, 179, 233, 258
consequential validity, 24
constructed response (CR), 177, 182, 228, 230-233, 236
Constructing Written Test Questions (NBME), 182, 191
content validity, 17, 23, 83, 152, 181, 209
context specificity, 129-130, 134-135, 141
continuing medical education (CME), 5, 213, 266
contracts, 8, 54, 147-148, 255-256
conversation/communication/dialogue, 4-5, 19-20, 27-28, 32-40, 44-47, 50, 53, 61, 64, 66, 80, 83-84, 86, 89, 91, 97, 99, 102, 106, 113-116, 118-123, 147-148, 155-156, 164, 168, 170, 172, 177, 201, 204, 212, 214, 216, 231-232, 235, 241, 243, 258-259
converting evaluations into grades, xi, 16, 18-19, 155, 239-249, 265
Conway, Patrick H., 116
Cook, David A., 24, 268
Corbett, Eugene C., 99

Core Entrustable Professional Activities for Entering Residency (CEPAER), 223-224
corrective feedback, 97, 163-164, 170-171
criterion-based evaluation, 13, 17, 87, 100, 102, 187, 219, 244-246
Crossing the Quality Chasm (IOM), 113
Cuddy, Monica M., 186, 188
cultures, 9, 38-39, 99-100, 118, 148, 163, 172-173, 224, 239, 258
curriculum, vii-viii, 2, 9, 13, 16, 23-25, 27-31, 33-34, 36, 39-40, 43, 47, 59, 62-63, 66-68, 71, 74, 87, 99, 108, 113-114, 116, 119, 122, 127, 141, 151, 153-154, 159, 177, 180-181, 206, 209-210, 213, 216-217, 223, 228, 230-231, 237, 239, 251, 257, 259, 264-265, 267-268
Cusimano, Michael D., 236
cut (or cutoff) point, 16, 235-236
dean's letter, 7, 149, 245
decision making, 21, 61, 72-73, 78, 97, 127-129, 135, 150, 152, 184-185, 202, 229, 251, 253, 255, 261
definition of professionalism, 147-150, 152-153, 155
descriptive evaluation, x, 6, 19, 72, 77-91, 249
developed locally, 4, 6, 66, 89, 91, 99, 141, 177, 180-183, 191, 228, 230, 234, 237
developmental frameworks/models/approaches, 13, 19-22, 32, 73-75, 108, 147, 150
Dewey, John, viii
dialogue/conversation/communication, 4-5, 19-20, 27-28, 32-40, 44-47, 50, 53, 61, 64, 66, 80, 83-84, 86, 89, 91, 97, 99, 102, 106, 113-116, 118-123, 147-148, 155-156, 164, 168, 170, 172, 177, 201, 204, 212, 214, 216, 231-232, 235, 241, 243, 258-259
dichotomous grading, 13, 16-18, 20, 115-116, 119, 204, 252
dimension-by-method blueprints, 71-72
direct borderline method, 236
direct observation, x, 7, 14, 22, 34, 61-62, 64, 66-67, 72, 79, 97-108, 128, 166-167, 172, 200-201, 203, 248, 264
direct observation of competence (DOC), 104-105
disciplinary issues, 5, 149, 254-255
disciplinary versus academic, 254-255
DOC training, 104-105
Donabedian, Arvis, 28-30
Donabedian Model, 28-30
Donahue v. Copiague, 257
Dougherty, Denise, 116
Downing, Steven M., 23-24, 142, 236
Dreyfus, Hubert L., 221
Dreyfus, Stuart E., 221
Dreyfus model, 61, 221
due process, 252-256, 259-261
Ebel method, 236
educational activities, 28-30, 32-33, 54, 217
educational impact, 28-30, 32, 34, 66, 140, 154, 181, 204, 219, 264
educational inputs, 14, 28-32, 34, 36, 38-40, 47, 90, 199, 241-242
educational malpractice, 256-257
educational outcomes, 30, 32, 34, 219, 266
educational outputs, 28-33, 38-39, 163
educational processes, 15, 35, 163, 210
educational research, 16, 27, 32, 116-117, 263, 265-267
educational systems, 27-28, 34-35, 38-39, 71, 75, 264
educational technology, 210-211
educator (in RIME), 17, 19, 64, 74-75, 86-87, 245
Eisner, Elliot W., 77
electives, 59, 61, 66-68, 84, 228, 230
end-of-life (EOL) communication, 114, 119, 121, 147, 159
Ende, Jack, 164
Engel, George L., 98
entrustable professional activities (EPAs), 32, 43, 59-60, 63, 219, 221-224
error, 23, 64, 78, 84, 97-100, 113, 116, 163-165, 215, 233-234
Eva, Kevin W., 165-167, 171
evaluation (as opposed to assessment), 13-15
evaluation bias, 6, 43, 45-47, 55, 77, 100, 154, 241

evaluation of medical/clinical/diagnostic procedures, vii, x, 7, 16, 43, 64, 72, 74, 98, 113-123, 158, 193, 211-213, 224, 236
evaluation sessions, 85, 88-89, 108, 242-243, 246
evaluative judgments, 13-15
examination blueprints, 192, 198, 201
examination construction, 181, 198, 202
extended matching (Type R) questions (EMQs), 135, 142, 181, 191, 196-197
face validity, 24, 83, 142, 184, 241
faculty development, 27, 29-30, 32-33, 38, 64, 84, 88-89, 91, 100-101, 104-105, 107, 158, 260, 269
faculty generated examinations (FGEs), 175, 178, 180-182, 198, 228-237, 248
failing grades, vii, xi, 16, 18, 50, 52-53, 56, 79, 81, 116, 180, 188, 206, 230, 236, 240, 245-246, 249, 251-261
Family Educational Rights and Privacy Act (FERPA), 46, 258-259
feasibility, 13, 23-24, 40, 54, 63, 79, 87, 89, 107, 156, 176, 182, 199, 210, 215-217, 236
feedback, vii-viii, 1-3, 8, 14-15, 27-28, 30-32, 37-38, 40, 44-46, 59, 61, 64, 71, 75, 77, 79-81, 84-85, 87-90, 97, 100, 102, 105-108, 114, 116, 120-122, 128, 149-150, 154-158, 163-173, 179, 203-205, 215, 223, 229, 231, 241, 246, 264, 266-267
feedback for faculty, 27, 171-172
feedback from faculty, 40, 46, 87, 154, 158, 169, 203
Fitch, Michael T., 118
fixed-standard evaluation, 13, 17-18, 240, 244-246
Flaim v. Medical College of Ohio, 254
formal evaluation sessions, 88, 242, 246
formative evaluation, x, 9, 13, 15-16, 38, 44, 61-65, 71, 89, 91, 107, 128, 141, 149, 151-154, 156-158, 163, 166, 176, 213-215, 223, 228, 230, 260, 264, 266
forward feeding, 43-45, 68
Fourteenth Amendment (U.S. Constitution), 252, 254
fourth year (MS4), 17, 22, 59-60, 62-63, 66, 87, 118, 122, 205, 213, 218, 236, 253
frame of reference training (FoRT), 32, 65, 85, 88, 99-100, 103-105, 108
frameworks, 4, 15, 20-22, 32-33, 36, 38, 62-63, 72-73, 78-79, 86-90, 116, 121-122, 221, 239-240, 244, 260
free text paragraph, 132, 138-139, 142
free text questions, 137-138, 142
Gage, Nathaniel Lees, 28
Gigante, Joseph, 167
Gingerich, Andrea, 100
Ginsburg, Shiphra, 82, 153
Gold Humanism Honor Society (GHHS), 156
Good, Mary-Jo DelVecchio, 9
Gorman v. University of Rhode Island, 255
Govaerts, Marjan J., 78, 100
Graber, Mark L., 98
grade average, 18, 50, 74
grade conversion, xi, 16, 18-19, 155, 239-249, 265
grading, 5, 9, 13-19, 37, 52, 71-72, 79, 84-85, 89, 91, 138, 166, 177, 179, 181, 187-188, 203, 232, 234-235, 237, 239-242, 244-249, 251-254, 256-257, 259, 261, 264-265
graduate medical education (GME), ix, 5, 22, 24, 29-30, 33, 37, 68, 71, 74, 108, 213, 219, 224, 260-261, 265
graduation, 50, 52, 59-60, 62-63, 66, 68, 102, 114, 118, 256
graduation competence/competencies, 59-60, 62
Green, Michael L., 75
Griffith, Charles H., 186
Hanson, Janice L., 78
Hawthorne effect, 155
Hemmer, Paul A., x-xi, 72, 247
Herbers, Jerome E., 99
high-risk students, vii, x, 27, 49-56, 264
Hodges, Brian, 78
Hofstee, Willem K.B., 120, 179, 236
Hofstee method, 120, 179, 236
Holmboe, Eric S., x, 72, 106, 223
Holtzman, Kathleen Z., 188
horizontal evaluation models, x, 28-32, 35, 213
illness scripts, 131-133
importance of feedback, 163-164

in-clerkship examinations, 188
information sharing policies, 46-47
Institute of Medicine (IOM), 97, 113
institutional policies, 46-47, 50, 255, 259, 261
interpreter (in RIME), 17-20, 25, 34, 59, 62, 74-75, 86-87, 245
interrater reliability, 51, 64, 82, 115, 138, 140, 142, 183, 205, 228, 230
Iobst, William, 104
item banking, 108, 236-237
Jha, Vikram, 153
judicial deference, 253-254
just-in-time training, 213, 218
Kalamazoo Consensus Statement, 122
Kalet, Adina, 99
Katsufrakis, Peter, 104
key features, 115-116, 131-134, 137-138, 142, 177-178
Klamen, Debra A., 85
Klass, Daniel J., 72-73
knowledge organization, 131-133
knowledge-skills-attitudes (KSA), 19-22, 61-62, 72-73, 77, 83, 87-88, 103, 219, 231, 239
Kogan, Jennifer R., 99-100, 106
Kübler-Ross, Elisabeth, 171
Kuder-Richardson formulae (KR-20, KR-21), 230, 234-235
LCME Standard ED-31, 168
lead-in questions, 136, 191-192, 194-197
learner experience, 1-3, 8, 16, 39, 46, 59-63, 66-68, 121-122, 150, 154, 158, 163, 166, 168, 178, 183-184, 187, 202, 221, 224, 244, 268
learner motivation, 1, 9, 51, 79, 148, 177, 183, 229, 246
learning climate, 1, 108, 165, 167
learning objectives, 61, 63, 67, 148, 166, 172, 177, 180, 209-210, 244
legal concepts, xi, 24, 81, 251-261, 265
letters of recommendation, 7, 51, 90, 245
Lewin, Linda Orkin, 140
Liaison Committee on Medical Education (LCME), 1-2, 39, 60, 113, 147-148, 163, 168
locally developed, 4, 6, 66, 89, 91, 99, 141, 177, 180-183, 191, 228, 230, 234, 237
Lynch, Deirdre C., 153
Lyons, Oliver, 157
Lypson, Monica Lenore, 98
Macy Model, 122
manager (in RIME), 17, 19, 34, 59, 62, 74-75, 86-87, 244-245
mannequins, 6, 203, 211-213
mastery learning, 1, 17-18, 25, 39, 53, 61, 74, 87, 98, 113-119, 121-122, 158, 200, 213-215, 218, 221, 231, 235-236, 264, 266-267
matching item questions, 139, 191, 196-197
Mazor, Kathleen M., 157
McGaghie, William C., x, 71, 85, 116-117
measurements, 2-3, 9, 13, 16, 18, 22, 30, 33-34, 43, 49-50, 55-56, 78, 114, 119-121, 135, 152, 159, 210-211, 214, 267
Medical College Admission Test (MCAT), 5, 49-51
medical error, 64, 97-100, 113, 116
Medical Schools Objectives Project (MSOP), 118
Medical Student Performance Evaluation (MSPE), 90-91, 149
Mennin, Stewart, 38
Michigan v. Ewing, 251-253
milestones, 3, 13, 20, 22-23, 32, 35, 39, 43, 63, 68, 73-75, 108, 172, 176, 219-223, 257, 266
Miller, George E., 9, 21, 61-62, 209-210
Miller's levels, 61, 209
Miller's pyramid, 62, 210
Miller's triangle, 21
mini clinical examination exercise (mini-CEX), 64, 77, 83, 85, 99, 101, 105-107, 142, 155
minimal passing score (MPS), 115-116, 119-122, 179, 249
minimum passing level (MPL), 116, 179, 215, 229
Missouri v. Horowitz, 253-254
motivation, 1, 9, 51, 79, 148, 177, 182-183, 200, 229, 246
multisource assessment, 153, 155-157

multiple choice questions (MCQs), vii, x, 4, 16, 18-19, 24-25, 30, 46, 53, 73, 128, 130, 135-136, 142, 175, 177-178, 180-183, 185, 191-199, 205, 211, 228, 230-234, 236, 265
Nabors, Christopher, 108
narratives, 16, 18-19, 46, 51, 77-80, 85, 88-90, 107, 158, 223
National Board of Medical Examiners (NBME), x, 16, 33-34, 49-50, 52-53, 175, 177-183, 186-188, 191, 194, 199, 228, 230, 233-234, 244, 246-249, 253
National Board of Medical Examiners Subject Test (NBME shelf exam), 16, 33-34, 49-50, 52-53, 175, 177-183, 186-188, 191, 194, 199, 228, 230, 233-234, 244, 246-249. 253
National Residency Match Program (NRMP), 218
NBME subject examinations, 16, 33-34, 49-50, 52-53, 175, 177-183, 186-188, 191, 194, 199, 228, 230, 233-234, 244, 246-249, 253
Nedelsky method, 236
Netherlands, 100
Next Accreditation System (NAS), 22, 68, 219
Noel, Gordon L., 99
Norcini, John J., 105, 142
normative evaluation, 3, 8, 13, 17-18, 100, 187, 240, 245-247, 249
objective evaluation, 4
objective structured clinical examination (OSCE), vii, x, 4-5, 7, 16, 19, 34, 49, 53, 61-62, 64-66, 73, 99, 142, 153, 157-158, 175, 180, 183-184, 202, 211, 228, 230-232, 234-236, 244, 246-248
observation by faculty, 51, 85, 98-101, 108
observation-rating-feedback process, 107
observation-reflection-action, 15, 249
observations about learners, 15, 36
one-best-answer questions, 136, 180-182, 184, 191, 194-196
One-Minute Preceptor, 167
oral examinations, 7, 67-68, 139-140, 142, 175, 180, 182-183, 187, 228, 230, 248
Outcomes Logic Model, 28-29, 33
outputs, 28-33, 38-39, 163
P-MEX, 155-156
Pangaro, Louis N., x-xi, 86
Paranjape, Anuradha 167-168
Pass/Fail cutoff, 18, 99, 106, 205, 235-236, 251-252
patient management problems (PMPs), 129-131, 133
patient safety, 5, 55, 113, 118, 123, 218, 266
peer assessment, 79, 155-156
performance appraisal, 77, 229
performance criteria, 103
performance dimension training (PDT), 102-104, 108
performance evaluation, x, 43-44, 72, 77-91, 149, 242, 244, 246, 249, 264
performance feedback, 3, 166
personalized mentoring, 44, 61
physician-patient relationship, 4-5, 86, 153, 259
policies, 43-44, 46-47, 50, 53, 55, 113, 117, 122, 239-240, 246, 254-257, 259, 261, 265
portfolios, 8, 52, 61, 65-68, 153, 158
post-clerkship, x, 27, 34, 44, 46, 59-68, 177, 261, 264
post-clerkship assessments, x, 27, 34, 59-68, 264
post-encounter exercise, 203
pre-clerkship assessments, 16, 34, 37, 49-56, 62, 67, 261, 264
pre-clerkship variables, x, 27, 49-56, 264
predicting, 1-3, 24, 49-56, 83, 89-90, 99, 117, 130, 153, 159, 206, 243
predictive validity, 24, 50, 52-56, 89, 99, 153
preparedness for residency, 60, 218-219
pretests, 53-54, 115-116, 119, 121, 139
privacy, 19, 45-46, 55, 164-165, 170, 199, 258
procedural due process, 252, 254, 259
procedural skills, 4-5, 9, 79, 113-114, 117-118, 122, 183, 215, 218, 264
procedures (medical/clinical/diagnostic), vii, x, 7, 16, 43, 64, 72, 74, 98, 113-123, 158, 193, 211-213, 224, 236
process versus product, 13, 16, 22, 28, 30, 34, 38
professional development portfolios, 153, 158
professional knowledge, 4

professional relationships, 4-5, 72, 107, 150, 152, 155, 171
professionalism, vii, ix-x, 4-5, 18, 20, 38, 47, 49-51, 54, 62, 66, 78-79, 90, 117, 147-160, 169-171, 231, 233, 254, 259, 264
proficiency, 4, 7, 9, 17-22, 25, 32, 34, 47, 73-74, 130-131, 177, 212, 214, 221
program effectiveness, 1-2, 4
program evaluation, 27, 29, 31, 33, 152
psychometric evaluation of tests, 77-78, 135-137, 178, 181, 215, 228, 234-235
Pygmalion effect, 45
quality improvement (QI), 4, 28-29, 31, 38, 67, 260
quality management, 28, 265
quantified evaluation, 7, 18, 40, 49, 54, 73, 77-78, 83, 89, 151, 201, 204, 229, 237, 239, 241, 247, 249, 264
quantitative evaluation methods, 13, 16, 18-19, 22, 46, 152, 155, 159, 240
rating scales, 7, 66-67, 77, 79, 82-83, 105, 115, 206, 211, 214, 234
recall questions, 142, 177-178, 191-192, 199, 231
Reflection Evaluation for Learners' Enhanced Competencies Tool (REFLECT), 154
reliability, 5-6, 13, 19, 23-24, 38, 40, 51, 54, 63-64, 67, 78, 81-84, 86, 90, 98-99, 105-107, 115, 129-131, 134-138, 140-142, 149, 152-153, 155, 157, 175-176, 178, 181-183, 185, 202-203, 205-206, 214-216, 228-231, 234-235, 237
reporter (in RIME), 17, 19-20, 25, 34, 55, 59, 62, 74-75, 86-87, 98, 244-245
reporter-interpreter-manager-educator (RIME), 17-20, 25, 32, 34, 55, 59, 62, 64, 74-75, 86-90, 98, 239, 243-246
residency, ix, 2, 14, 20, 22, 25, 33-34, 37, 44-46, 53, 59-63, 66-68, 71, 73-75, 79-80, 82-83, 87-91, 97-99, 101-102, 105-107, 114, 119-122, 152-153, 155, 157, 159, 167, 169-172, 176, 179, 185, 188, 206, 213, 218-219, 221-224, 233, 239, 241-243, 245-246, 249, 251, 256
RIME (reporter-interpreter-manager-educator), 17-20, 25, 32, 34, 55, 59, 62, 64, 74-75, 86-90, 98, 239, 243-246
Ringsted, Charlotte, 78
Rothman, Arthur I., 236
safety, 5, 29, 55, 113, 118, 123, 217-218, 259, 266
scalar grading, 13, 16-17, 252
Schein, Edgar H., 38
Schuwirth, Lambert, x, 72
Scottish Doctors Learning Outcomes, 4
script concordance testing (SCT), 135-137, 142, 175, 180, 184-185
scripts, 131-133, 135-137, 175, 184-185, 204
second-hand feedback, 169-170
SEGUE communications tool, 106-107, 122
self-assessment, 49, 106, 157-158, 166, 168
self-evaluation, 155, 168
semantic qualifiers, 132, 134
setting standards, xi, 23, 115, 120, 179-180, 182, 215, 229-237, 265
sharing student information, viii, x, 27, 43-47, 55, 264
shelf examinations, 16, 33-34, 49-50, 52-53, 175, 177-183, 186-188, 191, 194, 199, 228, 230, 233-234, 244, 246-249, 253
simulation, vii, xi, 2, 4-6, 21, 31, 33, 49, 65-66, 73, 85, 115-122, 131, 175-176, 184, 191, 196, 201, 203-205, 209-224, 265, 267-268
simulation technologies, vii, xi, 4, 176, 209-224, 265, 267-268
simulation-based assessments, 65, 115, 176, 211-215, 217-218, 224
simulation-based mastery learning (SBML), 116-118
single stem (Type A) item questions, 191, 194, 197
situativity, 134
skill retention, 117-118
social responsibility, 24, 44-45, 147-149, 151, 160, 218, 268
Society for General Internal Medicine (SGIM), 180
Society for Simulation in Heathcare (SSH), 212
Society of Teachers of Family Medicine (STFM), 24
specific, timely, objective, with a plan (STOP), 167
specificity, 50, 53, 56, 90, 129-130, 134-135, 137, 141, 164, 198, 202, 205

SPIKES, 121-122
standardized patient (SP) assessment, 46, 97, 176, 183, 200-206
standardized patients (SPs), x, 2, 4, 8, 19, 31, 73, 46, 97, 104, 115-116, 122, 135, 141, 157, 176, 183-184, 200-206, 211-212, 216, 230, 232-234, 265
standards in examinations, xi, 115-116, 215, 229-237, 265
stem questions, 191, 194-195, 197
structured assessments, 175-176, 263
structured clinical observation (SCO), 107, 167
structured reflection, 153-154
student anxiety, 1, 45-46, 121, 204
subinternship, 34, 37, 59-60, 63-65, 67, 87, 178, 202, 213
subjective evaluation, 5, 13, 18-19, 77-78, 136, 151-152, 183, 201, 251
substantive due process, 252
summative evaluation, x, 9, 13, 15-16, 18-19, 27, 37-38, 49, 61-63, 65, 91, 128, 140, 149, 151-152, 154, 156, 158, 163, 166, 168-169, 176, 202, 213-214, 216, 228, 230-231, 235-236, 239, 241, 260, 264
Supreme Court cases, 251-254
Swanson, David B., 142, 191-192
Swick, Herbert M., 148
syllabus, 13, 24-25, 29, 31, 237
synthetic frameworks/models/approaches, 13, 19-22, 32, 73, 75, 87
systems of assessment, x
Szmulowicz, Eytan, x, 72, 122
Takayama, Hiroo, 240, 245
task trainers, 203, 211-213
technical skills, 4-5, 9, 147, 203-204, 231
test administration, 23, 89, 119, 140, 178-179, 181-184, 188, 198-199, 204-205, 228-230, 233-235, 237
test items, 175, 230, 233, 236-237
test security, 178, 233-234, 237
testing, 43, 53, 115, 117, 119, 121, 135-136, 138, 142, 156, 181, 184-185, 188, 202, 205-206, 228-230, 234, 237, 254
think-aloud protocol, 140
third year (MS3), 17, 22, 25, 87, 119, 184, 186, 213, 231-232, 257
timeliness of feedback, 84, 164, 167, 215
Tonesk, Xenia, 80
translational science, 116-118, 221, 267
undergraduate medical education, ix, 1, 4-5, 39, 43, 114, 211, 218-219, 266
United Kingdom, 9, 100, 117, 156
United States Medical Licensing Examination (USMLE), 2, 4, 16, 49-54, 60, 99, 178, 183, 186, 188, 191, 206, 234, 252
validity, 13, 17, 19, 23-24, 50, 52-56, 61, 63-64, 67, 78-79, 83-84, 89, 99, 105-106, 131, 134, 137, 140, 142, 151-153, 156-157, 178, 181, 183-184, 186, 203, 205-206, 209-210, 215, 229-233, 237, 241-242, 244-245
van de Ridder, J.M. Monica, 163-164
van der Leeuw, Renée M., 172
van der Vleuten, Cees P.M., 142
variables, x, 27, 31, 49-56, 59-60, 68, 74, 99-100, 107, 115, 142, 183, 185, 215, 264
variance, 23, 31, 50-51, 98, 106, 140, 157-158, 185, 187, 230, 232-235, 237, 241-243
variance among teachers, 106, 157-158, 241-243
Veloski, Jon, 152
vertical evaluation models, x, 28, 32, 34-36
virtual case platforms, 141
virtual patients, 135, 141, 213
virtual reality, 6, 211, 213
weakest link models, 13, 18
weighting of grades, 63, 72, 177, 183, 187-188, 243, 247
weighting of items, 119, 183, 187-188, 241
Whitcomb, Michael, 99
White, Byron, 255
Williams, Reed G., 85
workplace assessments, x, 37, 46, 62, 64, 71-72, 77-91, 239, 263-264
written examinations, x, 22, 34, 52, 71, 119-121, 138, 177-178, 181-183, 191-199, 228
Yeates, Peter, 100
Yedidia, Michael J., 122